COURSE INSTRUCTIONS
IMPORTANT: Read these instructions *BEFORE* proceeding!

HOW TO EARN CONTACT HOURS

To earn contact hour(s) and receive a certificate of completion, you must read the entire cours~
score of 70% or higher, and complete the course evaluation. **Unless otherwise indicated, c**
for up to 1 year from the date on which this course was purchased.

FINAL EXAM

Enclosed with your course book you will find a FasTrax Answer Sheet and a FasTrax Instructio.   ~et. Use the Answer
Sheet to answer all of the final exam questions that appear in this course. FasTrax Answer Sheets are preprinted with your
name and address and the course title. If you are completing more than one course, be sure to record your answers on the
correct corresponding answer sheet.

Use blue or black ink to completely fill in the circles on the Answer Sheet. The FasTrax grading system will not read pencil.
If you make an error, you may use correction fluid (such as Wite-Out®) to correct it. If the course has fewer than 100 questions, leave any remaining answer circles on the Answer Sheet blank.

You must score 70% or higher in order to pass this course. Should you fail to achieve the minimum required score, an additional Answer Sheet will be sent to you so that you may make a second attempt to pass the course. You will be allowed three
attempts to pass this course. After three failed attempts, your file will be closed.

COURSE EVALUATIONS

The course evaluation provided in this course book is a required component of the course and must be completed and sub-
mitted with your final exam. Responses to evaluation statements should be recorded in the right-hand column of the Answer
Sheet, in the section marked "Evaluation." Your evaluation provides Western Schools with vital feedback.

To provide additional feedback regarding this course, our services, or to suggest new course topics, complete the Important
Information form found on the back of the Instruction Sheet. Return this completed form to Western Schools with your
Answer Sheet.

SUBMITTING THE FINAL EXAM AND EVALUATION

The Instruction Sheet provides detailed steps for submitting your completed Answer Sheet and Important Information form.
If you are mailing your Answer Sheet and Important Information form to Western Schools, we recommend that you keep a
copy as a back-up.

CHANGE OF ADDRESS?

In the event that your postal or email address changes prior to completing this course, please contact our customer service
department at 1-800-618-1670, or customerservice@westernschools.com, so that we may update your file.

WESTERN SCHOOLS GUARANTEES YOUR SATISFACTION

If any continuing education course fails to meet your expectations, or if you are not satisfied for any reason, you may return
the course materials for an exchange or a refund (less shipping and handling) within 30 days. Software, video, and audio
courses must be returned unopened. Textbooks must not be written in or marked up in any other way. Materials for courses
you have already received continuing education credit for will not be accepted.

Thank you for using Western Schools to fulfill your continuing education needs!

WESTERN SCHOOLS
P.O. Box 1930
Brockton, MA 02303
800-438-8888
www.westernschools.com

WESTERN SCHOOLS
STUDY TIME LOG

HOME HEALTH NURSING: A COMPREHENSIVE REVIEW OF PRACTICAL AND PROFESSIONAL ISSUES

INSTRUCTIONS: Use this log sheet to document the amount of time you spend completing this course. Include the time it takes you to read the instructions, take the pretest, read the course book, take the final examination, and complete the evaluation.

Date	Time Spent	
	Hours	**Minutes**
————————	————————	————————
————————	————————	————————
————————	————————	————————
————————	————————	————————
————————	————————	————————
————————	————————	————————
————————	————————	————————
————————	————————	————————
————————	————————	————————
————————	————————	————————
————————	————————	————————
————————	————————	————————
————————	————————	————————
————————	————————	————————
————————	————————	————————

TOTAL*

Hours   **Minutes**

* Please use this total study time to answer the final question of the course evaluation.

Home Health Nursing:
A Comprehensive Review of Practical and Professional Issues

3rd Edition

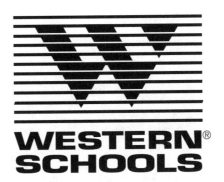

WESTERN® SCHOOLS

Original Author
Stephanie Mello, MS, MBA, RN, COS-C
Revised by
Lisa Gorski, MS, APRN, BC, CRNI, FAAN

30 contact hours will be awarded upon successful completion of this course.
Western Schools is accredited as a provider of continuing nursing education by the
American Nurses Credentialing Center's Commission on Accreditation.

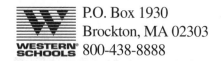 P.O. Box 1930
Brockton, MA 02303
800-438-8888

ABOUT THE ORIGINAL AUTHOR

Stephanie Mello, MS, MBA, RN, COS-C, is the chief operating officer at the Visiting Nurse Association of Southeastern Massachusetts, Inc. In addition to her current role, Stephanie serves as a senior associate consultant for OASIS Answers, Inc., located in Redmond, Washington, and is a member of the OASIS Certificate and Competency Board, Inc.

Stephanie Mello has disclosed that she has no significant financial or other conflicts of interest pertaining to this course book.

ABOUT THE THIRD EDITION AUTHOR

Lisa Gorski, MS, APRN, BC, CRNI, FAAN, has worked as a clinical nurse specialist in home health since 1985. She currently works for Wheaton Franciscan Home Health and Hospice in Milwaukee, WI. She also works as a consultant for OASIS Answers, Inc., providing clinical educational presentations on a variety of home health care topics. She is the author of numerous articles as well as four books and has presented on a variety of topics across the country. Her main areas of expertise include home infusion therapy and care of chronically ill adult patients. She was elected as the 2007–08 President of the Infusion Nurses Society and also serves on the Editorial Board for *Home Healthcare Nurse*. She participated on the committee to revise the American Nurses Association's *Home Health Nursing Scope and Standards of Practice*.

Lisa Gorski has disclosed that she has no significant financial or other conflicts of interest pertaining to this course book.

2ND EDITION SUBJECT MATTER REVIEWER & CONTENT EDITOR

Lisa Gorski, MS, APRN, BC, CRNI, FAAN

Nurse Planner: Amy Bernard, MS, BSN, RN-BC

Copy Editor: Jaime Stockslager Buss, MSPH, ELS

Indexer: Sylvia Coates

ISBN: 978-1-57801-407-1

WESTERN SCHOOLS
COURSE EVALUATION

HOME HEALTH NURSING: A COMPREHENSIVE REVIEW OF PRACTICAL AND PROFESSIONAL ISSUES

INSTRUCTIONS: Using the scale below, please respond to the following evaluation statements. All responses should be recorded in the right-hand column of the FasTrax answer sheet, in the section marked "Evaluation." Be sure to fill in each corresponding answer circle completely using blue or black ink. Leave any remaining answer circles blank.

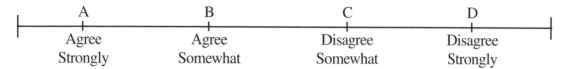

A	B	C	D
Agree Strongly	Agree Somewhat	Disagree Somewhat	Disagree Strongly

OBJECTIVES: After completing this course, I am able to

1. Discuss the major events that have shaped home health care today.
2. Discuss the American Nurses Association's *Code of Ethics for Nurses*.
3. Apply the six standards of practice to home health nursing.
4. Relate the nine standards of professional performance to home health nursing.
5. Describe the key components of a home health agency.
6. Apply the Outcome and Assessment Information Set (OASIS) to patient scenarios.
7. Describe how OASIS data can be used to measure patient outcomes.
8. Discuss payment mechanisms for home health care reimbursement.
9. Identify the rules that govern the provision of Medicare home health services.

COURSE CONTENT

10. The course materials were presented in a well organized and clearly written manner.

11. The course content was presented in a fair, unbiased and balanced manner.

12. The course expanded my knowledge and enhanced my skills related to the subject matter.

13. I intend to apply the knowledge and skills I've learned to my nursing practice. (Select the appropriate response below.)

        A. Yes   B. Unsure   C. No   D. Not Applicable

ATTESTATION

14. By submitting this answer sheet, I certify that I have read the course materials and personally completed the final examination based on the material presented. Mark "A" for Agree and "B" for Disagree.

COURSE HOURS

15. Choose the response that best represents the total number of clock hours it took to complete this **30 hour** course.

        A. More than 32 hours   B. 28–32 hours   C. Less than 28 hours

Note: To provide additional feedback regarding this course, Western Schools services, or to suggest new course topics, use the space provided on the Important Information form found on the back of the FasTrax instruction sheet included with your course.

CONTENTS

BOXES, FIGURES, AND TABLES

PRETEST

1. Begin this course by taking the pretest. Circle the answers to the questions on this page, or write the answers on a separate sheet of paper. Do not log answers to the pretest questions on the FasTrax test sheet included with the course.

2. Compare your answers to the PRETEST KEY located at the end of the Pretest. The pretest key indicates the chapter where the content of that question is discussed. Make note of the questions you missed, so that you can focus on those areas as you complete the course.

3. Complete the course by reading the chapters and completing the exam questions at the end of each chapter. Answers to these exam questions should be logged on the FasTrax test sheet included with the course.

Note: Choose the one option that BEST answers each question.

1. During the earliest part of the 19th century, nursing care in the United States was primarily provided by

    a. religious groups whose vocation was to alleviate the physical and spiritual suffering of man.

    b. nurses trained in the Florence Nightingale School of Nursing.

    c. middle-class women who could afford the formal education and training required by law.

    d. lower- and working-class women, functioning as lay nurses.

2. The first visiting nurse services were established by

    a. local and state departments of health to combat infectious disease.

    b. wealthy and upper-class women to meet the unique needs of their communities.

    c. hospital administrators as a means to increase the capacity of inpatient beds.

    d. nurses to assure a professional practice environment.

3. A code of ethics

    a. is a legal document.

    b. provides a detailed explanation of the services that one can expect.

    c. applies to nurses regardless of the practice setting or policies of an employer.

    d. is not directly applicable to day-to-day or routine activities.

4. A patient's right to confidentiality

    a. can never be violated regardless of the situation or circumstance.

    b. is an inalienable human right.

    c. does not apply to patients receiving home health care service because all of the team members have to know all patient-related details to establish an appropriate plan of care.

    d. is only valid between a patient and his or her doctor or lawyer.

5. Each nurse must be accountable for his or her own practice and must be adequately prepared to carry out every function that he or she is asked to perform. If a nurse is asked to carry out a function that he or she is not adequately prepared for, the nurse should

   a. complete the function as assigned.

   b. complete the function and then report dissatisfaction about the assignment to the agency's administrator.

   c. avoid attempting to carry out the function and jeopardizing the patient's well-being.

   d. report the unsafe practices of the agency to the state licensing board.

6. The term "information system" refers to

   a. the agency's computer system.

   b. information that is transmitted electronically from a referral source or physician.

   c. the patient's medical record or database.

   d. only agencies that have a complete electronic medical record.

7. According to the American Nurses Association, advocating for the patient, teaching self-care skills, and incorporating evidence-based knowledge into practice are responsibilities typically associated with

   a. only nurses functioning in advanced practice roles.

   b. only nurses functioning in generalist roles.

   c. licensed practical nurses' responsibilities.

   d. both nurse generalists and advanced practice registered nurses.

8. In home health care, best practice identification

   a. is not a realistic expectation due to the number of social variables.

   b. is solely the responsibility of the management team and advanced practice nurses.

   c. serves to establish standards that provide clear direction related to the provision of patient care.

   d. can only be accomplished when the agency seeks expertise from a hospital or nursing school faculty.

9. The role of the professional nurse in home care includes addressing issues of resource utilization and cost of care because

   a. patients have an inalienable right to health care.

   b. the nurse must carefully balance the cost of care with the amount of reimbursement and services provided.

   c. patients without insurance should receive less care than insured patients.

   d. patients have the right to be informed about the risks, benefits, and cost of their care.

10. The Conditions of Participation

   a. outline the basic organizational and oversight structure for certified home health care agencies.

   b. are optional for agencies that were established before 1965.

   c. are optional for agencies that were established as a result of the Stagger's lawsuit.

   d. are only applicable to not-for-profit home health care agencies.

11. The collection and analysis of standardized patient data allows the Centers for Medicare & Medicaid Services to

    a. penalize agencies with poor outcomes.

    b. provide financial rewards to agencies that achieve the best patient outcomes.

    c. identify agencies with best practices.

    d. prevent agencies with poor performance from participating in the Medicare home health care program.

12. Regulations require agencies to incorporate the Outcomes and Assessment Information Set (OASIS) items into their comprehensive patient assessment tools. The regulations also mandate that agencies

    a. reorder the questions so that they flow within the agency assessment document.

    b. do not take liberties with the punctuation or wording of any of the questions.

    c. eliminate the MO prefix, which delineates the OASIS item as a mandatory question.

    d. read the question to the patient and ask the patient to choose the answer that best describes his or her status.

13. The OASIS User's Manual instructs the home health care nurse to answer based on the

    a. patient at his or her worst.

    b. patient at his or her best.

    c. patient's ability at least 50% of the time.

    d. patient's status most of the time on the day when the patient assessment is being conducted.

14. A patient is admitted with shortness of breath with minimal exertion. On discharge, her shortness of breath occurs only when walking more than 20 feet. This type of patient outcome is considered

    a. an improvement in status or functional ability.

    b. a negative patient outcome because her shortness of breath is not completely resolved.

    c. null since the patient's shortness of breath remained unchanged upon discharge.

    d. a stabilization outcome since the patient is stabilized.

15. The implementation of OASIS has enabled agencies to measure

    a. patient satisfaction.

    b. referral source satisfaction.

    c. both aggregate and individual patient outcomes.

    d. staff efficiency.

16. The ability to benchmark an agency's performance is important because

    a. an agency can gain a competitive edge by identifying weaknesses in the performance of other agencies.

    b. it allows the agency to set realistic patient outcome goals.

    c. clinicians with poor performance can be identified and disciplined.

    d. the best performers will no longer be required to complete The Joint Commission and the Department of Public Health surveys.

17. The Medicare Prospective Payment System (PPS) is based on

   a. an agency's ability to attract patients who will result in the highest reimbursement.

   b. an agency's ability to avoid accepting patients who will result in low reimbursement or require high levels of service.

   c. an agency managing a balance of profitable and losing episodes.

   d. the number of visits provided to the patient.

18. The fee-for-service reimbursement structure

   a. always requires the completion of the OASIS.

   b. generally allows the visiting clinician to control the number of visits the patient will receive.

   c. generally requires that the number of visits provided to the patient be controlled by the insurance company or case reviewer.

   d. always results in a profitable PPS episode for the agency.

19. The determination of reasonable and necessary care depends on the

   a. physician's definition.

   b. nurse's definition.

   c. individualized and unique needs of the patient.

   d. written request from the referral source.

20. A condition that would disqualify a patient from receiving Medicare home health services is

   a. the patient's ability to pay for services.

   b. the patient's inability to visit a physician's office at least every 6 months.

   c. the absence of a caregiver in the home.

   d. the patient's need for home health services on a daily basis with no endpoint in sight.

PRETEST KEY

1.	d	Chapter 1
2.	b	Chapter 1
3.	c	Chapter 2
4.	b	Chapter 2
5.	c	Chapter 2
6.	c	Chapter 3
7.	d	Chapter 4
8.	c	Chapter 4
9.	d	Chapter 4
10.	a	Chapter 5
11.	c	Chapter 6
12.	b	Chapter 6
13.	d	Chapter 6
14.	a	Chapter 7
15.	c	Chapter 7
16.	b	Chapter 7
17.	c	Chapter 8
18.	c	Chapter 8
19.	c	Chapter 9
20.	d	Chapter 9

INTRODUCTION

This course is intended to meet the needs of nurses who practice in home health care by providing a comprehensive review of both practical and professional issues. This course will provide the inexperienced home health care nurse with the information necessary to develop the skills associated with a successful home health care practitioner, while the experienced home health care nurse will find opportunities to review the basics and reflect on the professional implications of practicing in this complex setting.

As with any subject of study, it is important to start at the beginning. For that reason Chapter 1 describes the evolution of home health care as we know it today. Although the role of the home health nurse has evolved over the past three centuries, home health nurses today essentially have the same role as the caregivers in the 1700's: teaching people to care for themselves in their own environments.

Home health care nurses are invited guests in the homes of their patients. They develop relationships with patients who are vulnerable and often in a "needy" or dependent state. As a result, home health nurses are at risk for blurring the lines of professional practice. This course will highlight the societal and professional expectations and standards associated with home health care nursing.

Regardless of the practice setting, no nurse functions in a vacuum. Every nurse is part of a team aimed at improving the health of patients. Like nurses who practice in facilities (such as hospitals, nursing homes, and clinics), home health nurses are only one part of a very complex, although somewhat invisible, system. Although home health nurses deliver their care in thousands of homes every day, they must recognize that there is an entire organizational structure behind them providing support.

This course is further intended to provide the reader with an overview of the federal regulations and requirements that govern the delivery of home health care and that must be considered by the field nurse when planning and delivering effective and efficient patient care.

CHAPTER 1

EVOLUTION OF
HOME HEALTH CARE

CHAPTER OBJECTIVE

At the completion of this chapter, the reader will be able to discuss the major events that have shaped home health care today.

LEARNING OBJECTIVES

After studying this chapter, the reader will be able to

1. identify Florence Nightingale's contribution to and influence on the practice of home health care.

2. recognize the accomplishments of Lillian Wald and her impact on modern home health care.

3. discuss the evolution of the Red Cross and its influence on home health care.

4. list examples of federal legislation that have impacted the home health care industry.

INTRODUCTION

The terms "home health nurse," "public health nurse," and "community health nurse" are commonly used interchangeably. Although the entire nursing profession's roots are community-based, home health, public health, and community health nursing are distinct areas of practice. However, some agencies and their nurses serve the function of all within a single community or geographic area. For the purpose of this course, home health care is a cadre of services for patients who are disabled, are chronically or terminally ill, or are recovering from acute illnesses.

Home health care agencies typically provide skilled, nursing, home health care aide, social, or rehabilitative services. Depending on the unique needs of the patient, any combination of these services may be provided. Regardless of which service the patient requires, the goal of home health care is to provide the services necessary to restore the patient to an optimal level of function within the limits of his or her capacity. Home health nurses achieve this through the assessment of patients in their own environments, understanding the impact that the environment has on a patient's well-being. These nurses mobilize and coordinate both agency and community resources that are necessary to safely maintain patients in their own homes for as long as the patients wish.

The nursing profession in the United States can trace its roots back to the late 1700s. Long before the existence of a formal health care system and schools of nursing, lay nurses provided in-home care to their families, friends, and neighbors.

As people immigrated from rural villages to large urban centers in the 1800s, public health nurses began providing care in many communities. The Women's Suffrage Movement of the 1920s expanded the rights of and opportunities for women, and the nursing profession provided them with a forum to exercise these newfound freedoms. As American culture evolved from its Puritan colonial past to a modern diverse society, the practice of nursing also advanced to meet the needs of the patients and communities.

For over two centuries, home health care has evolved yet remains ready to meet the needs of communities and citizens. To understand the role of home health care today and recognize the potential of the future, one must understand from where this profession and industry emerged.

THE 1700s

During the 1700s, care of the sick was the responsibility of religious groups whose vocation was to alleviate physical suffering and tend to the spiritual needs of patients. Suffering and illness were believed to be the result of evil spirits or retribution from God for one's misdeeds. Due to ignorance, fear, and superstitious beliefs, the infirm were ostracized and segregated from their communities and families.

The Boston Dispensary, founded in 1796, was one of the earliest health care organizations in the United States. It was organized around the following three principles:

- Care of the sick could be provided in the patient's home, preventing the pain caused by separation and segregation from one's family and community.

- The home was the least expensive environment in which to provide care.

- Care of those who needed charity could be provided in a confidential and respectable way.

(Greenleaf, 1898)

The Boston Dispensary provided organization to lay caregivers, who remained the primary providers of health services. In 1801, the Boston Dispensary became incorporated and formed the first Visiting Doctors Association, where many

well-known physicians were trained. In 1886, the Instructive Nursing Association was established as part of the Boston Dispensary; it later evolved into what is now known as the Boston Visiting Nurse Association (Greenleaf, 1898).

1800–1880

The period from 1800 to 1880 is characterized by two major events in American history. The American Civil War, fought from 1860 to 1865, marked the beginning of the Industrial Revolution. These events, coupled with the teachings and publications of London's Florence Nightingale, greatly influenced the development and advancement of formalized nursing and home health care during this period.

Influence of Florence Nightingale

Florence Nightingale, born in 1820, was raised by an affluent British family. As a young adult, she was interested in many of the social questions and ills of British society. Consistent with the social norms of the era, her family refused to allow her to pursue her interests in nursing because it was not considered a suitable profession for educated, well-bred women (Lewis, n.d.).

In an effort to distract Florence from her desire to work in nursing, her family sanctioned a tour of Europe with family friends. While in Germany, Florence met the superintendent of the Kaisersworth School for Nurses, who served to heighten her interest in caring for the ill and the poor. Contrary to her family's wishes, Nightingale remained in Germany, where she received 3 months of formal nurse training. Upon her return to Britain in 1853, she qualified for the position of Superintendent at the Institute for the Care of Sick Gentlewomen in Distressed Circumstances (Lewis, n.d.). Nightingale remained in this position until she was recruited by the British military during the Crimean War.

In 1854, Britain, France, and Turkey declared war on Russia. During this time, the British military was highly criticized by the British press for its inadequate care of soldiers and military casualties. Florence Nightingale was placed in charge of introducing female nurses into military hospitals in Turkey. Initially, physicians were not responsive to the presence of nurses in military hospitals; however, as they became overwhelmed by the number of casualties, the contributions of nurses were welcomed. The work of these 38 nurses resulted in improvements in the environment and morale in hospitals and barracks (Florence Nightingale Museum Trust, n.d.).

In 1860, the Florence Nightingale's Training School for Nurses was established. Nurses in training (probationers) received 1 year of experience on the wards of St. Thomas Hospital. Once nurses completed their formal training, they staffed hospitals in Britain, Europe, and the United States.

Although Nightingale oversaw the training of the probationers, during this time she also wrote *Notes on Nursing: What It Is and What It Is Not,* which outlined her observations and concepts of nursing and patient care (Florence Nightingale Museum Trust, n.d.). In this publication, Nightingale theorized that although an important role of nurses was to care for the sick, it was more important that they care for the well in an effort to prevent sickness all together. She also wrote about the notion that nurses should not be educated and managed by hospitals and doctors. Instead, she advocated for a "matron of nurses" who would be responsible for the education and practice of nurses (Lewis, n.d.). In addition, she published many writings about health care organizations and health care systems.

It was Nightingale's concept that organized nurses into geographic districts to provide home health care in Britain's neighborhoods and communities. This model was later expanded to the cities of the United States as a means to combat communicable diseases and other social ills of the 19th century.

Florence Nightingale was the recipient of many "firsts." In recognition of her wartime efforts, she was the first female appointed to the Royal Commission of the British Army and the first female fellow of the British Statistical Society (Florence Nightingale Museum Trust, n.d.). However, her greatest accomplishment was to advance the standing of nursing from an undesirable endeavor for the well-bred and educated to a profession that continues to have the highest ethical and moral standards (Florence Nightingale Museum Trust, n.d.).

Industrial Revolution

During the earliest part of the 19th century, the growth of American cities was phenomenal. People immigrated from rural towns and villages and from European countries in search of employment in American factories. These growing cities lacked hospital beds and adequate housing and were complicated by cultural and linguistic differences. During this expansion, great strides were being made in the advancement of both the arts and sciences. Class distinction and separation was common. Women of the middle and upper classes were not allowed to work outside of the home. Instead, they were expected to pursue artistic and philanthropic endeavors.

Nursing care in the early part of the 19th century was provided by working- and lower-class women. They were untrained and functioned as lay nurses, despite the lack of any formal health care system. Lay nurses were generally employed by individuals to assist in the care of a sick family member. Home care was provided by one or two lay nurses, who usually worked for a family 24 hours a day, 6 or 7 days a week. Early public health services were provided by volunteers, or if the community was lucky, services were provided under the direction of at least one trained nurse.

This period of nursing in the United States was informal and unregulated. Organized nurse training was not available until 1872, when the first two schools of nursing opened in Philadelphia and Boston (Timeline of nursing history, 2010). It was not until 1873 and the opening of three additional schools that the principles of infection control taught and published by Florence Nightingale were incorporated into the curricula.

The growing cities of the 1800s created environments of poverty, inadequate sanitation and food storage, and poor personal hygiene. These factors, coupled with crowded conditions, accelerated the spread of infectious and communicable diseases. Morbidity and mortality from these conditions was high among the very young and the very old. To combat these conditions, New York City established the Division of Child Hygiene in 1880 and hired "trained" nurses to reduce infant mortality (MetLife, n.d.). These public health nurses made home visits and taught mothers and their families how to provide sanitary environments for their infants.

Recognizing the benefits of having trained nurses, many communities began to support the establishment of a public health nurse service, and the demand for formally trained nurses grew. In addition to working for agencies supported by local governments, trained nurses were also employed by local visiting nurse services. During this era, wealthy and upper-class members of society provided the financial resources necessary to secure and support the development of their local visiting nurse services. Each organization was structured in a manner that met the needs of the community in which it was located, and the scope of each agency's service was often dictated by the interests of the group or individuals providing the financing. For example, the District Nurse Association of Fall River Massachusetts was incorporated for:

> The purpose of promoting the social and physical well-being of the citizens of Fall River; supplying the needy with necessary articles; providing medical, surgical and nursing attendance and means of instruction; and, in general, doing what may be done for improving social conditions in the city of Fall River.
>
> (Certificate of Corporation provided by the Commonwealth of Massachusetts to the District Nurse Association of Fall River, April 12, 1912)

1880–1929

By 1890, 21 visiting nurse associations (VNAs) existed in the United States, and the number was growing rapidly. Although these organizations became more sophisticated in structure, their purpose remained largely the same as it was in the 1800s: to care for the physically ill and the poor.

Poverty and infectious disease continued to plague citizens. By 1909, tuberculosis was responsible for hundreds of deaths on a daily basis. Metropolitan Life, a life insurance company for working families, found itself paying approximately 20% of its claims to victims of tuberculosis (MetLife, n.d.). Haley Fiske, the vice president of Metropolitan Life at that time, announced that the company's philosophy was about to change. He stated that insurance is not merely a business proposition but a social program and then took an aggressive two-pronged approach to combat tuberculosis (MetLife, n.d.). First, in 1909, Metropolitan Life published and distributed a pamphlet titled *A War on Consumption* as a means to teach citizens methods to reduce the spread of the infection (MetLife, n.d.). The second and most notable endeavor it undertook was to collaborate with Lillian Wald, a nurse who was recognized for her commitment to social reform and the care of the city's poor.

Lillian Wald had already established and was directing the operations of the Henry Street Settlement House (later known as the Visiting Nurse Service of New York), thereby providing home visits to New York City residents (Profiles in Caring, n.d.). She convinced Metropolitan Life executives to participate in a 3-month pilot program to evaluate the effectiveness of in-home nursing services in the reduction of deaths related to tuberculosis. The pilot was so successful that Metropolitan Life extended its home care benefit to policyholders in many American cities. Metropolitan Life employed a nursing force of its own to deliver care in areas where there were no organized visiting nurse services. In addition to tuberculosis, nurses treated policyholders for such common ailments as diphtheria, influenza and smallpox.

The success of these programs supported Metropolitan Life's expansion of the home health care benefit to over 20 million policyholders in 7,000 cities (MetLife, n.d.). At the height of the program, home care was provided free of charge to approximately 35 out of every 1,000 Metropolitan Life beneficiaries. By 1924, more than 3,000 communities could boast of having their own visiting nurse services. Other insurance companies, such as John Hancock in Boston, began similar programs.

As Metropolitan Life was expanding the availability of home health care to its policyholders, the American Red Cross also recognized the benefit of community-based nurses and began developing a national nursing service. The American Red Cross had already demonstrated its ability to train and mobilize nurses to care for casualties of war. Under the guidance of Clara Barton, Red Cross nurses were successful at reducing the spread of infection and alleviating the pain and suffering of soldiers during the Spanish-American War. Nurses found the conditions of the soldiers and the camps deplorable. One nurse reported "desperately sick fever patients, United States soldiers on United States soil were lying on the cots between heavy military blankets, no sheets, no pillows, no towels, no mosquito netting, although they were being tormented beyond words by mosquitoes, flies and sand fleas" (American Red Cross , n.d.-a).

Army officers and President McKinley recognized that without the help and contribution of the Red Cross nurses, the entire military operation would have been at risk. Recognizing the success of the Nurse Corps, the Red Cross changed its focus toward developing a program to assure that there would be a volunteer nurse in every American community. The administration of the Red Cross envisioned a legion of Red Cross nurses that could be mobilized in times of crisis, such as with floods, fires, or wars.

Jane A. Delano, the superintendent of the Army Nurse Corps, was charged with the development of a Red Cross nursing service. Despite the lack of trained nurses nationwide, by the time the United States entered World War I, there were 18,000 nurses ready to serve their country (American Red Cross, n.d.). Although many nurses remained in the United States, nearly 9,000 served war casualties in American field hospitals in France (American Red Cross, n.d.). The nurses who remained in the United States were responsible for assuring the health and sanitation of more than 50 American Army and Navy bases (American Red Cross, n.d.).

Between October and November of 1918, the home health nurses who were so successful at combating the tuberculosis epidemic in 1909 were once again put to the test. The influenza epidemic of 1918 stretched the resources of every health care provider in the cities, suburbs, and counties. Unlike the tuberculosis epidemic, the influenza epidemic began and ended in roughly 8 weeks. Cooperative efforts between Red Cross nurses and the Visiting Nurse Service were responsible for limiting the devastating influenza epidemic of 1918.

Permellia Murnan Doty, Executive Secretary of the Nurses Emergency Council in 1918, described how communities mobilized all able-bodied individuals to assist in hospitals, clinics, and homes. Communities organized headquarters from which all operations were directed. Radio announcements and handbills instructed volunteers where to report for assignment. Doty wrote:

"For this work, women were needed who were not only willing to take care of the sick but also to help with household affairs. It was, of course, a good deal of a risk to send untrained women about whom we knew so little into the homes to care for desperately ill people, but under the circumstances it was the only thing to do." (Doty, 1919, p. 951).

In the article "A Retrospect of the Influenza Epidemic," Doty described the conditions in which visiting nurses found patients and their families. She stated,

"Nurses were finding many households where whole families were ill, or perhaps a mother and several children, without anyone to give them even the simplest nursing care. Some patients were critically ill. Because of the prejudice against hospitals, which was doubtless accentuated during the epidemic by reports of so many deaths in institutions, it was necessary that someone be found to stay with the sick in the homes since many people refused to allow their friends and relatives to be taken to the hospital." (Doty, 1919, p. 954).

Despite the heroic efforts of nurses during the influenza epidemic, more than 675,000 American lives were lost (American Red Cross, n.d.-b).

At the end of the influenza epidemic, the home health nurses returned to their roles as health educators and direct care providers. They continued to teach about modes of disease transmission, prevention, and infant and child care and also provided direct care to the acutely ill. During this period, the model of having one nurse care for many families evolved as the most efficient means for a limited number of professional nurses to have the greatest impact on the communities they served. Also during this time, the services of professional nurses were sought to staff hospitals, to work for private businesses, and to care for private individuals. The services of visiting nurses were also frequently requested by other community-based or social-service organizations that identified people in need of health care services. Box 1-1 contains the

response of the administrator from one agency to one such request.

1930–1954

Between 1930 and 1940, there was a major shift in the provision of health care in the United States. This post–World War II era saw the rapid advancement of science and the subsequent decline of infectious disease as the major health problem. Instead, the growth of chronic and acute illnesses emerged.

The shift from community-based to hospital-based health care was rapid. Although more costly, hospital care was available to all social classes and became the primary source of health care for American citizens.

The availability of hospital care diminished the need for home-based services. By the early 1950s, Metropolitan Life eliminated its home health benefit, and the American Red Cross closed its national nursing service. However, local VNAs that were previously established continued to receive financial support from charitable donors and local governments. These visiting nurse services carried on their tradition of providing infection control and healthy lifestyle education, caring for the poor, and addressing the social ills in their communities.

1955–1964

Hospital costs that resulted from caring for the growing number of chronically ill and elderly patients had risen dramatically. By 1955, the value and cost savings associated with home health care services was once again sought and care began to shift back to the community. The health care system once again began to recognize that the patient's own home was perhaps the most efficient place for care. This realization spawned the development of hospital-based home health agencies and community-based homemaker services, in addition to

BOX 1-1: LETTER

February 19, 1915

Dear Sir:

I have your letter of February 17th, and before submitting it to the Board of Managers should like to know more definitely what your proposition covers.

We (the Fall River District Nurse Association) undertake to care for all persons in the City needing nursing attention so far as time of our nurses will allow. Various corporations pay the expense of five nurses; the Anti-Tuberculosis Society pays the expense of another; the Union Hospital contributes $1200 a year, thus obliging us to care for discharged patients requiring dressings and other service in their homes; the Metropolitan Life Insurance Company pays 50 cents a visit: and it is, of course, our first duty to see that the work which we undertake for this is satisfactorily performed. After this is done, the nurses give their attention to calls coming from individuals, making a charge of 50 cents per visit when the patients are able to pay, but otherwise rendering free service. As result of all these activities, our corps of ten nurses is already fully occupied, and we cannot see how we can undertake any further obligations without adding to our nursing force, and this we are unable to do without addition to our funds.

We recognize the importance of following up discharged patients, by inducing them to return to clinics, in accordance with instructions, and also by rendering such nursing care as may be necessary at the homes, and should be very glad to assist in this work if we had nurses available, but we cannot see how it can be accomplished unless the expense of such work is covered.

It has been our experience that patients may be discharged from the hospital, if properly cared for at the home, at an earlier date than would otherwise be possible, with resulting good to the patient and economy to the hospital; and we also believe that may be accomplished more economically and efficiently by a district nursing service than by a single nurse because of the acquaintanceship of each nurse in her district and the saving of travel. We do not know how many such cases would develop from the City Hospitals. If only a few and the Hospital were willing to take the chance of a nurse's time being available, the Board of Managers would probably be glad to authorize us to do what we could. But even a call to induce a patient to report at a clinic often requires much time for persuasion, and a nursing call requires even more time. Our nurses are able to make between eight and nine visits a day on the average; and the cost for each nurse, including supplies and carfare, approximates $800.00 a year.

Yours truly, L.

(*Note.* From Visiting Nurse Association of Southeastern Massachusetts, 502 Bedford Street, Fall River, Mass 02777, n.d.. Reprinted with permission.)

the visiting nurse services that already existed. All of these agencies continued to depend on the generosity of charitable organizations and private foundations for funding. In addition, some funding was received from town and city governments as a means to care for their citizens.

1965–1987

The demand for home health care by the growing number of patients was beyond the scope and resources of most agencies. Despite the generosity of philanthropic endeavors, agencies could not meet the needs of all who required care. In 1965, in an effort to meet patient needs while reducing costs, the federal government enacted Medicare legislation that established a home health benefit for beneficiaries. The Medicare home health benefit would ignite the most significant growth of home health care services to date. The original benefit provided financial reimbursement for the provision of skilled nursing care. Due to patient needs, coverage was later expanded to provide services of the medical social worker; physical, speech and occupational therapist; and home health aide.

To participate in the Medicare reimbursement system, agencies must be certified by a process outlined by the Centers for Medicare & Medicaid Services (CMS), formerly the Health Care Financing Administration. Initially, only not-for-profit organizations could be certified to receive reimbursement for providing home health care services to Medicare beneficiaries.

Medicare home health benefits were primarily available only to people over 65 years of age; however, the CMS required each state to provide a home health benefit to qualified elderly and the poor through their state-funded Medicaid programs. Finally, the Older Americans Act of 1965 solidified the home health benefit, as it required both the federal and state governments to design programs to assist and support elders to remain in their homes and avoid costly facility-based care and institutionalization.

Initially, reimbursement was intended for home health services that were the result of at least a 3-day hospital stay. For beneficiaries to be eligible, they had to be strictly homebound and the services had to be short-term and recuperative in nature. These criteria severely limited the utilization of this benefit by Medicare beneficiaries. At this time (1965), approximately 1,275 organizations were certified by Medicare to provide home health services to Medicare beneficiaries (Reichley, 1999).

The growth in the number of certified agencies from the inception of the Medicare certification in 1965 to the 1980s and 1990s was phenomenal. In testimony provided to the House Commerce Subcommittee on Health and Environment, Bruce Vladeck, Administrator of the CMS, estimated that the number of agencies certified to receive Medicare reimbursement in 1982 was approximately 3,125 (Vladeck, 1997). Many of these agencies were small, local organizations that provided care to friends and neighbors.

Recognizing this growth, and the expense implications associated with it, the CMS implemented new policies aimed at slowing the proliferation and certification of new home health care agencies. In essence, this policy would reduce the availability of rapidly expanding home health services, hence curbing the growth.

The CMS used medical record review as a mechanism to "teach" home health care providers to properly administer the Medicare benefit. Although the CMS always conducted a limited amount of medical record review, more stringent medical review policies and procedures were implemented. Claims were reviewed from both a clinical and technical perspective.

The decision to review a claim required the home health agency to photocopy and mail a portion (usually 1 month's documentation) of the medical record to the CMS. Records were then evaluated for indicators, such as the reasonableness and necessity of services. If a Medicare reviewer did not agree that the services provided by the agency were reasonable and necessary, the reviewer had the authority to deny payment for the claim.

1987–1996

In 1987, as a result of a public outcry related to reduced access to home care services, a congressional delegation led by senators Harley Staggers and Claude Pepper filed and won a lawsuit against the CMS. This resulted in an easing of the restrictions used by CMS to govern and control the home health industry (Reichley, 1999). The easing of medical review policies, the elimination of the 3-day hospital stay eligibility requirement, and the broadening of homebound criteria and certification requirements ignited a growth in the home care industry that the CMS would find problematic in the 1990s.

Until the Stagger's lawsuit, all Medicare-certified home health care providers were required to be not-for-profit organizations. One of the unanticipated effects of the easing of the certification restrictions was the entry of for-profit providers into the home health care field. In addition, easing of the restrictions and decreased medical review encouraged home health agencies to provide large numbers of visits to beneficiaries. An agency would bill the CMS for every visit it provided to the beneficiary, and the CMS would reimburse up to $120 for each nursing visit. This visit-based reimbursement system created an incentive to provide large numbers of visits to Medicare beneficiaries. Unfortunately, these circumstances led to the proliferation of less-scrupulous agencies that defrauded the Medicare trust fund.

In his testimony to the Subcommittee on Health and Environment in March of 1997, Bruce Vladeck asserted that approximately 25% of all home health claims were inappropriate or outright fraudulent (Vladeck, 1997). Vladeck provided examples of unscrupulous providers who billed for services provided to patients who were deceased and agencies that billed Medicare for services that were never provided to beneficiaries who never existed (Vladeck, 1997). He cited examples where foreign nationals obtained Medicare certification and had Medicare payments sent to their countries of origin without ever providing any patient care.

1997–2000

By the mid-1990s, the industry peaked to over 10,000 home health providers. In an effort to again curb the growth of and spending on home health services, the CMS introduced the concept of a prospective payment system (PPS).

Changing from a visit-based reimbursement system to a PPS was not a new concept. During the 1980s, hospital systems shifted from a fee-for-service system to a diagnosis-related group (DRG) reimbursement system, as did the nursing home industry in the early 1990s. Simply stated, under a PPS a provider receives a fixed dollar amount to provide care for a patient based on the severity of the patient's clinical status for a finite period of time.

The Balanced Budget Act, signed by President Clinton in August 1997, put the home health industry on notice that effective October 1, 1997, reimbursement would be capped. The period from October 1, 1997, to October 1, 2000, was characterized by a system known as the interim payment system (IPS). The IPS was designed to limit the amount the CMS would pay to an agency regardless of the number of visits it provided to the patient. These limits were intended to prepare the home health care industry for the transition to PPS, which became effective October 1, 2000.

Provisions mandated by the Balanced Budget Act and enforced by the CMS were based on the perception that the home health industry was fraught with fraud (Vladeck, 1997). The Balanced Budget Act provided a multitude of strategies to reduce fraud and abuse. To meet the outlined objectives, agencies had to:

• alter billing practices

• secure surety bonds

• undergo increased scrutiny of medical records

• withstand increased payment denials

• institute the electronic transmission of clinical data to both state and federal agencies

• administer changing interpretations of beneficiary eligibility criteria

• reduce services

• cut the costs of operations.

As a result, the home care industry perceived that it was under siege. From 1997 to 2000, over 4,000 agencies closed. Those that remained open hoped that the implementation of the PPS would provide both regulatory and financial relief. To survive, agencies had to change quickly to maximize efficiency. Only 6,000 agencies were successful in making these rapid, widespread changes.

2000 TO CURRENT

Since October 1, 2000, the CMS has reimbursed home health care agencies for services to beneficiaries via the PPS. In general, after the clinician completes the patient assessment, the agency receives one payment to manage all of the patient's home health care for the next 60 days. Although some agencies have fared well in this system and even managed to generate a profit, the Balanced Budget Act of 1997 requires Congress to evaluate the rates paid to home health agencies on a regular basis. As a result, agencies have endured several additional cuts in reimbursement since the implementation of PPS.

SUMMARY

Through the efforts of nursing matriarchs like Florence Nightingale, Lillian Wald, Jane Delano, and countless others, the cost effectiveness of home health nursing was demonstrated. For over 100 years, home care nurses have been able to improve the physical and social health of individual citizens and the community. This model of providing health care was so profound that its influence continues to shape the delivery of home health care services in the 21st century.

EXAM QUESTIONS

CHAPTER 1
Questions 1-6

Note: Choose the option that BEST answers each question.

1. Florence Nightingale's greatest accomplishment was to

   a. organize home health care nurses into geographic districts.

   b. publish *Notes on Nursing*.

   c. advance the standing of nursing from an undesirable endeavor to a profession that continues to have the highest ethical and moral standards.

   d. establish the Florence Nightingale Training School for Nurses.

2. Lillian Wald convinced the executives of the Metropolitan Life Insurance Company to participate in a 3-month pilot program to

   a. evaluate the effectiveness of in-home services in the reduction of tuberculosis-related deaths.

   b. treat common ailments such as diphtheria, influenza, and smallpox.

   c. teach mothers how to provide care to their newborn babies.

   d. conduct physical assessment prior to issuing a life insurance policy.

3. Clara Barton was most noted for mobilizing American Red Cross nurses to

   a. care for victims of natural disasters.

   b. inoculate citizens of large cities against tuberculosis.

   c. teach principles of sanitation and hygiene to people living in rural communities.

   d. care for soldiers wounded at war.

4. After World War II, the American health care system experienced rapid advancement in technology and sciences, which increased the

   a. number of home health care agencies.

   b. availability of hospital care.

   c. amount of Medicare payments for home health care services.

   d. number of proprietary agencies in the home health care industry.

5. In 1965, the Older Americans Act required both federal and state governments to design programs to assist and support elders with remaining in their homes. To qualify, beneficiaries were required to

   a. have experienced at least a 3-day hospital stay prior to the initiation of home health care services.

   b. be in need of services from at least two professional disciplines.

   c. have a primary care provider who would provide assistance to the elder.

   d. agree to a 10% copayment for all services received.

6. In August of 1997, in an effort to curb expenses and reduce fraud and abuse in the home health care industry, President Clinton signed into law

   a. Staggers lawsuit.

   b. Medicare Home Health Benefit.

   c. Balanced Budget Act.

   d. DRGs.

CHAPTER 2

CODE OF ETHICS FOR NURSES

CHAPTER OBJECTIVE

At the completion of this chapter, the reader will be able to discuss the American Nurses Association's (ANA) *Code of Ethics for Nurses.*

LEARNING OBJECTIVES

After studying this chapter, the reader will be able to

1. identify the purpose of the ANA's *Code of Ethics for Nurses.*

2. recognize the patient's right to self-determination and the professional nurse's responsibility with regard to his or her own opinions and judgments.

3. list three examples that demonstrate the home health nurse's ability to advance nursing knowledge and professional practice.

4. identify the risks associated with delegation of patient care activities to ancillary staff.

5. recall the characteristics of a professional relationship.

INTRODUCTION

A code of ethics is a set of "imperatives formulated as statements of personal responsibility and identifies elements of such a commitment" to a profession or organization (Association for Computing Machinery [ACM], 1992, p. 1). An ethics code describes the expectations and values of an individual or organization and serves to address many, but not all, issues a professional is likely to face (ACM, 1992).

The first statement of ethics for nursing can be traced back to the late 1800s, when Lystra Gretter wrote "The Nightingale Pledge" (see Box 2-1). Between 1893 and 1950, a number of nursing organizations authored various codes of ethics for nursing; however, it was not until 1950 that the ANA drafted the *Code of Ethics for Nurses* that is widely accepted today. The practice of nursing has significantly evolved over the last 50 years. The *Code of Ethics for Nurses* has also evolved and has been revised to reflect the changes in nursing practice; however, the fundamental concepts of ethical nursing practice and behavior have endured.

The ANA's 2001 *Code of Ethics for Nurses with Interpretive Statements* consists of nine provisions that outline the conduct that is expected of every nurse. Like all ethical codes, the *Code of Ethics for Nurses* is intended to serve as a framework for decision making, conduct, and practice. Although not a legal document, the *Code of Ethics for Nurses* represents the promise that all professional nurses make to the patients they care for. It is similar to a contract between business partners. It succinctly outlines the services that the patient should expect and will receive.

The Nightingale Pledge
Lystra Gretter 1893

I solemnly pledge myself before God and in the presence of this assembly, to pass my life in purity and to practice my profession faithfully. I will abstain from whatever is deleterious and mischievous, and will not take or knowingly administer any harmful drug. I will do all in my power to maintain and elevate the standard of my profession, and will hold in confidence all personal matters committed to my keeping and all family affairs coming to my knowledge in the practice of my calling. With loyalty will I endeavor to aid the physician, in his work, and devote myself to the welfare of those committed to my care. (McDonald, n.d.)

The *Code of Ethics for Nurses* serves to remind nurses that the privilege of caring for patients and their families is not one that should be taken lightly. These expectations apply to nurses regardless of the policies of an organization or setting of practice and are applicable in the day-to-day activities of every nurse.

THE PROVISIONS

The ANA's *Code of Ethics for Nurses* has nine provisions. Each general provision is further clarified by a subset of interpretive statements. The role of the nurse as it relates directly to patient care is outlined in the first three provisions. It is important to note that, for the purposes of the *Code of Ethics for Nurses,* the "patient" may be defined as an individual, a family, or an entire community.

Provisions Four, Five, and Six outline the nurse's obligation to cultivate and develop his or her own practice. These provisions address issues of clinical competence, professional growth, and the individual's responsibility to exert influence on health care systems and organizations in an effort to maximize the quality of nursing care provided within these institutions.

Finally, Provisions Seven, Eight, and Nine outline the obligations that each nurse has to support and advance the agenda of the nursing profession. In essence, these provisions delineate the obligation that each individual nurse has to the entire body of professional nurses. While Provision Seven requires the nurse to develop and advance nursing knowledge, Provisions Eight and Nine describe the nurse's role in initiatives to influence and improve health on local, national, and international levels.

Society holds the profession of nursing to the highest ethical standards; therefore, nurses must also hold themselves and their nurse colleagues to the standards outlined in Table 2-1. Adherence to these provisions and standards has allowed nurses to remain the most respected and trusted health care providers today.

CASE STUDY

The case study of Mrs. Smith will demonstrate application of the first three provisions outlined in the *Code of Ethics for Nurses*.

Mrs. Smith is an 80-year-old patient with congestive heart failure (CHF). She was referred to your home care agency after experiencing three hospitalizations for CHF in the last 2 months. Your clinical manager has assigned her case to you.

As you approach Mrs. Smith's home, you note that she lives in a residential suburban neighborhood and her home appears to be reasonably well kept. As you go up the six stairs to her front door, you note that although the stairs seem safe, there is no handrailing. When you knock on the door, you hear a distant voice say, "Come in."

As you enter the home, a number of cats scamper out of the way and disappear into other rooms, blending in among a large volume of clutter. The

TABLE 2-1: ANA CODE OF ETHICS FOR NURSES

Provision One

The nurse, in all professional relationships, practices with compassion and respect for the inherent dignity, worth, and uniqueness of every individual, unrestricted by considerations of social or economic status, personal attributes, or the nature of health problems.

Provision Two

The nurse's primary commitment is to the patient, whether an individual, family, group, or community.

Provision Three

The nurse promotes, advocates for, and strives to protect the health, safety, and rights of the patient.

Provision Four

The nurse is responsible and accountable for individual nursing practice and determines the appropriate delegation of tasks consistent with the nurse's obligation to provide optimum patient care.

Provision Five

The nurse owes the same duties to self as to others, including the responsibility to preserve integrity and safety, to maintain competence, and to continue personal and professional growth.

Provision Six

The nurse participates in establishing, maintaining, and improving health care environments and conditions of employment conducive to the provision of quality health care and consistent with the values of the profession through individual and collective action.

Provision Seven

The nurse participates in the advancement of the profession through contributions to practice, education, administration, and knowledge development.

Provision Eight

The nurse collaborates with other health professionals and the public in promoting community, national, and international efforts to meet health needs.

Provision Nine

The profession of nursing, as represented by associations and their members, is responsible for articulating nursing values, for maintaining the integrity of the profession and its practice, and for shaping social policy.

Note. From *Code of Ethics for Nurses with Interpretive Statements,* by American Nurses' Association, 2001, Silver Spring, MD: American Nurses Publishing. Reprinted with permission.

patient calls once again, "Who's there? Come on in so I can see you."

Once you enter the room, you see Mrs. Smith. She is lying in a hospital bed with her head elevated. You note that the bed itself is in a raised position. Placed all around her on various tables and in the bed are her medication bottles, various foodstuff, reading material, bottles of water, bottles of what appear to be alcoholic beverages, and personal hygiene products.

Mrs. Smith appears to be angry and states, "I have been sitting on this bed pan since the ambulance brought me home." You recall that your refer-

ral documents state that Mrs. Smith left the hospital yesterday afternoon.

Once you find a reasonably clean place to set down your nursing bag, you use your waterless soap to wash your hands and put on gloves so you can assist Mrs. Smith off of the bedpan. As you do, you notice that her bed linens are soiled and recognize the odor as urine. She remains in a hospital gown, and it appears that she has not had any personal care for at least 24 hours. You note that it is remarkable that she has not suffered any breakdown in her skin on her back or buttocks.

When you enter the bathroom to empty the bedpan, you realize that what first appeared to be only clutter now appears to be hazardous. The facilities are not clean, and cat excrement is on the floor in various places.

When you return to the bedroom, you begin your assessment of Mrs. Smith and her environment, realizing that none of this information is on your hospital referral. Mrs. Smith readily tells you that she lives alone and has an "aide" who usually helps her out but that the aide has not shown up since she got back from the hospital.

When you query her about additional help, she gets angry once again and states, "Yeah, I got kids, and not one of them is good for anything." You quickly realize that this line of questioning is upsetting to Mrs. Smith. Before you can move on to another topic, she asks, "Are you just like the rest of them, coming in here and wanting to know my business?"

You then change the subject to something that you hope will be less upsetting to Mrs. Smith. You begin to explain to her that your agency received a request from the hospital to evaluate how she is managing at home. You explain to her that you are a registered nurse and that her doctor has requested an assessment of her cardiac condition.

PROVISION ONE

By evaluating the case of Mrs. Smith, it is clear to see how the provisions of the Code of Ethics for Nurses can be applied to the day-to-day practice of the home health nurse. Provision One requires that, "The nurse provides services with respect for human dignity and the uniqueness of the client unrestricted by considerations of social or economic status, personal attributes, or the nature of health problems" (ANA, 2001, p. 7). Provision One also dictates that the need for health care is universal, and nursing care must be delivered without prejudice. When planning a patient's care, the nurse must consider the lifestyle and value system of the patient and customize care to meet that individual patient's needs.

Although Mrs. Smith's current lifestyle and value system may not be conducive to what is considered a healthy environment, it is clearly her choice. The *Code of Ethics for Nurses* does not require the nurse to condone or agree with a patient's choice, it does however require the nurse to provide care to the patient regardless of the patient's choices (ANA, 2001). Unless breaking a local law, if Mrs. Smith chooses to keep 20, 30, or even 100 cats in her home and allow them to roam freely across all surfaces, it is her right to do so.

As the nurse standing in her bedroom, you can identify a number of interventions to "improve" the conditions of Mrs. Smith and her home. Unless declared incompetent, it is up to Mrs. Smith to dictate what type and how much help or care she is willing to receive. It is your obligation to provide her with information to help her exercise her right to self-determination and choose the care and interventions that she feels are appropriate for her needs.

Self-determination, a term that is frequently used in clinical settings, is defined as a patient's "moral and legal right to determine what will be done with their own person; and

- to be given accurate, complete, and understandable information in a manner that facilitates an informed judgement;
- to be assisted in weighing the benefits, burdens, and available options in their treatment including the choice of no treatment;
- to accept, refuse, or terminate treatment without deceit, undue influence, duress, coercion, or penalty; and
- to be given necessary support throughout the decision-making and treatment process."
(ANA, 2001, p. 8)

Unlike nursing care provided in a clinic, physician's office, hospital, or long-term care facility, home health care is provided to a patient in his or her home and the locus of control changes from the organization to the individual patient. The patient determines how he or she will live and what he or she will have for dinner – whether or not the selection is within his or her dietary restrictions. It is not uncommon for a home health nurse to characterize the choices that a patient has made as right, wrong, good, or bad. However, an experienced home health nurse realizes that characterization of patient choices is fruitless. The competent home health nurse realizes that patients make these choices despite receiving the best care, information, and instruction, and it is the nurse's obligation to work within these choices.

Mrs. Smith is clear in her decision to remain in her current environment, stating, "I have lived in this house all my life. I was born here, I had my children here, and I will die here. These cats keep me company all day and night. They are all I have left." At first blush, these choices may seem "bad" or "poor;" however, when you take the time to hear Mrs. Smith's words, you realize that her home and her cats are her personal treasures.

Provision One of the *Code of Ethics for Nurses* requires nurse respect for the worth and dignity of the individual applies irrespective of the nature of the health problem (ANA, 2001). In the case of Mrs. Smith, this creates an immediate difficulty for you. Through your education and experience, you know that Mrs. Smith's condition will continue to deteriorate if she remains in her current situation. At the very least, you anticipate pressure sores due to poor nutrition and immobility, exacerbations of CHF, as well as potential complications related to her alcohol intake. The question here is: What intervention, if any, can be implemented in caring for Mrs. Smith?

Provision One requires that you provide appropriate care to Mrs. Smith, even if her home environment is distasteful. You must ensure, to the best of your ability, that decisions you make related to Mrs. Smith's care safeguard her well-being and safety. This becomes a critical moment in the home visit of Mrs. Smith. What would you do?

- Leave Mrs. Smith's home and call your supervisor to discuss the concerns that you have about Mrs. Smith's living situation.

- Apologize to Mrs. Smith for upsetting her with the questions you have asked, and attempt to continue the visit by beginning her physical assessment.

- Inform Mrs. Smith that her unwillingness to be more cooperative and her obvious displeasure with you makes her inappropriate for home care services, and move on to your next patient.

The first and second options are reasonable and would not conflict with Provision One of the code. Depending on the experience of the home health nurse and agency policy, the nurse may choose one or both of these strategies to complete the visit with Mrs. Smith. The third option, deciding that Mrs. Smith is not appropriate for services because of the nurse's discomfort with the patient and environment, would violate Provision One.

PROVISION TWO

Provision Two requires that the nurse collaborate with other members of the health care team and defines *collaboration* as the "concerted effort of individuals and groups to attain a shared goal" (ANA, 2001, p. 10). In the case of Mrs. Smith, a number of opportunities exist for collaborative care.

In all likelihood, Mrs. Smith would benefit from a physical therapy evaluation to address safety issues and improve her ability to get out of bed. Perhaps if she could tolerate aggressive therapy, she might eventually be able to maneuver around her home with a walker or cane.

Referral to a medical social worker would be appropriate to help identify additional community-based services, such as adult day care or adult foster care, that might be mobilized to reduce Mrs. Smith's isolation. You must also consider whether Mrs.

Smith would benefit from a visit by a registered dietician, who could evaluate her eating habits, make suggestions to improve her nutrition, and minimize complications such as fluid retention. As the nurse assigned to Mrs. Smith's case, it is your obligation to make the appropriate referrals and coordinate her care so that the goals established for her are met.

PROVISION THREE

The third provision outlined in the *Code of Ethics for Nurses* obligates nurses to "safeguard the client's right to privacy by judiciously protecting information of a confidential nature" (ANA, 2001, p. 10). The right to privacy is described as an inalienable human right. You now have to determine if Mrs. Smith's situation places her in such jeopardy that it should be reported to the local bureau of elder services for a formalized "elder at risk" assessment or to the local board of public health for evaluation of the conditions inside her home.

Although Mrs. Smith has clearly made some poor lifestyle choices, you have to consider that it is her right to make them. Mrs. Smith has already stated that she is not interested in allowing outsiders to "know [her] business." Although involving elder services seems like the "right" thing to do, you must consider your rationale for making or not making the decision to report Mrs. Smith's living situation. During your conversation with Mrs. Smith, she was able to answer all questions appropriately (even though she was a little angry and upset), and she demonstrated her ability to understand and follow directions. Her competence to make decisions does not appear to be an issue.

Is Mrs. Smith's home environment so hazardous that it should be reported to the local board of health or health agent? The decision to disclose protected health information to those not directly involved in Mrs. Smith's case is a serious one. It is not likely that Mrs. Smith would give you permission to contact either the bureau of elder services or the board of health; therefore, doing so would certainly be against her wishes.

If you make the decision to report Mrs. Smith's situation, Provision Three requires that you disclose only the information necessary for her treatment and well-being. For example, if you decide to report the conditions inside Mrs. Smith's home to the board of health, only information related to the home environment should be disclosed – not her apparent alcohol use and estrangement from her family. In Mrs. Smith's case, would you:

- report Mrs. Smith's home environment to local authorities?

- report Mrs. Smith's condition to the bureau of elder services?

- do neither and instead continue to assess her and build a therapeutic relationship?

If you decide that Mrs. Smith is appropriate for the home health care services provided by your agency, you must also consider how much of your assessment, observation, and interaction with Mrs. Smith is necessary to document in her medical record. How much should be discussed with the other members of the home health team? How much should you report to Mrs. Smith's physician?

Provision Three also requires you to consider the state of Mrs. Smith's home in light of the aide who should be assisting her with her personal care and homemaking. Could the house be in such disarray because of the few days Mrs. Smith was hospitalized? Is the disarray the result of Mrs. Smith's refusal to allow the aide to perform the necessary homemaking duties?

You decide to continue your assessment of Mrs. Smith. You ask her which agency her aide is from and whether this agency has been notified about her return from the hospital. Mrs. Smith states, "I have the number right here. They told me my girl would be here today, but she hasn't come yet." Mrs. Smith continues, "She is supposed to be here from 9 to 11 in the morning and then come back at night. Sometimes she can't come back at night so I sign her papers and stay in bed all day. If she is coming back, she gets me up into the wheelchair and I can go sit in the living room for the day. Once she said she was coming back and never showed up. I had to spend the night in the wheelchair. Boy, that was a tough night."

Your experience tells you that there is something questionable about the services being provided to Mrs. Smith by her aide. At the very least, you recognize that Mrs. Smith is at the mercy of this aide and her inconsistent service. As a result of this brief assessment and conversation, you begin to formulate your plan of care and decide:

• Mrs. Smith is appropriate for admission to the services of your agency.

• Social work services are necessary to sort out the issues around the lack of community-based support for Mrs. Smith.

• You are obligated to inform the agency that employs the aide about what appears to be substandard performance and uncertain attendance.

Once you have decided to admit Mrs. Smith to the agency's caseload, you explain to her the services that your agency provides and the services requested by the hospital. You also explain to her which services she is eligible for and what her insurance will pay for. You explain that, as part of the admission process, you must ask her a few more questions and complete a physical assessment. You provide her with a copy of the agency's Patient's Rights and Responsibilities form and tell her that once you get through all of this paperwork, you will leave copies of it for her for future reference. Once she agrees, you explain that she has to sign a consent for treatment form and other agency paperwork required by home health care regulations.

You make a note to contact the agency that provides the aide to inform them of the lack of attendance of their worker. Past experience reminds you

that many aides are paid when visit documentation includes a patient's signature. Clearly, if Mrs. Smith signs the forms in advance of receiving service, the agency is potentially paying the aide for services that were not provided. You are also aware that this accusation has serious consequences for the aide and the aide's agency; however, the *Code of Ethics for Nurses* requires you to act on questionable or uncertain practices. Your options are:

• Call the agency that provides the aide to Mrs. Smith and inform them that your agency will now be involved in Mrs. Smith's care.

• Plan your next visit to coincide with the visit of the aide to conduct your own assessment of the care she is providing to Mrs. Smith.

• Plan to discuss the situation with your clinical manager when you return to the agency.

At this point, you realize that you have made significant progress in the planning of Mrs. Smith's care. You have identified several problems but have not yet conducted a physical assessment. You explain to Mrs. Smith that her physician has ordered a cardiopulmonary assessment and medication compliance assessment and has also requested that you perform a generalized home safety assessment. You explain that you would like to complete her physical assessment, and she agrees.

You have already noted that Mrs. Smith is alert and oriented. She is able to communicate her needs and follow directions. She has gross and fine motor control of her upper extremities, as evidenced by her ability to hand and receive items to and from you and by her ability to sign her name. You know that she can move both of her legs because she used them to roll in the bed and lift her buttocks off of the bedpan. She denies any numbness, tingling, or weakness in any of her extremities.

Her pupils are equal and reactive to light. You note that she has two pairs of glasses, one of which she has worn the entire time you were in the house, except when she changed to another pair to read and sign her name.

Mrs. Smith is able to move her head and neck from side to side, and as you palpate these areas, you do not feel any lumps or masses. You notice a denture cup on the bedside table and question her about her teeth and her ability to swallow both liquids and solids. She informs you that she has a full set of dentures and has never had any trouble swallowing as long as she has a good "swig of water."

You assist Mrs. Smith in sitting upright. You listen to her lungs and note diminished breath sounds at the bases. Mrs. Smith also has a slight expiratory wheeze, but she denies shortness of breath or a cough.

You observe that Mrs. Smith's mucous membranes are moist. During the assessment, you smell a faint odor of alcohol but decide that you will ask her about this later. Mrs. Smith's apical pulse is 58 beats/minute and regular, as is her radial pulse. You are not able to identify any abnormal heart sounds. Her blood pressure is 158/94 mm Hg on her right arm and 162/92 mm Hg on her left arm.

Mrs. Smith's bowel sounds are present in all four quadrants. You question her about a scar on her right upper abdominal quadrant, and she states, "They took something out a long time ago, probably before you were born." You measure Mrs. Smith's abdominal girth, explaining that because she is unable to stand on the scale, this measurement might help to identify early signs of CHF.

You assess Mrs. Smith's lower extremities. You note that her skin is very dry and scaly. You are unable to palpate her pedal pulses, and you notice bilateral pitting edema with a 10- to 15-second capillary refill time. Although the color of her feet is good, they are cool to the touch. You also note the presence of nickel-sized blackened areas on both of Mrs. Smith's heels. You ask her how long she has had them, and she states, "I never knew I did. Are

you pulling my leg?" You ask her for a mirror, and show them to her. She denies any pain in either heel.

You ask to look at Mrs. Smith's prescriptions. She begins to hand you the prescription bottles that are on the left side of her. As she hands you the bottles, she explains, "This one is my heart medication. I take it once a day. This little one is for my pressure. They say I got high blood pressure, you know. I take it in the morning. I have bad cholesterol. I am supposed to take this one three times a day, but I don't. It is very expensive so I cut it in half and take one in the morning and one at night."

Mrs. Smith continues to hand you five additional bottles, which include acetaminophen, docusate sodium, and other over-the-counter drugs. As she hands them to you, you compare them to the list provided on your hospital referral. You ask Mrs. Smith, "Do you take a fluid pill?" She states, "Oh, that one. That one is a devil. I have it here somewhere." Mrs. Smith looks on the table next to her bed and retrieves two additional prescription bottles. One you recognize as sublingual nitroglycerin, and the other is Lasix. "Here they are. Doctor Jones wants me to take them every day, but how can I? As soon as I take them I have to use the pan. I have to use it and use it. It's not easy for me, you know. And if my girl doesn't come or comes late…well, I am in big trouble." You now realize that you are beginning to see the source of Mrs. Smith's recidivism.

PROVISION FOUR

As a professional nurse, you understand that you are entirely responsible for your actions and judgments. Due to the complexities of Mrs. Smith's case, you request a case conference to assist in the development of an appropriate plan of care. Provision Four of the *Code of Ethics for Nurses* requires that when the patient's needs are "beyond the qualifications and competencies of the nurse, consultation and collaboration must be sought from qualified nurses, other health professionals, or other appropriate sources" (ANA, 2001, p. 17).

As part of your plan of care, you consider utilizing the following services:

- a certified wound-ostomy-continence nurse to address Mrs. Smith's skin integrity

- a cardiac nurse to evaluate the medication plan and increase Mrs. Smith's overall compliance

- the services of a psychiatric nurse to help you address Mrs. Smith's feelings of anger and lack of trust.

Every nurse "is responsible and accountable for individual nursing practice and determines the appropriate delegation of tasks consistent with the nurse's obligation to provide optimum patient care" (ANA, 2001, p.16). As noted earlier, society's trust of professional nurses is the result of the standards that nurses established for themselves in day-to-day practice. Provision Four requires every nurse to accept accountability for his or her own practice. For the home health nurse, there are many obvious examples of being accountable for one's own practice.

In the case of Mrs. Smith, you have to make a judgment about whether to make a report to the Bureau of Elder Services. Although that decision seems benign, consider the potential results. A report to the Bureau of Elder Services might require you to:

- Violate the trusting relationship that has begun between you and Mrs. Smith. If the Bureau does not substantiate the concerns and thereby does not intervene, will you be able to rebuild the trust that is necessary for a therapeutic relationship?

- Disclose not only protected health information but also very personal and intimate details about Mrs. Smith's current living situation and personal life, such as her estrangement from her children.

- Witness Bureau intervention, which could result in Mrs. Smith being unwillingly removed from her home and being placed in a long-term care facility.

Any of these scenarios is a possibility, and as the home health nurse initiating the process you are also accountable for the outcome.

As defined by the ANA, "Accountability means to be answerable to oneself and others for one's own actions" (ANA, 2001, p. 16). It means providing an explanation or rationale to oneself, to clients, to peers, to the nursing profession, and to society. The decision to report Mrs. Smith's unsafe or "at risk" situation to the Bureau of Elder Services may be easily rationalized to your peers, the profession and even society, but how do you rationalize it to Mrs. Smith and will your rationale matter to her? On the other hand, a decision not to report Mrs. Smith's situation may be easily rationalized regarding Mrs. Smith, but what about your accountability to your peers, profession, and society? It is important to understand that the *Code of Ethics for Nurses* may or may not exceed the requirements of law. You, as a professional nurse, must be familiar with the *Code of Ethics for Nurses,* agency policy, and the laws and regulations governing nursing practice in your state.

Would you report Mrs. Smith to the Bureau of Elder Services? Would your agency require you to? What guidance or direction does your licensing board or state laws provide?

Provision Four also offers guidance to the nurse related to issues of delegation. Delegation is a phenomenon that affects nurses in virtually every practice setting, including home health care. Delegation is a reality that has resulted from changes in the health care delivery system due to financial pressures to reduce costs. The delegation of nursing care by the professional nurse does not diminish the nurse's accountability for the care actually provided to the patient. Furthermore, the professional nurse is responsible for the competence of the health care worker to whom the care is delegated and must be sure that the individual is competent to carry out the assigned patient care. The *Code of Ethics for Nurses* points out that "employer policies or directives do not relieve the nurse of accountability for making judgments about the delegation of nursing care activities" (ANA, 2001, p. 17).

When considering issues of delegation, nurses commonly think of hospitals and other facility-based care environments. Another important issue of delegation relates directly to the area of home health care aides (HCAs). In some states, HCAs are allowed to insert indwelling urinary catheters, perform venipunctures, give medications, and change dressings. Identification of tasks that can be delegated is governed and regulated by each state, and every home health nurse should have a thorough understanding of these regulations.

Consider the case of Mrs. Smith. At this point, numerous patient care tasks have been identified, which may or may not be delegated to an HCA. As the nurse in Mrs. Smith's home, consider which of the following tasks you would delegate:

- Due to Mrs. Smith's inability to remove the wrapper, you ask the HCA to change Mrs. Smith's Nitro-Patch after her bath.

- Mrs. Smith has a treatment order for debridement of the necrotic areas on her heels. As part of the HCA's plan of care, you instruct the aide to change the outer dressing on both heels every day and to report any drainage that has come through the dressing.

- Mrs. Smith's care requires the level of peripheral edema to be measured every other day. As part of the HCA's plan of care, you instruct the aide to measure the edema and notify you if an increase occurs.

The issues related to Mrs. Smith's case are not uncommon in home health care. Any seasoned home care nurse can readily provide examples of similar cases and scenarios. What is important to understand is that, in every case, the provisions of the *Code of Ethics for Nurses* are applicable and can provide guidance to the nurse.

The first four provisions describe the values and commitment required of all professional nurses. The situation and circumstances of Mrs. Smith are fairly common and each nurse should explore his or her decision-making processes and rationales when faced with similar scenarios.

PROVISION FIVE

As noted earlier, Provisions Five, Six, and Seven address "boundaries of duty and loyalty" (ANA, 2001, p. 6). Provision Five outlines the nurse's obligation to cultivate and develop his or her own practice and knowledge base.

As a professional nurse, it is not likely that you have forgotten the rigors of nursing school. However, you must also acknowledge that learning is a lifelong endeavor; if learning stopped when you graduated from nursing school, you would not be able to function as a professional nurse today. Remember, what you learned in nursing school was the very minimum required to take state licensing exams. Provision Five requires nurses to maintain competence in nursing and states: "Nurses are required to have knowledge relevant to the current scope and standards of nursing practice, changing issues, concerns, controversies, and ethics" (ANA, 2001, p. 18). This provision outlines the obligation that each nurse has to actively seek new knowledge and incorporate that knowledge into the delivery of patient care.

Many states require professional nurses to continue formalized education through completion of contact hours or continuing education units; however, many states have no such requirement. The absence of a state regulation does not relinquish professional nurses from their obligation to continue to expand their knowledge.

The practice of nursing is dynamic and evolving. The scope of nursing is shaped by advancement of nursing knowledge and by influences of the health care delivery system. This ever-changing environment is not without risk for the professional nurse. As previously stated, each nurse is accountable for his or her own practice – regardless of the setting or circumstance. Each nurse must be adequately prepared to carry out every function that he or she is being asked to perform. If a nurse is inadequately prepared to complete a function, he or she must not attempt to carry out the function and jeopardize the patient's well-being.

The most obvious examples of this in home care are usually related to specific tasks, such as changing of an Unna boot dressing or maintenance of an epidural catheter for pain management. Certain tasks are better addressed by other disciplines or by nursing specialists.

Provision Five also introduces the concept of "wholeness" of character and preservation of integrity as crucial to the nurse's ability to demonstrate ethical decision-making. In the earliest days of formalized nursing, only "right" or "good" people were allowed into the profession. The "rightness" and "goodness" of individuals was judged by nursing leaders, who were primarily educators or administrators. Nursing leaders were revered and occasionally used their authority to exert influence on the personal and professional lives of the nurses they encountered. For example, nurses trained in hospital-based schools of nursing were required to live on campus, could not be married, and were even subjected to weekly weigh-ins (C. Cardoza, personal communication, November 18, 2002).

In the 21st century, nurses are as diverse as the patients and communities they serve. Nurses have both personal and professional identities, and the process of becoming a nurse requires an individual to accept and integrate the values of nursing outlined in the *Code of Ethics for Nurses* into his or her existing value structure. Achieving this and understanding integration is especially important in the nurse-patient interaction.

To illustrate this point, consider a patient who requests your personal opinion about a health or personal issue. Almost every nurse has been asked:

- "Do you think my doctor is doing the right thing?"
- "What would you do if you were in my place?"
- "Do you think I should get a second opinion?"
- "Do you think I did the right thing?"

Although you are likely to have a personal opinion about each of these questions, in answering them, you must recognize that your role as a nurse represents a "knowing" opinion and may exert unintentional influence on the patient's decision. When you, as the nurse, are placed in this position, it is always better to assist patients to clarify their own expectations and guide them to make informed decisions.

PROVISION SIX

The privilege of autonomous practice and self-regulation increases the nurse's responsibility to ensure that the practice setting is "conducive to high quality nursing care" (ANA, 2001, p. 20). In fact, Provision Six specifically states: "All nurses have a responsibility to create, maintain, and contribute to environments that support the growth of virtues and excellences and enable nurses to fulfill their ethical obligations" (ANA, 2001, p. 20). For the purpose of this passage, "virtues" are defined as nursing actions that promote well-being, health, and independence of a patient. Working in home health care, nurses will find unique professional opportunities to participate in initiatives to enhance the practice of nursing.

Although most home health care agencies work within the medical/disease model, nursing is the primary service provided. Unlike many other practice settings, home health care is organized to provide and support the provision of nursing care. There are often many opportunities for the nurse to participate in committees and task forces that are organized to improve the conditions of the work setting and improve the quality of patient care. Participation on committees that address issues such as safety and infection control fulfills the nurse's obligation to contribute to an environment conducive to high-quality nursing service and patient care.

Provision Six puts the responsibility for maintaining and improving health care environments squarely on the nurse's shoulders. It requires each nurse to participate in collaborative relationships with colleagues and peers that work to identify and solve issues related to the practice setting and working conditions. Provision Six states: "Acquiescing and accepting unsafe or inappropriate practices, even if the individual does not participate in the specific practice, is equivalent to condoning unsafe practice. Nurses should not remain employed in a facility that routinely violates patient rights or requires nurses to severely and repeatedly compromise standards of practice of personal morality" (ANA, 2001, p. 21).

Although these statements may initially seem severe, consider them from the patient's perspective. The trusting relationship that exists between society and the nursing profession should never be compromised. If a professional nurse participates in unscrupulous behavior or is employed by an unscrupulous provider, he or she is directly responsible for undermining the trusting relationship that has developed between society and the nursing profession over the last 200 years.

Examples of unsafe or inappropriate practices in home health care might include:

- discharging a patient because his or her required care is too costly

- performing a task for which the nurse does not have the clinical skill or there is no clinical procedure (e.g., blood transfusions)

- performing duties that are beyond the scope of nursing practice or limited by the state licensing board (e.g., sharp debridement of wounds).

Clearly, no nursing professional wants to be associated with an organization that routinely denies a patient's right to participate in the care planning process, self-determination, or informed consent.

The *Code of Ethics for Nurses* acknowledges that, for some nurses, collective bargaining may be a mechanism to change organizational practice. If collective bargaining is used, the collective bargaining agreement must "be consistent with the profession's standards of practice, the state law regulating practice, and the *Code of Ethics for Nurses*" and "balance the interest of patients and nurses" (ANA, 2001, p. 22).

PROVISION SEVEN

Provision Seven outlines the professional nurse's responsibility to participate in activities that advance nursing knowledge and professional practice. Reading this provision might make you, as a nurse, question how this can possibly be an individual responsibility. Is not the advancement of knowledge best left to nursing educators and researchers?

Unfortunately, many nurses are so consumed by the activities of daily practice that they do not realize how often they participate in knowledge development and professional advancement. In an effort to improve patient outcomes, home health care agencies have instituted specialty or disease management teams. Participation on these teams enables nurses to share the latest research and then utilize and apply it to patient care.

For example, the *Clinical Practice Guidelines* published by the Agency for Healthcare Research and Quality (formerly known as the Agency for Health Care Policy and Research) discourages the use of solutions, such as Dakin's solution or acetic acid, for wound packing. Although these treatments were commonly used in the past for treatment of infected wounds, the home health nurse now recognizes that this treatment is a detriment to wound healing and therefore seeks treatment alternatives.

On occasion, a home health nurse has the opportunity to participate in or conduct nursing research. Given this opportunity, the nurse is obligated to ensure that the participant's rights are protected and that all of the necessary approvals are received.

In the advancement of nursing knowledge and professional practice, nurse educators must also adhere to the *Code of Ethics for Nurses* by ensuring that individuals eligible to take licensing exams have "demonstrated the knowledge, skills, and commitment considered essential to professional practice" (ANA, 2001, p. 2).

Many home health agencies are privileged to provide a clinical experience for nursing students. Whether the experience is observational or one in which the student conducts independent home visits, it is the home care nurse's obligation to give honest and constructive feedback to the student and the instructor. A home health care nurse might think that providing a clinical experience for a student nurse seems burdensome. However, at the end of the day, week, or semester, many nurses find the experience rewarding and recognize it as one way to meet their obligation to participate in the development and advancement of the profession. Some home health care agencies also offer nurses the opportunity to participate in a preceptor or mentoring program for new employees. Participation in these types of programs also provides nurses with an avenue to fulfill their professional obligations.

PROVISION EIGHT

The long standing relationship between the public and the nursing profession is highly valued. Each nurse bears the responsibility to be aware of and knowledgeable about major threats to health and wellness in his or her community. Nurses who support and participate in civic and political initiatives have the unique opportunity to educate the public to make informed choices about health and health-related issues, such as poverty, homelessness, domestic abuse, and violence.

As discussed in Chapter 1, the efficiency of a district nurse included having knowledge of the issues that families, neighborhoods, and entire communities were facing. Modern home health nurses continue to have the same level of knowledge; however, they are also aware of the services available to address these issues.

Do you know:

- Which churches in your community have an active parish nurse program?

- Does your city or town have a woman's shelter?

- Do homeless people sleep in your parks and alleys? If so, are there places where they can seek shelter from inclement weather?

- Does the nurse at the local high school distribute condoms?

- Where can members of your community get a flu or pneumonia vaccine?

- Is there an individual or group that provides holiday meals to homebound elders and shut-ins?

- Are the children in your town at risk for asbestos or lead poisoning?

PROVISION NINE

Provision Nine acknowledges that nursing has a long-standing commitment to social reform and requires nurses to work through professional associations and affiliations to identify political solutions to local, national, and international health and social problems. While working with these groups, individual nurses should seize the opportunity to meet with and educate their local, state, and federal representatives and senators about the issues that effect the health and welfare of the community. Participating at this level empowers nurses and nursing organizations to shape the health care delivery system, health care reimbursement mechanisms, and health-related social issues.

ADDITIONAL CONSIDERATIONS

Professional Boundaries

The *Code of Ethics for Nurses* establishes expectations with regard to professional boundaries and impaired practice. Although these issues are not unique to home health care, nurses who practice in this setting face challenges in maintaining these standards. The ANA defines a professional relationship as one that "has as a foundation, the purpose of preventing illness, alleviating suffering, and protecting, promoting and restoring the health of patients" (ANA, 2001, p. 11).

Like all practice settings, home health care provides the professional nurse with pros and cons. The concept of one patient and one nurse is probably the most appealing characteristic of home health nursing. For some nurses, it is this same appeal that can jeopardize the ability to maintain professional boundaries and limits.

Many agencies are organized in such a way that one nurse is assigned to a group or caseload of patients for whom he or she is responsible. In addition to providing direct hands-on care, the nurse is also responsible for the coordination of agency- and community-based services for his or her caseload. This case management role fosters the development of an intimate and long-term relationship between the nurse and the patient. Nurses in home health care often report that this level of involvement leads to job satisfaction and professional fulfillment. However, for some nurse, it also lends itself to the compromise of professional boundaries and limits.

Most agencies have policies and procedures designed to minimize the blurring of professional boundaries and limits. Nurses who violate these poli-

cies may be subject to progressive discipline or termination from the agency. Depending on the severity of the violation, nurses may also be subject to a report being filed with their state board of nursing.

The failure to maintain professional boundaries and establish limits is usually an insidious process. Home health care nurses who have difficulties with professional boundaries do not necessarily realize that a problem has developed until it is too late. By the time the problem is recognized, the nurse has great difficulty changing the behavior, especially with a "favorite" patient or family. After all, once a nurse has exceeded the limits of professional boundaries, how would he or she tell the patient that the behavior cannot continue?

It is true that, on occasion, a patient will tug at your heartstrings; however, as a professional nurse, you are expected to provide care that is compassionate while remaining within the professional boundaries outlined in the *Code of Ethics for Nurses*. It is not uncommon for you, the nurse, to be the only person a patient sees in a day or even a week. As the home health nurse, you may be the only person who knows that one, two, or three of your patients will spend an entire holiday alone, without the company of family or friends. In all likelihood, you will encounter patients who will challenge your ability to maintain these boundaries.

The *Code of Ethics for Nurses* clearly states that the nurse is solely responsible for maintaining the professional relationship, and if a jeopardizing situation arises, "the nurse should seek assistance from peers or supervisors or take appropriate steps to remove him/herself from the situation" (ANA, 2001, p. 11). Table 2-2 provides a list of warning signs that individually or in combination could signal the home health nurse that he or she is at risk for compromising professional standards.

The following scenarios are intended to highlight potential violations of the standards of professional boundaries. If you were the nurse in Mr.

TABLE 2-2: BREECH OF PROFESSIONAL BOUNDARIES WARNING SIGNS

- Checking voice mail or email on days off
- Calling the agency to "check on things" while on vacation
- Forgetting that the patients to whom you are assigned to case manage do not "belong" to you
- Expecting that, if you change jobs, you will be allowed to transfer patients to the new agency
- Thinking that none of your colleagues can do the job as well as you can
- Visiting a patient on your day off or after regular working hours
- Introducing your family members or children to a patient
- Purchasing groceries, prescriptions, or other items for a patient
- Taking a patient to your home
- Representing yourself as the patient's friend or caregiver
- Providing services beyond those that are reasonable or necessary

Donovan's or Mrs. Smith's case as they are outlined below, what would you do?

Mr. Donovan

Mr. Donovan is an elderly patient who has a history of cardiac disease and diabetes. He is also deaf and mute. Until recently, he was independent and able to get around the city using public transportation. The home health plan of care requires the nurse to assess his cardiac status twice each week. Mr. Donovan communicates to you that he would like you to stop at a local candy store to pick up some diabetic chocolates before your next visit, and he hands you a ten-dollar bill.

How would you respond to this simple request from a patient who has no other means of obtaining this very small pleasure? After all, he has lost his independence and you will be going right by the store. In fact, that store is right in your district and you must go by it two or three times a day. What harm could possibly come from granting this request?

Mrs. Smith

Consider the case of Mrs. Smith, who was discussed in depth earlier in this chapter. You may recall she had multiple readmissions to the hospital for management of CHF exacerbations. On one of your visits, you identify that she is beginning to retain fluid again. She states that she has been following the diet and fluid restriction that the registered dietician planned for her. She also tells you that she has no money to refill her prescriptions and will not have any money until her check comes late next week. She ran out of her diuretic 3 days ago.

What would you do? Would you call her pharmacy and ask them to send her a few pills until her check comes? Would you call her physician and ask him or her if he or she has any free samples in the office that you could go and pick up for Mrs. Smith? Perhaps you could pay to have her prescription refilled just this once.

In both of these cases, the "correct" answers can be found by considering the role of the professional nurse in home health and the definition of a professional boundary. Would your decisions meet the objectives of these directives?

IMPAIRED PRACTICE

Addressing a colleague whose practice is impaired as a result of drug or alcohol use is the most difficult professional experience that a nurse will encounter. According to Dunn (2005), approximately 10% of nurses abuse alcohol or drugs. Historically, the highest incidence of chemically dependent nurses has been found in emergency and critical care. The *Code of Ethics for Nurses* outlines the responsibility of every nurse "to protect the patient, the public, and the profession from potential harm when a colleague's practice, in any setting, appears to be impaired" (ANA, 2001, p. 15). Every nurse is bound by duty to act when he or she identifies a colleague who is practicing while impaired.

Although the incidence of chemical dependence and impaired practice is not readily documented in home health care, this does not mean that they are not issues. Home health care is one of the fastest growing practice settings for nurses. The autonomy and independence of home health care creates an environment where a chemically dependent nurse could function with a low risk of being detected.

Outlined below is the case study of Nancy Nurse. Consider this scenario and identify the point at which your professional duty would require you to intervene.

Nancy Nurse

Nancy Nurse has 20 years of nursing experience, and many of the nurses in your agency know her from working with her in previous settings. She has been assigned to the same district of the city where you work. During her orientation, you have an opportunity to talk with her every day, and your clinical nurse manager tells you that she expects the two of you to cover each other's patients for days off and vacations.

After a couple of months of working with Nancy, you realize that she has fallen asleep during a staff meeting. You ask her if she is okay. She tells you that she is having marital and other personal problems that have diminished her ability to get enough sleep, but other than that, she is fine.

The nurses who work in your district customarily meet one day a week to have lunch at a local diner. You arrive just after Nancy, and notice her sitting in her chair. Before she gets out, you notice she takes a couple of sips of what appears to be

mouthwash and places a fresh piece of gum in her mouth. Come to think of it, Nancy is always chewing gum or eating candy or mints.

On another day, Nancy comes into the office early one morning, and you note a faint odor of alcohol on her breath. Although you do not mention it to her, she later tells you that she had a few drinks the night before to relax after fighting with her husband. She tells you she is worried that someone might notice and asks if you can still smell alcohol on her breath. You minimize the issue by telling her, "Not really."

After a few months of working with Nancy, you notice one day that her speech is slurred, and she appears to be having difficulty concentrating. When you ask her about her behavior, she informs you that she has a number of newly diagnosed medical problems, her physician is currently adjusting her medication regimen, and she must be experiencing side effects.

While conducting a routine home visit, you mistakenly lock your keys in your car. You call the agency to inform your clinical nurse manager and to ask if someone could bring you the spare key that you keep in your desk. Your clinical nurse manager tells you that someone will bring it out shortly. Unbeknown to you, Nancy was in the office at the time of your call and arrives with your spare key. When she opens the door of her car to get out, two beer cans fall to the sidewalk. She explains that her husband was returning them to the recycling center. She says he must have dropped them in the car, and they rolled under her seat.

Nancy has completed the probationary period just in time for her to cover some of your patients while you are on vacation. When you return, you get report from Nancy, and she tells you that nothing unusual happened while you were away. However, when you see your patients, they tell a different story and make subtle comments about Nancy. Mr. Ellis is one of your patients who tells you, "I am glad you're back. My medications were all messed up when you were gone. I even ran out of my pain medication. Good thing that other nurse called the pharmacy, picked them up, and straightened them out for me."

Later in the week, you visit Mrs. Flannigan. Her plan of care includes the prefilling of liquid morphine into individual spill-proof cups. She tells you that her back pain had gotten much worse while you were on vacation and that Nancy called the physician to arrange for her to begin taking twice the amount of medication. She reports that she feels much better today and thinks that she could go back to the previous dose.

Finally, Mrs. Gagnon tells you, "I think that other nurse looked in my medicine cabinet in the bathroom. She was taking a long time in there. You never take that long, and you never close the door when you go in to wash your hands. When my daughter knocked on the door to see if she was alright, she thought she heard a pill bottle hit the floor. When that Nancy came out, she said she was taking one of her own medications because she has high blood pressure. My daughter and I felt very funny about her. Please don't send her back."

Considering these examples, Nancy's behavior has clearly been questionable. However, the true behavior of a chemically dependent nurse would unlikely be as obvious. It is more realistic to expect the behavior to be subtle and insidious. Recognizing that the *Code of Ethics for Nurses* requires nurses to protect patients, the public, and the profession, what would you do when faced with a nurse who might be practicing while impaired? Most practice settings have policies and procedures that provide guidance on the reporting of this sensitive issue. These policies should be stringent enough to protect all parties, while providing an environment that is conducive to the professional nurse's treatment, recovery, and return to work.

In the area of home health care, some additional issues must be considered. When Mr. Ellis

reported that Nancy called the pharmacy and then picked up and delivered his medications, you must question if she returned with all pills that were dispensed by the pharmacy. What if the correct number of pills was delivered, but Nancy substituted plain Tylenol for the Tylenol with codeine the patient usually receives?

Is it a coincidence that Mrs. Flannigan experienced an exacerbation of her back pain while you were on vacation? Would you be surprised to find out that it took twice as much morphine to restore her comfort? Would you recognize that her remaining doses of prefilled morphine appear to be lighter in color than you remembered and seem somewhat watery in consistency? Is it possible that Mrs. Flannigan's morphine had been diluted with water and half of a bottle removed from her home?

In the case of Mrs. Gagnon, is it possible that Nancy looked through the medicine cabinet and removed something? Could she have removed an entire bottle of medication or even just a few tablets?

It is clear that if Nancy switched, diluted, or outright stole a patient's medication for her own use, in addition to the impaired practice issues that you suspected, you also have issues of theft. Will the theft of patient medications require that Nancy's behavior be reported to the state board of nursing or the local police? Will her nursing license to practice be suspended while she receives treatment for her chemical dependency, or will she lose her license as a result of diverting or stealing patient medications? Will Nancy's position at the agency be held for her while she receives treatment, or will she be forced to resign her position? Should she practice in home health care after she completes her treatment, or do the autonomy and independence of home health care create situations that might jeopardize her recovery? Will she be subject to criminal prosecution?

How will you feel if Nancy's behavior is only coincidental, and you falsely accuse her of practicing while impaired or diverting patient medications? If you decide not to report Nancy, how will you rationalize your decision if a patient suffers needlessly or is hurt as a result of Nancy's clouded judgment?

As stated earlier, addressing a colleague's issue of impaired practice or chemical dependency is the most difficult professional decision a nurse may face. The employer and the nurse reporting these issues must do so in a manner that preserves the dignity of their colleague and respects that person's right to confidentiality.

SUMMARY

The *scope of nursing* is defined as the "protection, promotion, restoration of health; prevention of illness; and alleviation of suffering in the care of clients, including individuals, families, groups, and communities" (ANA, 2001, p. i). On any given day, home health care nurses find themselves caring for patients and families along this continuum. The *Code of Ethics for Nurses* is the yardstick by which all nurses, regardless of their area of practice, are measured. The goal of nursing is to "support and enhance the client's responsibility and self-determination to the greatest extent possible" (ANA, 2001, p. i), and the home environment poses unique challenges that are not always anticipated or easily overcome.

CHAPTER 2
Questions 7-20

Note: Choose the option that BEST answers each question.

Consider the case of Mrs. Rodrigues when answering questions 7 through 10.

Mrs. Rodrigues is an 87-year-old patient who lives in a poor, inner-city neighborhood. You are going to see Mrs. Rodrigues to administer her evening dose of antibiotics. When you turn down Mrs. Rodrigues' street, you notice that many of the houses are run-down. Some even have their doors and windows boarded up and look uninhabited. When you reach Mrs. Rodrigues' address, you slowly drive past the house because you are not sure if you have the correct address. Once you double-check the address, you realize that you are at the right location and that the porch light is on. The street is empty and it is dark outside. Although you are uncomfortable with the neighborhood, you do not feel threatened or perceive any safety risks.

7. The *Code of Ethics for Nurses* requires you to

    a. complete the visit and suggest to Mrs. Rodrigues that she find a "better" neighborhood to live in.

    b. call your manager and refuse to complete the visit because of your discomfort.

    c. respect human dignity and the uniqueness of Mrs. Rodrigues, unrestricted by considerations of social or economic status.

    d. suggest to your manager that referrals for patients similar to Mrs. Rodrigues be declined.

Mrs. Rodrigues tells you that most of the houses on the street are empty, and she suspects that homeless people sometimes stay in them. She says, "Sometimes, those boys even sell drugs on the corner." She tells you that she never walks down the street anymore; if she needs to leave her home, she calls a cab because it is "safer." She reminisces that she and her family have lived in their house for almost 100 years and tells that her great-grandfather built the house for the family, so she could never leave it.

8. Provision One of the *Code of Ethics for Nurses*

    a. requires a nurse to condone and agree with a patient's choices regardless of whether those choices jeopardize the patient's safety.

    b. requires that a nurse not form an opinion about a patient's circumstances regardless of what they are like.

    c. does not provide any guidance for a nurse when it comes to differing opinions.

    d. does not require a nurse to condone or agree with a patient's choice but does, however, require the nurse to provide care regardless of the patient's choices.

9. By remaining in her home, Mrs. Rodrigues

   a. is exercising poor judgment.

   b. shows a sign of incompetence.

   c. is jeopardizing her ability to receive services.

   d. is exercising her right to self-determination.

   Based on your conversation with Mrs. Rodrigues, you get a sense that she is sad and might be somewhat depressed. Without any friends or neighbors, she is isolated at the very least. You make a note of these findings and plan to discuss this issue further with your manager and the team assigned to this district. You consider whether Mrs. Rodrigues would benefit from attending adult day care for socialization.

10. Provision Two of the *Code of Ethics for Nurses* requires you as the nurse to

    a. collaborate with other team members in an effort to attain the goals of Mrs. Rodrigues' care plan.

    b. notify elder-at-risk services to address the poor choices that Mrs. Rodrigues is making.

    c. discharge Mrs. Rodrigues from your agency's caseload because you are not supposed to support a plan of care that is unsafe or jeopardizes patient safety.

    d. document your findings and leave Mrs. Rodrigues information regarding who will be conducting the morning visit.

11. The realities of practicing in home health care make Provision Four of the *Code of Ethics for Nurses*

    a. impossible to uphold.

    b. necessary and a common occurrence.

    c. outdated and not applicable.

    d. unrealistic and rarely done.

12. When an HCA is assigned to a case, the nurse is responsible for his or her supervision because

    a. the home health plan of care is signed by a physician and contains an order to conduct supervision visits at least every 2 weeks.

    b. agency policy requires it.

    c. every nurse is responsible and accountable for individual nursing practice and determines the appropriate delegation of tasks; therefore, it is the nurse's obligation to ensure that optimum patient care is being provided.

    d. the patient's plan of care or condition may change.

13. The first four provisions outlined in the *Code of Ethics for Nurses* describe

    a. values and commitments required of all professional nurses.

    b. nurses' role in policy and procedure development.

    c. boundaries of duty and loyalty.

    d. nurses' obligation to continue to develop their practice and acquire continued education.

14. The responsibility to create, maintain, and contribute to an environment that supports growth and excellence in nursing is typically

    a. an administrative function.

    b. the responsibility of every professional nurse.

    c. a situation that results when the nursing staff is unionized.

    d. not a realistic expectation.

15. Participation in nursing research activities, a preceptorship with a new staff member, or a performance improvement team

    a. is considered going "above and beyond" the duties typically associated with a professional nurse.

    b. is not practical for most professional nurses.

    c. requires knowledge and skills only associated with advanced practice nurses.

    d. is the responsibility of all professional nurses, as outlined in Provision Seven of the ANA's *Code of Ethics for Nurses.*

16. Working in districts affords the home health care nurse an opportunity to learn about the needs of the community and the services available to meet patient needs. Provision Eight of the *Code of Ethics for Nurses* identifies that the professional nurse bears the responsibility to

    a. support political candidates that the agency's administration recommends.

    b. support and participate in civic and political initiatives designed to improve the health and wellness of the community.

    c. remain apolitical.

    d. run for public office whenever possible.

17. Provision Nine of the *Code of Ethics for Nurses* requires the professional nurse to

    a. recognize that health and social problems faced by local communities are basically irreversible.

    b. recognize that without increased economic opportunities, the nursing profession is powerless to affect meaningful change.

    c. "think globally and act locally."

    d. work through professional associations and affiliations that are committed to identifying political solutions to local, national, and international health and social problems.

18. A professional relationship is one that "has a foundation, the purpose of preventing illness, alleviating suffering, and protecting, promoting, and restoring the health of patients" (ANA, 2001, p. 11). Home health care nurses who violate this expectation

    a. are not at risk for breaching professional boundaries.

    b. are not subject to the same consequences due to the uniqueness of the home health practice setting.

    c. may be subject to progressive discipline, termination, or action by the state board of licensure.

    d. respond to a higher standard and therefore cannot be held to this standard.

19. Visiting a patient on your day off or while you are on vacation or providing services beyond those that are reasonable and necessary are examples of

    a. a conscious decision to be kind.

    b. lack of confidence in your professional skills.

    c. lack of confidence in the skills of the staff covering in your absence.

    d. potentially exceeding professional boundaries.

20. The number of nurses who are chemically dependent is estimated to be

    a. 5%.

    b. 10%.

    c. 15%.

    d. 20%.

CHAPTER 3

SCOPE AND STANDARDS OF HOME HEALTH NURSING PRACTICE

CHAPTER OBJECTIVE

At the completion of this chapter, the reader will be able to apply the six standards of practice to home health nursing.

LEARNING OBJECTIVES

After studying this chapter, the reader will be able to

1. define the terms *information system, data,* and *database.*

2. differentiate between an outcome and an expected outcome.

3. discriminate between a nursing plan of care and a home health plan of treatment.

4. list four patient rights.

5. list three patient responsibilities.

INTRODUCTION

The American Nurses Association (ANA) defines a *standard* as a "norm that expresses an agreed-upon level of excellence that has been developed to characterize, to measure, and to provide guidance for achieving excellence in practice" (ANA, 1986, p. 21). Standards of practice represent the expectations for the personal and professional integrity of nurses. The ANA published the first *Standards of Home Health*

Nursing Practice in 1986. This publication outlined 12 standards that, as a whole, represented the complex nature of home care nursing. These original standards included structural (agency-related), process (nurse-related), and outcome (patient-related) criteria for each of the standards.

In 1999, the standards were revised, consolidated, and renamed the *Home Health Nursing: Scope and Standards of Practice.* This revision eliminated the structural components of the standards and defined and recognized home health care nursing as a unique and distinct area of nursing practice. This document is organized into six patient-focused "Standards of Care" and eight "Standards of Professional Performance."

In 2005, the ANA convened a group of home health nurses who volunteered to review and revise the 1999 document so that it more closely reflected home health nursing practice in the 21st century. In October 2007, the new standards were published. A notable change in the 2007 revision is expansion of the role of the advanced practice nurse (master's-prepared clinical nurse specialists and nurse practitioners) in home health care. For the purposes of this course, the discussion in this chapter focuses on the Standards of Care for the nurse generalist (standards 1 to 6), and the Standards of Professional Performance (standards 7 to 15) will be covered in Chapter 4.

Regardless of the setting, the goal of nursing can be defined as the promotion of a patient's optimal level of function within the limits of his or her disease process. Nurses achieve this goal through the implementation of an organized nursing process.

The home health care nurse focuses on the patient and his or her interactions with family, care-givers, and the community. The repertoire of home health care nursing skills includes assessment, intervention, teaching, counseling, managing and mobilizing resources, and providing direct care – all in a patient's home.

DATA COLLECTION AND INFORMATION SYSTEMS

Before discussing the Standards of Care, it is important to clarify some of the terminology used in this chapter. The Standards of Care frequently use the terms *data* and *information systems,* which are not commonly used by nurses to describe patients or patient-related issues. For many nurses, these terms are more easily related to computers than patients.

To provide context for these terms, consider that nursing is both an art and a science. All scientific endeavors require data to be collected and organized in a manner that maximizes its usefulness. For the purposes of this discussion, *patient data* refers to patient information, and *information systems* refers to medical records.

All home health care nurses collect patient data and enter it into their agency's information system. The information systems found in home health care are rapidly evolving. Although the majority of agencies continue to utilize paper-driven patient information systems, most are actively investigating electronic medical record systems. Regardless of the type of information system used, at the very least, the system must provide patient data that is easily accessible, organized, and current while protecting patient confidentiality.

STANDARDS OF CARE

Each of the six Standards of Care is simply stated and includes measurement criteria to clarify and define it. Like all professional standards, the ANA Standards of Care are organized in a manner that makes them easily applicable to the day-to-day practice of every home health care nurse. Below is a discussion of each of the standards. Illustrative patient examples are provided where applicable.

Standard 1: Assessment

Standard 1 requires that "the home health nurse collects comprehensive data pertinent to the patient's health or the situation" (ANA, 2007, p. 29). Every nurse-patient relationship begins with an assessment. The nurse usually begins the day by calling all of the patients he or she intends to see that day. Even a simple phone conversation can provide clues to the home health care nurse. The nurse can evaluate the patient's hearing and cognition. While waiting for the front door to be opened, an astute home health nurse evaluates how long it took the patient to answer the door. Did the nurse have to knock or ring the bell more than once? If so, was it because that patient has a hearing deficit? Did the patient actually come to the door or just holler for the nurse to come in? Why did the patient not come to the door? Is the patient's mobility limited? If the patient did manage to get to the door, did he or she do it in a reasonable time? If not, would the patient be able to get out of his or her home in an emergency, such as a fire?

Once the patient opens the door to the home health care nurse, the assessment process continues. Every detail of the patient and the environment are observed and "stored" by the nurse for later use. The nurse uses many sources of information in the assessment process.

In the case of Mrs. Smith, presented in Chapter 2, your first source of patient data was provided by the hospital's discharge forms and referral information. It was immediately clear to you that this information was incomplete and inadequate.

When reconsidering the case of Mrs. Smith, you remember that, from the outside, her home appeared to be well-kept and orderly. However, once you entered the home, you realized that there was no way the hospital or any other referral source could have anticipated the condition of the inside of Mrs. Smith's home.

As data are collected, they are prioritized based on the patient's most immediate needs. In the case of Mrs. Smith, you determined that her inability to complete activities of daily living (ADLs) and instrumental activities of daily living (IADLs) were her most urgent issues. The majority of the first visit with Mrs. Smith was spent collecting data related to the presence of a caregiver, the adequacy of the care provided, and the lack of other social supports.

The ongoing collection of data is necessary for the nurse to establish a nursing diagnosis, identify expected outcomes, plan, intervene, and then evaluate the patient as he or she reacts to his or her environment, disease process, and interventions.

When conducting an assessment, the nurse collects and records data related to the patient's physical status, including current and past history. Information related to the patient's psychosocial status, economic status, environment, religion, and culture is also collected. The nurse is responsible for assessing the patient's ability to perform ADLs and IADLs. The Joint Commission (formerly, the Joint Commission on Accreditation of Healthcare Organizations [JCAHO]) (2006) defines a comprehensive home health nursing assessment as one that includes an assessment of:

- The patient's problems, needs and strengths
- The patient's prognosis, diagnosis, physical findings including medical history
- Age-specific and gender-specific findings
- Laboratory results

- Prescribed and over-the-counter medication
- Any identified symptoms of pain
- The patient's nutrition status and dental function
- Functional status, including mobility, continence, independence in activities of daily living and ability to operate and maintain equipment
- The patient's psychosocial status, including emotional barriers to treatment, cognitive limitations, memory and orientation
- History of chemical dependency
- Cultural and religious practices
- The patient's wishes regarding care, treatment and end of life decisions
- The home environment
- Equipment
- Preventative and periodic health screening
- The patient's family or support system and the care they are capable of and willing to provide
- The patient's and family's educational needs, abilities, motivation and readiness to learn
- Anticipated discharge needs.

(p. PC-9)

In 1999, the Centers for Medicare & Medicaid Services (CMS) mandated the use of a standardized assessment tool for home health care: the Outcome and Assessment Information Set (OASIS). OASIS is a tool that requires the home care nurse to collect data at several points in time. These data are then used to determine the outcome of the care that was provided to the patient. Chapters 6 and 7 provide in-depth discussions of the OASIS documents and their value in measuring outcomes and quality in home health care.

To collect comprehensive patient data, the home health nurse uses standardized models of data collection in addition to OASIS. In an effort to streamline the process and reduce the time burden, many agencies have incorporated standardized mini-assessments throughout the OASIS assessment. For example, assessment of a patient's cognition might be expedited by having the home health nurse complete an abbreviated mental test examination (see Box 3-1).

The usefulness of the data collected by the nurse is measured by ensuring that the database (medical record) is comprehensive and accurately reflects the patient's status. In essence, the database provides a detailed picture of the patient that allows the nurse to proceed to the development of the nursing diagnosis.

Standard 2: Diagnosis

The second standard of care encompasses the formulation and integration of patient data into nursing diagnoses. In home health care, the nurse formulates nursing diagnoses that are based on the patient's current status, as derived through the data collection process. Nursing diagnoses must take into account the patient's needs while respecting his or her right to self-determination.

BOX 3-1: ABBREVIATED MENTAL TEST SCORE

This is a quick and easy test that can be used in the consultation.

Each question scores one point.

1. Age ☐
2. Time to nearest hour ☐
3. An address (for example, 42 West Street) to be repeated by the patient at the end of the test ☐
4. Year ☐
5. Name of hospital, residential institution or home address, depending on where the patient is situated ☐
6. Recognition of two persons (for example, doctor, nurse, home help, etc.) ☐
7. Date of birth ☐
8. Year first world war started ☐
9. Name of current president ☐
10. Count backwards from 20 to 1 ☐

Total score _____

A score of less than six suggests dementia.

If you think someone has dementia:

- Use the abbreviated mental test score (above). This is only a rough guide to diagnosis.
- Carry out routine blood tests.
- If in doubt, refer to specialist – a general psychiatrist, geriatric psychiatrist, or neurologist depending on age of patient and who is available locally.

Note. Adapted from *Dementia Tutorial: Diagnosis and Management in Primary Care. A Primary Care Based, Education/Research Project* by T. Austin. Retrieved from http://www.ehr.chime.ucl.ac.uk/display/demcare/Abbreviated+Mental+Test+Score

One way to validate your nursing diagnoses is to ask the patient to state what they hope to accomplish as a result of your nursing visits. Once again, consider the case of Mrs. Smith. As a result of the nursing assessment, a number of nursing diagnoses could be established. Examples of some diagnoses that might be appropriate for her include

- Alteration in skin integrity related to decreased mobility, decreased circulation, and compromised nutritional status

- Knowledge deficit related to medication management evidenced by lack of compliance with physician-ordered plan

- Decreased ability to cope as evidenced by alcohol use and minimal social support

- Potential for injury related to inability to safely transfer out of bed.

Once nursing diagnoses have been formulated, the nurse must validate the diagnoses with the patient to ensure that they represent the patient's perspective of his or her needs. An inexperienced home health nurse can easily become overwhelmed with the number of issues he or she perceives to be problematic. In many cases, from the patient's perspective, the issues identified by the nurse are not problematic at all. When these differing perspectives are not resolved, the nurse and the patient will lack the coordinated effort required to meet goals. This results in both the nurse and the patient becoming frustrated and dissatisfied. The nurse may deem the patient "noncompliant" and the patient may request another caregiver due to a personality conflict or complaints about the nurse's skills. To illustrate this point consider the case of Mrs. King.

Mrs. King

You have been assigned to admit Mrs. King to your agency's services. Mrs. King's physician has requested skilled nursing to teach her how to prepare and administer insulin. When you approach her home, you hear loud voices. It sounds like Mrs. King is arguing with someone. After you ring the doorbell, the apartment becomes quiet.

An elderly lady answers the door; she is in a bathrobe and looks as if she has not combed her hair, even though it is 2:30 p.m. She asks, "Are you the nurse who called? Come on in." As you enter, you observe that the small apartment is spotless, except for clutter on one small end table near a reclining chair. An elderly man is sitting in the chair and appears angry and upset.

Mrs. King states, "Ignore him. He is all bark and no bite."

Mr. King shoots back, "Yeah, that's right. I'm all bark, all bark! If I had a bite, you'd be in trouble."

"Trouble?!" shouts Mrs. King, "I have had nothing but trouble since I married you." Mrs. King turns to you and says, "I have had nothing but trouble since I married him in 1945. Look at him. He is a no good, lazy slob."

At this point, you interrupt Mrs. King and try to redirect her to the reason for your visit. She turns her attention to you and says, "Fifty-two years, four kids, and eleven grandchildren with him. Can you believe it? Okay, let's get on with it."

During your visit, the bickering between Mr. and Mrs. King continues intermittently. From the living room, Mr. King listens to your conversation with Mrs. King and occasionally interjects a comment, which results in an unpleasant rebuttal from Mrs. King.

As a result of your visit, it is clear that you will establish a nursing diagnosis or two related to Mrs. King's diabetes, but what about the relationship between Mr. and Mrs. King? Would you establish a nursing diagnosis to address their relationship? Does either of these individuals appear to be a victim of domestic abuse or violence? Is their constant bickering a problem that requires intervention, or has their 52-year marriage always been filled with bickering and unkind words? If you establish a nursing diagnosis to address their relationship, would Mrs. King be inclined to agree or would she more likely want to focus on learning to administer and manage her insulin independently?

Standard 3: Outcomes Identification

The *Standards of Home Health Nursing Practice* require the nurse to identify patient-related outcomes. For the purposes of this chapter, the term *outcomes* is used to describe a change in the patient's health status between two points in time. Because most home health care services are provided on an intermittent, short-term basis, it is imperative that care be focused on the achievement of patient outcomes within the identified time frames.

Expected outcomes are established at the start of the patient's care and are based on the patient's assessment and diagnoses. They are identified through the collaborative efforts of the nurse, the patient, the physician and other members of the health care team. Because these outcomes provide direction for all interventions, they must be measurable, realistic, and attainable.

Although the identification of patient outcomes appears to be easily achieved, it provides some interesting challenges for the home health care nurse. Achievement of an outcome may take weeks or even months of intensive intervention. The nurse must consider who will be providing reimbursement for the home health care services and assist the patient in understanding the limitations or restrictions that may be placed on the level of services provided.

The home health nurse cannot avoid addressing the issues of cost and insurance coverage. Both the ANA's and The Joint Commission's standards require the nurse to acknowledge the cost of patient care.

In most inpatient facilities, reimbursement details are addressed by the admissions or billing departments as part of the application or screening process. In most home health care agencies, some preliminary reimbursement screening occurs when the referral is taken. A more thorough evaluation of

the patient's insurance and ability to qualify for home health care services cannot be achieved until the nurse actually makes visits the patient's home. Home health care is one of the few practice settings in which the nurse who provides the direct patient care is also responsible for evaluating and substantiating that the patient meets the criteria of his or her insurance plan. In addition, the nurse has the responsibility of informing the patient of what the estimated financial liability is if the insurance company refuses to pay for the services or if a co-payment is required for each visit. In fact, agencies accredited by The Joint Commission are required to provide the patient with an actual dollar amount in writing. To illustrate this point, consider the case of Mr. Highland.

Mr. Highland

Mr. Highland is a 75-year-old man who was admitted to your agency after the repair of an inguinal hernia. He developed a postoperative wound infection and now requires skilled nursing to manage his wound. Mr. Highland's primary insurance is Medicare, and he meets all the criteria necessary to receive home health care services.

Once Mr. Highland's plan of care is established and certified by the physician, your agency will receive one episodic payment from Medicare to provide his services for the next 60 days. Based on his clinical needs and the physician's order, Mr. Highland will require daily nursing visits to change his dressing and assess the status of the infection and the healing of the wound. Because daily nursing visits will most likely exceed Medicare's reimbursement, you must work aggressively to promote wound healing, resolve the wound infection and reduce the frequency of nursing visits.

If Mr. Highland's insurance is provided by another insurance company, perhaps one with a limited home health care benefit, you will have to discuss his progress toward the outcomes with a case reviewer every week or two to obtain further authorization for visits. You will have to provide written documentation and justification as to why it would be inappropriate to delegate Mr. Highland's care to a friend or family member or for him to do the dressing himself.

If his insurance plan only includes coverage for six or eight visits each quarter, your expected outcomes might be very different. Your primary outcome may be to teach a friend or family member the dressing technique and signs and symptoms to report to the physician. If Mr. Highland has no one available to teach, you might have to get creative and teach him to change his own dressing while lying on his back using a mirror, or he may need to return to the physician's office for the dressing change.

Standard 4: Planning

The planning standard requires the nurse to develop "a plan that prescribes strategies and alternatives to attain expected outcomes" (ANA, 2007, p. 33). Each patient's plan of care must be customized to meet his or her specific and unique needs. Although many home health care agencies use care paths or protocols, just as many have abandoned these models of care delivery. To be effective, a care plan must be flexible enough to adapt to the unique needs of the patient while considering the effects of "patient beliefs, values, characteristics, and situation" (ANA, 2007, p. 33). This standard requires the home health nurse to base planning activities on evidence-based best practices.

Consider the care path for a patient who is hospitalized with a primary diagnosis of heart failure (HF). An acute inpatient plan of care for HF patients will likely include routine or standing orders for the administration of diuretics, blood work to monitor the patient's electrolytes and renal function, oxygen, and a chest X-ray. The nursing plan of care might include plans for vital sign monitoring, medication administration, monitoring of the patient's response to the diuretics, dietary teaching, a referral to home health care, and instructions to

follow up with the primary care physician. The patient's entire length of stay might be 2 or 3 days. The expectation might be that the same protocol be implemented for every patient with a primary diagnosis of HF who is admitted to the facility.

When an HF patient returns to the home environment, a number of factors that are not directly related to the patient's diagnosis may impact the plan of care, as were seen with the case of Mrs. Smith. The nurse must be able to identify and plan for simple barriers, such as:

- affordability of medications
- ability of the patient to obtain medications and adhere to the prescribed schedule
- ability of the patient to adhere to dietary restrictions
- the patient's willingness to comply with the prescribed plan of care.

From an inpatient perspective, these barriers are absurd. After all, the patient's medications are dispensed from the pharmacy and administered by the nursing staff at the frequency prescribed by the physician. Adherence to dietary restrictions is easily achieved. The patient's no-added-salt meals arrive from dietary promptly at 7:30 a.m., 12 noon, and 5:30 p.m. In addition, the nurse's aide makes rounds every hour to monitor and record the patient's intake and output. Can this structure be achieved in the patient's home as well?

At first blush, one might think the four barriers discussed above are not barriers at all but merely excuses and examples of the patient sabotaging the plan of care through noncompliance. In actuality, the reality for this patient at home might be something very different. The home health nurse must first ascertain whether the patient can afford to purchase the medications that have been prescribed. It is important to remember that many home health care recipients are on fixed incomes and spend a significant portion of that income on medications. Frequent changes in medication regimens result in wasted medicine and an increased burden on the patient's limited financial resources.

For homebound elders, obtaining medications might pose a serious and real barrier to following the plan of care. If a patient cannot drive or use public transportation, how can he or she obtain the medications? Does a pharmacy in the neighborhood make home deliveries? What if the patient uses a mail order system to obtain medications? Customarily, the patient has to order a 3-month supply to achieve a discount and then must wait 2 or 3 weeks for the medication to arrive. For a brittle HF patient, a 2-week wait could result in at least one additional hospitalization, another change in the medication regime, and the cycle continuing again and again and again.

Diuretic therapy can pose an additional challenge to the homebound elder, and an astute home health nurse will recognize this immediately. It is not uncommon for patients to manipulate their medication schedules due to frequent urination. Consider what 40, 60, or 80 mg of Lasix might do to a patient with limited mobility or severe joint pain. The case of Mr. Indeglia highlights this point.

Mr. Indeglia

Mr. Indeglia is a 74-year-old widower. He has no children and currently lives in an apartment complex that is restricted to elderly residents. In addition to his complex underlying medical problems, he has a history of degenerative joint disease and underwent a total hip replacement 6 months ago. He now uses a rolling walker at all times.

Mr. Indeglia was admitted to your agency after he suffered a myocardial infarction that resulted in right-sided heart failure. When you first visit him, you find that, although he appears medically stable, he also appears somewhat depressed. He tells you that he used to go to the community room every morning to have coffee and play cards with his "buddies." He then reveals that he now has problems with "holding his water" and once even had an "embarrassing accident." He states, "When I have to go, I had better be close to the bathroom, or look out! It's a terrible thing."

Because Mr. Indeglia had an indwelling urinary catheter in the hospital, you further inquire about whether he has pain or burning when he urinates so that you can rule out a urinary tract infection. He denies any symptoms.

You ask him to describe his daily routine before he went to the hospital and uncover that he was usually in the community room from 8:30 a.m. to 11:30 a.m. and then returned to his apartment for lunch and remained there until dinner. He tells you that, after the evening news, he always returned to the community room to watch evening television with his friends.

Recognizing that the effects of Lasix peak in 1 to 2 hours, you suggest to Mr. Indeglia that he alter the schedule of his medication and take his "fluid pill" with lunch instead of breakfast. You explain that this change will allow him to return to his old routine and join his friends in the community room without the risk of an "embarrassing accident."

Clearly, the discharge plan established for Mr. Indeglia by the hospital was medically appropriate; patients on diuretic therapy typically take their medication every morning. There is no way the nurse in the hospital could take into consideration the impact that one pill would have on this patient when he returned home. Would the nurse in the hospital be surprised to realize that the diuretic therapy could result in Mr. Indeglia's feelings of social isolation and depression?

Finally, it is important to discuss documentation of the plan of care. Whether the agency uses care paths or protocols, traditional nursing plans of care, or physician-certified plans of treatment, the nurse who establishes the plan of care is responsible for documentation in the medical record system regardless of whether the record is computerized or on paper. The documentation must "provide for continuity" of patient care and can be altered with the changing needs of the patient (ANA, 2007, p. 33).

Home health care regulations and reimbursement require that the plan of care be physician driven. All home health plans of care require a physician signature to verify and certify that the care is appropriate for the patient. These requirements force the nurse to organize patient care based on the medical diagnoses. Home health care regulations provide little room for nursing interventions that are not sanctioned by the physician.

Standard 2 requires that diagnoses be documented "in a manner that facilitates the determination of expected outcomes and plan of care" (ANA, 2007, p. 29). Since the plan of care is physician driven and developed in the medical/disease model of care, there is a general trend to move away from a separate list of nursing diagnoses or a nursing care plan. Nursing care that is not ordered by a physician can result in survey deficiencies from accrediting and regulatory bodies.

Once again, it will be useful to consider the case of Mrs. Smith to highlight this point. As a result of your assessment of Mrs. Smith and her environment, you identified that she would benefit from skilled nursing visits twice a week to evaluate her cardiac and environmental status. You include this on the plan of care that is sent to the physician for certification and signature.

On your third visit, Mrs. Smith appears short of breath and her peripheral edema has worsened. Because a previous patient required you to measure oxygen saturation with a portable pulse oximeter and you still have the equipment in your car, you decide to test Mrs. Smith's oxygenation as part of your assessment and you document the results in her medical record. Although this seems like a reasonable nursing intervention, you would be cited by The Joint Commission for providing care without physician orders.

From this example, it becomes easy to understand why it is risky to establish both a nursing and a medical plan of care in home health. Providing services that are not physician ordered or not providing services that are ordered will result in a quality of care citation from regulatory and accrediting agencies.

The organizing and documenting of patient care is complex in any setting. In home health care, these tasks are further complicated because, as discussed previously, the plan of care must be approved and certified by the physician. The way nurses plan, carry out, and document patient care is primarily the result of having to demonstrate the provision of skilled nursing care to the payer.

Information systems and medical records tend to be organized in such a way that the reimbursable skills are easily identified. In addition, the presence of a nursing plan of care separate from a physician-certified plan of treatment increases the potential for clinicians failing to obtain physician orders for every treatment. For this reason, many agencies have eliminated the traditional nursing plan of care and work off of a physician-certified plan of treatment.

The physician-certified plan of treatment is commonly known as "the 485." The 485 is a Medicare form that has been adopted by many home health care payers. (See Appendix A, CMS form 485.) It is a dynamic document that incorporates the changing needs of the patient. The plan of treatment includes goals and an outline of the interventions necessary to achieve those goals.

When planning care, it is imperative to respect the patient's right to self-determination. The patient, physician, family, and other members of the health care team must be considered (and sometimes consulted) when the nurse is establishing the patient's plan. Home care agencies require the patient to acknowledge in writing that he or she is aware of the plan of care and agrees to participate in the planning process. As part of the process, the nurse is responsible for establishing and informing the patient of the services that will be provided and the frequency at which they will occur. In addition, the patient has the right to be informed when the plan of care changes, including changes in visit frequency or additional services or disciplines that may be participating in the plan.

Although patients have the right to self-determination, the agency also has rights. When a home health plan of care is established, it is essentially an agreement between the patient and the agency. Requirements of patient rights vary from state to state. Tables 3-1 and 3-2 provide lists of patient rights and responsibilities.

Standard 5: Implementation

Although home health care is an extremely autonomous practice setting, Standard 5 requires the home health nurse to implement "individualized patient plan" in a safe and timely manner (ANA, 2007, p. 34).

Even though nurses do not require a physician to dictate the patient systems to be assessed, a nurse working in home care must be careful not to implement interventions that require a physician's order. As a rule of thumb, any time the nurse adds a new service or discipline, changes a visit frequency, or alters a treatment, a physician order is required. Failure to obtain an order means that the nurse is practicing out of their scope of practice and will result in denial of payment, subsequently jeopardizing the agency when it is surveyed. It is just as important for the nurse to recognize that failure to complete an intervention that was ordered by the physician will have the same negative consequences.

When reviewing the plan of care established for Mr. Indeglia, the expected interventions are clear. The nurse is to:

• Assess his cardiovascular status, medication compliance, nutrition, hydration, and diet

• Perform venipuncture every week to evaluate

TABLE 3-1: PATIENT RIGHTS

Patients have the right to:

• Be treated with dignity, respect, and consideration;

• Receive services regardless of race, color, sex, religion, disability, sexual preference, or ability to pay

• Have their home health care providers communicate with them in a language that they can understand

• Be free from physical and mental abuse and neglect

• Have their property treated with respect

• Be given complete and accurate information concerning their diagnosis, treatment, alternatives, risks, and prognosis

• Refuse treatment or medication without reprisal or discrimination, as well as be informed of the consequences of such actions

• Receive effective coordination and continuity of services

• Expect that their reports of pain will be believed, receive information about pain and preventative measures, and have concerned staff who respond quickly to reports of pain

• Confidentiality

• Access their medical records and bills

• Obtain information about the agency and its ownership.

Note. From Electronic Code of Federal Regulations. Title 42: Public Health. Part 484: Home Health Services, 2010, by Centers for Medicare and Medicaid Services. Retrieved June 24, 2010, from http://ecfr.gpoaccess.gov/cgi/t/text/text-idx?c=ecfr&tpl=/ecfrbrowse/Title42/42cfr484_main_02.tpl
Note. From Comprehensive accreditation manual for home care, 2006-2007, 2006, by Joint Commission on Accreditation of Healthcare Organizations. Oakbrook Terrace, IL: Author.

TABLE 3-2: PATIENT RESPONSIBILITIES

Patients have the responsibility to:

- Provide a safe environment for agency staff

- Provide the agency with accurate, complete, and timely medical and insurance information

- Inform their physician or nurse of changes in health, reactions to medications or instruction given to them regarding treatment

- Follow the plan of care as designed and determined by them and their care providers

- Promptly notify the agency if they are not going to be home for a scheduled visit

- Assume the costs for services and supplies not covered by insurance

- Ask their nurse what to expect regarding pain management.

Note. From *Electronic Code of Federal Regulations. Title 42: Public Health. Part 484: Home Health Services,* 2010, by Centers for Medicare and Medicaid Services. Retrieved June 24, 2010, from http://ecfr.gpoaccess.gov/cgi/t/text/text-idx?c=ecfr&tpl=/ecfrbrowse/Title42/42cfr484_main_02.tpl
Note. From *Comprehensive accreditation manual for home care, 2006-2007,* 2006, by Joint Commission on Accreditation of Healthcare Organizations. Oakbrook Terrace, IL: Author.

his prothrombin time, electrolytes, blood urea nitrogen, and creatinine

- Teach him signs and symptoms to report, energy conservation techniques, and an emergency plan.

These physician-certified interventions give clear direction to every nurse visiting Mr. Indeglia. Each nursing note should include documentation of the patient assessment, tasks performed, and teaching accomplished. In addition, the visit note should include Mr. Indeglia's response to the teaching and his progress toward the anticipated outcomes.

In 2007, this standard was expanded to reflect the home health nurse's role in coordination of care and patient teaching in addition to the provision of direct care (ANA, 2007, p. 35). The home health nurse spends a large part of her time coordinating the patient's care with other community-based providers.

As noted in the "Introduction," the goal of home health nursing is to "maintain or improve the quality of life for patients and their families/caregivers, or support patients in their transition to end of life" (ANA, 2007, p. viii). This goal cannot be accomplished alone. The home care nurse is a skillful negotiator and coach who is able to mobilize other services and providers necessary to meet the needs of the patient. Whether the nurse is coordinating

with a Meals On Wheels provider to deliver the patient's meals to a neighbor on the patient's dialysis days, assisting the patient to arrange for transportation service to physician appointments, or connecting an "at-risk" elder with a legal clinic, the home health nurse remains focused on supporting the patient to return to his or her most independent state. The home health nurse remains focused on the patient's discharge from home health services and strives to provide the patient with the resources necessary to navigate the complex health and human service delivery system.

Standard 5 has also been expanded to capture the home health nurse's responsibility to incorporate teaching about health promotion and safety (ANA, 2007, p. 36). Over the last several years, the home health industry has refocused on these areas, which have opened the door to hundreds, if not thousands, of patient education tools that incorporate disease-specific health and safety information. Many of these patient education tools are in the public domain and are available on the internet for use without special permission. Chapter 7, "Outcome-Based Quality Improvement and Outcome-Based Quality Monitoring" will provide a detailed discussion of these tools.

Standard 6: Evaluation

The final standard relates to the evaluation of a patient's progress toward the anticipated outcomes. This standard is clarified by five measurement criteria. Although an evaluation usually occurs at the completion of a task or process, evaluation of the patient's progress toward the outcomes is ongoing and should be documented systematically and in a timely fashion. The process of evaluation is ongoing, and it affords the nurse the opportunity to revise the diagnoses, expected outcomes, and overall plan of care based on the changing needs of the patient and the dynamics of the patient's living situation. As a result of ongoing evaluation, the nurse might find that the diagnoses, expected outcomes, and plan of care are appropriate, and only the interventions need to be revised. Consider the case of Mrs. Jones.

Mrs. Jones

Mrs. Jones is a 68-year-old patient who experienced a stroke and has residual right-sided hemiparesis. She is cognitively intact. Although she lives alone in her single-family home, her daughter stayed with her for the first 2 weeks following Mrs. Jones' return from the hospital. Her daughter has assisted Mrs. Jones with all of her ADLs and IADLs. Although Mrs. Jones has had occupational and physical therapy since her stroke, she is unable to complete her personal care independently. You are the nurse assigned to Mrs. Jones' case and are aware that she is a Medicare beneficiary, which qualifies her for home health care aide (HCA) services. Mrs. Jones is agreeable to this service, so you contact her physician and obtain an order and establish a plan of care for the HCA to follow.

At the time of Mrs. Jones' admission to the agency, one of her expected outcomes was to return to independence in all ADLs and IADLs within 1 or 2 months. However, the loss of her daughter as a primary caregiver represents a major change in her living situation, and a reevaluation of the expected outcomes is warranted. As the nurse assigned to Mrs. Jones' case, would you:

- Change the expected outcomes and begin planning for Mrs. Jones' permanent dependence in ADLs and IADLs?

- Extend the time frame to achieve the expected outcomes from 2 months to 4 months?

- Request a multidiscipline case conference to discuss realistic goals and establish new time frames?

Although the first option might seem like the most reasonable, Mrs. Jones' home health care benefits only provide for short-term, intermittent home care services. Therefore, as the nurse caring for her, you realize that the HCA services will not be available to her indefinitely. The planning for permanent dependence may require Mrs. Jones to change her current living environment, resulting in a transfer to an assisted living or skilled nursing facility. At the very least, altering the plan would require a discussion with Mrs. Jones to determine if this is the course of action that she would choose.

Extending the time frames for her to achieve the expected outcomes sounds like a reasonable option; however, with the change in the caregiver situation continuing on the same course, the plan of care might be inadequate. In this case, requesting a multidiscipline case conference to discuss realistic goals and establish new time frames is the best course of action for Mrs. Jones' plan of care. The multidiscipline approach, which includes the nurse, an HCA, occupational and physical therapists, and a medical social worker, allows each unique discipline to discuss Mrs. Jones' progress to date and formulate reasonable expectations for additional progress toward independence. As a team, the group can establish a new plan of care that is tailored to Mrs. Jones' current needs and then confer with the physician, the patient, and the family.

SUMMARY

Every patient admitted to home health care represents a unique set of circumstances and health-related issues. The ANA's Standards of Care provide home health care nurses with some basic guidelines for the day-to-day performance of their duties.

In all practice settings, the professional nurse has the responsibility of developing a plan of care. The plan of care is based on collected data, diagnoses, and expected outcomes. The plan of care is a dynamic document that provides a focus and direction for the implementation of the nurse's interventions as the needs of the patient change.

EXAM QUESTIONS

CHAPTER 3
Questions 21-33

Note: Choose the option that BEST answers each question.

21. The patient's medical record

    a. is not considered part of the agency's information system unless it is computerized.

    b. only becomes part of the information system after the patient is discharged from the agency and the record is archived.

    c. is part of the agency's information system regardless of whether it is in an electronic or paper medium.

    d. cannot become part of the large information system due to confidentiality and Health Insurance Privacy and Portability Act regulations.

22. The ongoing collection of patient data is

    a. not necessary due to the short home health length of stay.

    b. necessary for the nurse to establish nursing diagnoses, identify expected outcomes, plan, intervene, and evaluate the patient.

    c. only necessary if the nurse is concerned that the patient's case may be subject to litigation.

    d. only necessary in cases that require interdisciplinary collaboration.

23. A comprehensive database

    a. provides a detailed picture of the patient that allows the nurse to develop nursing diagnoses.

    b. can only be achieved when the agency uses computerized medical records.

    c. is in jeopardy if the agency utilizes a traditional (paper) medical record.

    d. is not a realistic expectation due to unique issues associated with the home health care setting.

24. The nurse uses the information recorded during the assessment to formulate nursing diagnoses. Once nursing diagnoses are formulated, the nurse must

    a. have the patient's attending physician verify them in writing.

    b. obtain approval from the agency's medical director.

    c. validate them with the clinical manager, supervisor, or quality assurance department.

    d. validate them with the patient to assure that they represent the patient's perspective of his or her own needs.

49

25. The most realistic expected outcomes are identified through the collaborative efforts of the home health care nurse, the physician, and the

    a. patient.

    b. patient's significant other or spouse.

    c. CMS medical review nurse.

    d. case reviewer.

26. Home health care is one of the few practice settings where the nurse who provides direct care is also responsible for

    a. evaluating and substantiating that the patient meets the criteria of the insurance plan.

    b. completing duties or services that are typically associated with ancillary services such as homemaking.

    c. achieving the expected outcomes.

    d. sharing the responsibilities for the patient's outcomes with other members of the health care team.

27. The patient's plan of treatment must

    a. be customized to meet the patient's specific and unique needs.

    b. follow the agency's care path.

    c. be based on a physician-certified protocol.

    d. only consider the patient's physical and physiological needs.

28. Home health regulations and reimbursement require that the plan of care be driven by the

    a. physician and the medical diagnoses.

    b. nurse and the nursing diagnoses.

    c. patient and his or her needs.

    d. Medicare guidelines.

29. In order to reduce the potential of failing to obtain physicians' orders for every treatment, some agencies work off of a physician-certified plan of treatment commonly known as the

    a. M0080.

    b. M0245.

    c. M025.

    d. 485.

30. Patients have the right to

    a. jeopardize the health and safety of agency staff by exercising their right to self-determination.

    b. require that the agency assign a nurse who is the same race, religion, or sex.

    c. be treated with dignity, respect, and consideration.

    d. manage the type and frequency of service that the agency will provide.

31. Patients have the responsibility to

    a. alter their own plan of care.

    b. provide a safe environment for agency staff.

    c. accept all treatments and services offered by the agency.

    d. protect their own personal health information by requiring the nurse to document a minimal amount of information and include only the information that the patient feels is necessary.

32. Each nursing note should include

    a. only documentation of the physician-ordered treatments.

    b. documentation of the patient's current condition.

    c. a minimum amount of information to avoid the legal risks associated with poor or excessive documentation.

    d. documentation of the patient's assessment, tasks performed, and teaching accomplished.

33. The process of evaluation

    a. is necessary only at discharge to evaluate if the patient's expected outcomes were met.

    b. is only necessary if the patient experiences an unanticipated change in condition.

    c. affords the nurse the opportunity to revise the plan of care.

    d. is not necessary due to the short length of a home health care stay.

CHAPTER 4

STANDARDS OF PROFESSIONAL PERFORMANCE

CHAPTER OBJECTIVE

At the completion of this chapter, the reader will be able to relate the nine standards of professional performance to home health nursing.

LEARNING OBJECTIVES

After studying this chapter, the reader will be able to

1. differentiate between the roles of the generalist nurse and the advanced practice nurse in home health care.

2. recognize the role of the home health care nurse in an agency's performance improvement activities.

3. specify the nurse's role in the identification and development of agency "best practices."

4. state the value of the performance appraisal process.

5. identify the standards related to the enhancement of the professional nurse's education and competence.

INTRODUCTION

The American Nurses Association's (ANA's) *Home Health Nursing: Scope and Standards of Practice* defines two levels of practice in home health care. The standards describe the generalist nurse as one who is preferably prepared at a baccalaureate level, whereas the advanced practice nurse possesses a Master of Science degree (ANA, 2007). Despite the recommendations of the standards, many of the registered nurses practicing in home health care today come from a variety of educational and clinical backgrounds. Like all practice settings, home health care agencies employ nurses with diplomas in nursing, associate degrees in nursing, and baccalaureate and master's degrees.

Regardless of his or her educational background, the generalist nurse's primary focus should be on the patient and his or her family. In addition to the responsibilities outlined in the Standards of Care discussed in Chapter 3, the nurse generalist is required to demonstrate skills in:

- advocating for the patient and his or her family with respect to self-determination

- participating in performance improvement activities

- educating and counseling the patient in relation to self-care activities and health promotion and maintenance

- incorporating "evidence-based multidisciplinary knowledge into their nursing practice" (ANA, 2007, p. 13).

In addition to all of the functions that the generalist nurse performs, the advanced practice nurse possesses substantial clinical experience with individuals, families, and groups. The objective of this chapter is to provide a basic overview of the ANA's Standards of Professional Performance.

Standard 7: Quality of Practice

Many regulatory and accrediting bodies require home health care agencies to monitor and improve the quality of the services they provide. The ANA standards specifically require home health care nurses to "systematically enhance the quality and effectiveness of nursing practice" (ANA, 1999, p. 13).

There are many opportunities for generalist nurses and advanced practice nurses to participate in quality initiatives in their agencies. Through the application of the nursing process, nurses at both practice levels have a role in and an obligation to assist the agency's management and performance improvement staff to identify "aspects of care that are important for quality monitoring" (ANA, 1999, p. 13). Although the perspectives of the generalist nurse and the advanced practice nurse may differ, both are necessary for meaningful and sustained improvement in the quality of patient care.

The generalist nurse represents the patient's perspective and provides the agency with an understanding of the impact changes in policy and process might have on the patient, whereas the advanced practice nurse must represent the patient and organizational impact of changes. These perspectives are equally important, and both the generalist nurse and the advanced practice nurse are in a position to exert substantial influence on both patient-related and organizational processes. Consider the example of Mary R.N. and My Town Visiting Nurse Association (VNA).

Mary R.N. and My Town VNA

Mary R.N. is a baccalaureate-prepared home health nurse with over 20 years of experience at My Town VNA. Over the years, she has developed a strong interest in the care and management of patients who require wound or ostomy care. As a participant on many agency committees, Mary sought an opportunity to discuss with agency management her thoughts and recommendations for improving care for this cohort of patients. By collaborating with the agency's advanced practice nurse and other management staff, Mary developed a proposal to present to the agency's administrative staff. The proposal convinced the administration that, through the use of a wound care team, the agency could achieve improved patient and financial outcomes.

The development of a wound care team required My Town VNA to change the agency's clinical structure and processes. Clinical resources were reallocated to enhance and develop a wound care team in a cost-efficient manner. The agency had to invest in the education and development of its clinical staff to meet this objective. Policies and procedures were reevaluated and amended to give clear guidance to all clinicians. When the wound care team members were identified and oriented, they participated in data collection to monitor the appropriateness and quality of wound- and ostomy-related nursing care. As the team grew, physical therapy, nutrition and social work disciplines were added.

Once the wound team was implemented, Mary decided to seek formal training related to the care of wound and ostomy patients and enrolled in a certification program. The agency's administration supported her initiative and granted her a scholarship to defray the cost of pursuing the wound, ostomy, and continence nurse certification (CWOCN). Mary completed her certification and continued her work at My Town VNA, actively working to improve the effectiveness of nursing care and the quality of life for wound and ostomy patients.

From the example above, it is clear that Mary was a self-motivated individual who had an understanding of her agency's structure, process, and mission. Through her thoughtful recommendations, she was responsible for igniting a major restructuring of her agency's entire nursing practice.

Historically, agencies organized their quality improvement activities around standards and recommendations of accrediting bodies such as The Joint Commission (formerly the Joint Commission on Accreditation of Healthcare Organizations [JCAHO]). Typically, agencies monitored quality improvement activities that were high volume, low volume, high risk, or problem prone (JCAHO, 2006). The home health care nurse had a responsibility and the ability to assist the agency in identifying the practice issues that meet these criteria. The agency typically took a task-oriented or patient-cohort approach to identifying the important aspects of care. Table 4-1 provides examples of tasks and patient cohorts that would be found in a home health care agency's quality monitoring program.

More recently, the Centers for Medicare & Medicaid Services (CMS) has begun to influence home health agency quality improvement initiatives with its focus on the publically reported outcomes described in Chapter 7. The CMS has reallocated federal resources to assist agencies in improving patient-related outcomes. Through the combination of The Joint Commission and CMS approaches to quality improvement, the home health care nurse has ample opportunity to be involved.

By participating in the collection and analysis of patient, and agency-related data, the home health care nurse can influence the development of recommendations to improve the effectiveness of nursing practice. Once recommendations are made, every nurse in the organization has a responsibility to implement them, even if they have to amend their practice to do so.

In the example of My Town VNA, the organization clearly made a commitment to implement a wound care team, which significantly changed the clinical structure and operations. The change required all wound and ostomy patients to be evaluated by a wound team nurse: if a patient met the agency's criteria, he or she would receive the services of the wound team on an ongoing basis. Agency policy would require the wound team nurse to co-manage all wound care patients with their primary clinicians. The wound team nurse was to revisit the patient at least once every 2 weeks to evaluate wound healing and make treatment recommendations, if warranted.

Initially, some of the agency's staff were resistant to the concept of a wound management team. However, the coordinated efforts of the agency's management team and improved patient outcomes convinced the staff of their professional obligation to change their practice to benefit their patients. Once the changes were framed from the patient perspective, the cooperation of all agency staff was achieved.

The nurse's participation in quality improvement processes has the potential to assist the agency in identifying "best practices." Through collaboration with other members of the home health care team, both the generalist nurse and the advanced practice nurse will find many opportunities to improve their practice and patient care.

TABLE 4-1: EXAMPLES OF TASK AND PATIENT COHORT GROUPS APPROPRIATE FOR QUALITY MONITORING		
Criteria	**Tasks/Skills**	**Patient Cohort**
High volume	Indwelling urinary catheter insertion and maintenance	Chronic obstructive pulmonary disease and congestive heart failure patients
Low volume	Unna boot dressing changes	Cystic fibrosis patients
High risk	Management of epidural and intrathecal catheters	Addicted or premature infants
Problem prone	Ostomy management	Psychiatric patients

Documentation of "best practices" in agency policies, procedures, and clinical guidelines serve to establish an agency standard that provides the home health care nurse with clear direction related to the provision of patient care. The implementation of a wound care team at My Town VNA resulted from the idea of a single nurse who recognized a weakness in the agency's process of care. By working with the agency's advanced practice nurse and clinical management, Mary was able to positively impact the care of hundreds of patients. One nurse committed to the delivery of quality care elevated the clinical practice and effectiveness of the agency's nursing staff and improved both patient and financial outcomes.

Standard 8: Education

Standard 8 requires each nurse to attain "knowledge and competency that reflects current nursing practice" (ANA, 2007, p. 43). This standard requires the home health nurse to be self-directed and self-motivated in the pursuit of the lifelong learning necessary to practice in home health care.

Although home health care regulations and standards require agencies to ensure that patient care is delivered by competent and skillful staff, it is not the sole responsibility of the agency. As in any practice setting, the home health care nurse must work to acquire knowledge and maintain competency and skills that support the services of the agency and the practice of nursing (ANA, 2007). Reconsider the case of My Town VNA. Is it practical for the agency to allow a single nurse to refuse to learn a new skill?

The ANA standards do not restrict or dictate the methods or settings that nurses should use to achieve continuing education requirements. Professional education may be achieved through continuing education programs, in-services, self-learning modules, seminars, or lectures or through the return to formal classroom education in a col-

lege or university setting. Standard 8 does compel the nurse to maintain competency in the areas of "interpersonal, technical, and information technology skills" (ANA, 2007, p. 43).

Standard 9: Professional Practice Evaluation

Standard 9 specifically requires the nurse to evaluate "one's own nursing practice in relation to professional practice standards, and guidelines, relevant statutes, rules and regulations" (ANA, 1999, p. 37). The process of self-appraisal allows the individual nurse to identify both strengths and weakness in his or her own practice. This process enables the nurse to develop a plan to either improve weaknesses or share strengths. In either case, this results in the overall advancement of the individual, the profession, and patient care.

In reality, having one's performance evaluated by a manager or peer can be an anxiety-provoking experience. However, it is important to recognize that professional growth and development cannot occur until each nurse takes the time to participate in the performance appraisal and self-evaluation process. Consider the example of Dr. Landry.

Dr. Landry

Dr. Landry is a new physician who has established a pain management practice in the same city as your agency. In addition to subcutaneous and intravenous methods, Dr. Landry also uses advanced techniques, such as epidural and intrathecal delivery systems to achieve pain control for his patients.

When your agency became aware of Dr. Landry's practice and methodology, it established an in-service education and competency assessment program related to the care and management of patients with epidural and intrathecal catheters.

Like many of the nurses in your agency, you are comfortable and competent with managing pain through common methodologies, but what about the new, more advanced techniques? Through the self-appraisal process, you recognize that failure to expand your knowledge in this area could be detrimental to your patients and career. As part of the self-appraisal process you ask yourself:

- If I have a patient who might benefit from a referral to the pain management clinic, would I avoid making it because I am not comfortable with their techniques and what might be required of me? Would I deprive my patient of a referral to the pain management clinic and allow my patient to suffer?

- If I make the referral and it results in the placement of an epidural or intrathecal catheter, what will I do? Will I explain to my patient that I do not have the skills to manage his or her pain anymore and request a transfer to another more skilled clinician?

- What happens when my agency begins to have more and more patients with these devices? Will the agency have to avoid sending me to these patients? Is that reasonable? What about coverage on weekends and holidays? Will I refuse to see these patients?

- What if all of the agency's nurses demonstrated the same unwillingness to develop their knowledge and skills? Who would take care of these patients?

In home health care, nurses should expect regular evaluations of their clinical and case management skills in the office as well as in the field. It is not uncommon for a nurse manager to conduct joint home visits to witness the nurse's interaction with the patient and family. Joint home visits provide an opportunity for the nurse's manager to see them "in action." The nurse manager will take this opportunity to evaluate clinical techniques, such as infection control, wound care, and venipuncture. The clinical nurse manager will also have an opportunity to witness the nurse's assessment, teaching, and communication skills.

In addition to the formal one-on-one performance appraisal system, the home health care nurse may be asked to participate in a peer review process. The intent of peer review is not to criticize or second guess one's actions. It is intended to provide nurses with insights into their performance, as it is perceived by their colleagues. Participation in the peer appraisal process should be viewed as a non-threatening and nonjudgmental opportunity for professional growth.

Standard 10: Collegiality

As previously discussed, the individual home health care nurse bears the responsibility of ensuring that their own practice and the practice of their peers is high quality and effective. Achievement of this goal can only be realized in an environment that is collegial and supportive in nature. Standard 10 requires each home health care nurse to interact "with and contribute to the professional development of colleagues" (ANA, 2007, p. 45).

It is important to recognize that the provision of constructive feedback and the sharing of knowledge and skills ultimately benefits patients and professional nursing practice. The complexity of the home health care system and the acuity of patients demands that the home health nurse develop relationships with colleagues from nursing and other disciplines. Understanding and exercising these relationships contribute to the professional development of the individual nurse.

To this end, Standard 10 outlines the nurse's responsibility to establish professional relationships that contribute to productive work environments and to the professional development of all team members. This standard holds the individual nurse accountable for his or her role in the creation of the organization's culture, encouraging every nurse to recognize and accept responsibility for achieving an effective and supportive work environment. The old saying, "If you are not part of the solution, you are part of the problem" could not be truer.

Standard 11: Collaboration

Standard 10 outlines the expectation for a collegial and productive work environment. Standard 11 extends the benefits of the collegial work environment to the realm of the patient. It requires the home health nurse to collaborate "with the patient, family, and others in the conduct of nursing practice" (ANA, 2007, p. 46).

The expectations outlined in Standard 11 are the foundation for the provision of quality and effective nursing practice. It is imperative that the home health nurse recognize the limits of his or her practice and collaborate with other health care professionals to ensure that the patient's needs are met. Consider the case of Mr. Corneau.

Mr. Corneau

Mr. Corneau is an 84-year-old patient with uncontrolled diabetes. His inability to control his diabetes has resulted in many complications. The latest and most serious complication is a right, below-the-knee amputation. As a result, he receives daily nursing visits for wound care on his right, below-the-knee amputation stump. In addition to nursing, he receives physical therapy twice a week for strengthening and home health care aide (HCA) services three times a week for personal care and assistance with showering.

Despite intensive home health services, the wound has not shown any improvement. In an effort to debride the wound, the physician is now ordering Mr. Corneau to attend an outpatient clinic for whirlpool treatments. At first glance, what seems like a very slight change in Mr. Corneau's plan of care requires you, his home health care nurse, to coordinate many changes, including:

- explaining to Mr. Corneau the benefits and risks of this treatment change

- coordinating transportation to the outpatient clinic

- rearranging the schedule and amending the

HCA's plan of care so that Mr. Corneau is dressed and ready for his appointments

- assisting Mr. Corneau in avoiding an insulin reaction by helping him to understand the importance of getting up early enough to eat an adequate breakfast;

- teaching him to adjust the times that he takes his pain medications and diuretics

- reminding Mr. Corneau to contact the agency that provides his homemaking and shopping service to change his scheduled time

- encouraging Mr. Corneau to contact the Meals On Wheels delivery service to have his meals delivered to a neighbor's apartment on Monday, Wednesday, and Friday, when he will be attending the outpatient clinic

- contacting the therapist at the outpatient clinic for updates and progress reports on Mr. Corneau's treatment and progress.

Mr. Corneau's case illustrates how one small change in a treatment plan can result in many changes for the patient. Unless the physician or nurse making treatment recommendations has had any exposure to home health care, they will not be aware of the repercussions of this small change.

The inclusion of additional disciplines into the plan of care does not diminish the nursing role or contribution. In fact, Mr. Corneau's case illustrates that the multidisciplinary approach to patient care heightens the need for the nurse to coordinate the patient's care and safeguard the patient's right to self-determination and informed decision-making.

Standard 12: Ethics

Chapter 2 provided an in-depth discussion of the *Code of Ethics for Nurses*. However, this standard further provides specific guidance for nurses working in home health care to incorporate "ethical principles into all areas of practice" (ANA, 2007, p. 47). This standard clearly requires the home health nurse to understand the statutes (laws) that protect patient confidentiality and rights. This standard puts the responsibility of maintaining therapeutic professional practice boundaries squarely on the nurse's shoulders. It mandates the individual home health nurse to protect both patients and professional nursing practice by requiring the reporting of "illegal, incompetent, or impaired practice" (ANA, 2007, p. 47).

Standard 13: Research

Unless directly participating in research initiatives, it is doubtful that the nurse will question: "What is the latest research in this area?" However, this standard requires the home health care nurse to "integrate research findings into practice" (ANA, 2007, p. 48). Standard 13 requires the nurse to utilize "the best available evidence, including research findings, to guide practice" (ANA, 2007, p. 48).

Through participation in continuing education and quality improvement activities and policy and procedure development, the home health nurse is exposed to the most current research information. This information is commonly presented in a way that it can be evaluated and incorporated into day-to-day patient care activities.

Does Standard 13 require that every nurse subscribe to and read journals of nursing research cover to cover? No. Although exposure to "pure" research is beneficial to every nurse's practice and critical thinking skills, this expectation is not realistic for every home health nurse. What is realistic is making a personal commitment to subscribe to and read journals, newsletters, or other professional publications that relate directly to the contemporary practice of home health nursing.

Despite the growth in home health care, there continues to be comparatively little research that is based in this practice setting. Nurses often have to evaluate research that was conducted in other practice settings to determine its applicability to home health care. Although many home health care resources exist in hard copy and on the world wide web, the *Home Healthcare Nurse* journal is the only peer-reviewed journal that is directed to both the generalist and advanced practice home health nurse. This journal is an excellent resource for addressing contemporary issues in home health care (C. Humphrey, personal communication, November 18, 2002).

Standard 14: Resource Utilization

It is naïve and unprofessional to think that the role of the professional nurse in home health should not include addressing issues of resource utilization and costs of care. Regardless of an individual nurse's comfort level in discussing these issues, patients have the right to be informed about the risks, benefits, and cost of the services they receive.

In the United States, health care and the availability of health insurance is not an inalienable right. In fact, the Department of Health and Human Services estimates that nearly 46 million Americans were uninsured in 2005 (United States Department of Health & Human Services, 2005). Further complicating the resource utilization issue is an additional 16 million underinsured people during the same time (Schoen, Doty, Collins, & Holmgren, 2005). A competent home health nurse has to demonstrate the ability to aid the patient in identifying services that will assist in the management of his or her health care needs within reimbursement restraints. Standard 14 requires the home health nurse to "consider factors related to safety, effectiveness, cost, and impact on practice in the planning and delivery of nursing services" (ANA, 2007, p. 449).

SUMMARY

The *Scope and Standards of Home Health Nursing Practice* published by the ANA provides the home health care nurse with expectations for the personal and professional integrity of nurses (ANA, 2007). This document states that "home health nurses will experience additional challenges as the home becomes more often the point of care delivery. Home health care nurses will be called upon to coordinate and deliver care unlike ever before" (ANA, 2007, p. 28).

For the purpose of discussion and illustration, this author separated the *Code of Ethics for Nurses* (discussed in Chapter 2) from the Standards of Care and the Standards of Professional Performance (presented in Chapters 3 and 4). In reality, this has been a simplified approach and the practice of home health care requires nurses who can integrate all of these expectations into their day-to-day activities.

Every patient, family, community, nurse, colleague, and employer of home health care nurses has the right to expect the level of practice outlined in these three chapters. Clearly, the expectations are high.

To some, home health care remains a setting where nurses with "less skill" practice or where nurses go when they do not want to work hard. Home health care nurses possess the same skills as many of the nurses practicing in the most advanced intensive care units. What the home health care nurse does not have is high-tech equipment to monitor the patient, another nurse who can be called from down the hall to "come take a look at this," a physician in the building, control of every minute of the patient's day, or visiting hours that allow the nurse to control the patient's interaction with family and friends.

What the home health care nurse does have is a set of sharp clinical and assessment skills, the ability to build consensus, and the ability to assist patients in reaching their full potential within the limits of their disease processes or disabilities. Are home health care nurses better than nurses who practice in other settings? Certainly not. Are home health care nurses less skilled than nurses who practice in hospital or clinic settings? Certainly not.

No matter what the background of the home health care nurse or whether he or she is a generalist or specialist, the standards described in this chapter apply equally. When agencies, managers, and peers recognize and promote the strengths of all nurses, patient care is optimized.

EXAM QUESTIONS

CHAPTER 4
Questions 34-42

Note: Choose the option that BEST answers each question.

34. Although most home care agencies employ nurses with varied educational backgrounds, the ANA's *Scope and Standards of Home Health Nursing Practice* recommends the minimum level of nursing preparation for a generalist nurse to be a(n)

    a. practical or vocational nursing license.

    b. diploma in nursing.

    c. associate degree and nursing license.

    d. baccalaureate degree in nursing.

35. The nurse generalist

    a. has no role in the agency's performance improvement activities.

    b. often represents the patient's perspective and provides the agency with an understanding of the patient impact of changes in policy and process.

    c. should only participate in performance improvement activities when requested.

    d. does not have the educational preparation to participate in performance improvement activities.

36. Many agencies organize their performance improvement activities around standards established by accrediting bodies. Agencies typically monitor activities that are

    a. high volume, low volume, high risk, or problem prone.

    b. performed by new employees.

    c. identified as problematic on surveys.

    d. delegated to HCAs or provided by contract employees.

37. By participating in the agency's performance improvement activities, the home health care nurse

    a. can reduce the number of visits he or she is required to make.

    b. can expect to be compensated at the management level.

    c. should take on management responsibilities.

    d. can influence the development of recommendations to improve the effectiveness of nursing practice.

38. The goal of a performance appraisal is to identify areas of practice that may be enhanced by additional education. Standard 8

    a. requires the nurse to acquire and maintain current knowledge and competency in nursing practice.

    b. requires that the nurse only participate in mandatory agency programs.

    c. requires the nurse to seek additional education only when mandated by the state licensing board.

    d. only considers attendance at formal college classes to be suitable additional education.

39. The process of self-appraisal

    a. includes peer review. ✕

    b. requires a managerial evaluation. ✕

    c. enables the nurse to develop a plan to either improve weaknesses or share strengths.

    d. requires verbal or written information provided by patients, their families, and physicians.

40. Standard 10 defines "collegiality" as

    a. an uncommon phenomenon only associated with nurses who practice in home health care.

    b. a phenomenon that is typically associated with nurses who practice in hospitals or other facility-based settings.

    c. individual nurse accountability for his or her role in the creation of the organization's culture.

    d. important only to nurses who are in college or have returned to college to continue their formal education.

41. Standard 11 requires the nurse to collaborate with all members of the home health care team, including the physician and payer. The goal of this collaborative effort should be to

    a. delegate distasteful tasks to other members of the team.

    b. ensure that the patient's needs are met.

    c. minimize the amount of time the nurse has to spend documenting and communicating the patient's plan.

    d. force the patient to find alternative mechanisms to meet his or her needs.

42. The home health care nurse

    a. cannot possibly participate in nursing research.

    b. cannot practice without an extensive knowledge of current nursing research.

    c. can utilize the best available evidence to implement the patient assessment and to plan care, interventions, and evaluation activities.

    d. should be expected to conduct at least one clinical trial upon receipt of a master's degree.

CHAPTER 5

AGENCY STRUCTURE

CHAPTER OBJECTIVE

At the completion of this chapter, the reader will be able to describe the key components of a home health agency.

LEARNING OBJECTIVES

After studying this chapter, the reader will be able to

1. list at least three strategies an agency may use to market its services.

2. list the three major functions of the intake department.

3. identify the role of each professional discipline customarily associated with clinical home care.

4. identify four major functions of an agency's fiscal department.

5. recognize the role of the quality assurance/performance improvement department.

6. recognize the primary function of the medical records component.

7. identify the role of the information systems component as it relates to all other agency components and departments.

8. list the five major functions of the human resources department.

9. state at least two reasons that Medicare certification is important to a home health agency.

INTRODUCTION

A small hospital may treat 5,000 inpatients in a year. A medium-sized home health agency may treat just as many. The primary difference between these settings is that the 5,000 patients treated by the hospital receive treatment at a single facility, whereas the thousands of home health patients receive services in many unique and individualized settings. Providing patient care in the home requires even the smallest agency to be complex and highly organized.

As discussed in Chapter 1, freestanding not-for-profit visiting nurse associations (VNAs) provided the majority of home health services until the 1980s. These organizations were community-based and, until 1965, primarily supported by the generosity of philanthropic citizens and organizations.

Due to economic pressures, hospital-based agencies emerged in the 1950s and 1960s. Hospital administrators recognized home health as both a financial and patient care opportunity. In theory, hospital-based agencies could function as an extension of the hospital's services. Once a patient was discharged from the inpatient setting, home health kept the patient "connected" to the organization.

The Staggers lawsuit of 1987 gave entrée to proprietary organizations into the home health arena. Large national corporations developed strategic plans that included participating in the home health industry. This was accomplished by opening numerous branch offices in hundreds of cities and towns. Examples of these organizations can be found in any community in the United States.

In 2000, Fazzi Associates, Inc., a home health consulting and research firm, facilitated the 3M National Expert Design Project. The goal of the project was to identify the key components and departments common to all home health organizations (Fazzi Associates, 2000). This national project was funded by the 3M Company, the National Association for Home Care, and Fazzi Associates, Inc. and included the participation of many industry leaders and experts. As a result of this effort, the following eight components/departments were identified as common to all home health organizations regardless of the agency's size, structure, or mission.

MARKETING

Home health is a highly competitive business. All agencies are dependent on new patient referrals to survive. The 3M National Expert Design Project identified marketing as a key organizational component (Fazzi Associates, 2000). The summary report defined *marketing* as the component "dedicated to increasing referrals by implementing a marketing plan that targets an appropriate case mix for the agency. The marketing component is also the one (not the only one) that has a responsibility of developing and maintaining positive relationships with referral sources" (Fazzi Associates, 2000, p. 11).

The marketing of agency services typically occurs using a wide range of methods. Advertising agency services in print or on the radio or television might be the first thoughts of an agency's marketing strategy. If it is, you might think, "Well, my agency could certainly improve in this area." However, the 3M National Expert Design Project describes the agency's marketing strategy as one that must be "dedicated to increasing referrals" (Fazzi Associates, 2000, p. 11). With that being

said, one must question if using these traditional methods are effective mechanisms to increase the number of patients referred to the agency. An agency's marketing plan should be much more strategic in nature and target those who provide referrals to the organization, such as hospitals, physician offices, insurance companies, and other health and human service providers in the community. The development of positive, productive working relationships with key individuals in each of these organizations may be the agency's primary and most effective marketing objective.

Marketing strategy can be influenced by a number of issues, such as the agency's mission, its scope of services, and changes in the local or regional community. Understanding the mission and scope is necessary for those in charge of the agency's marketing endeavors. For example, recall from Chapter 2 the case of My Town VNA and the issues related to the use of epidural and intrathecal pain management. Before the agency decided to train all of its staff to clinically manage these patients, it had to decide if the provision of care to these patients was within the agency's scope of services and consistent with the agency's mission. My Town VNA determined that the provision of epidural pain management services was within the agency's mission and scope and dedicated the resources necessary to train the staff to care for these patients. In this case, the allocation of agency resources to increase the clinical competence of the staff provides an example of how the agency sought to develop and maintain a working relationship with Dr. Landry as a new referral source.

Although agencies may have one person or department responsible for the development of a marketing plan, this task cannot be done in isolation. In essence, every clinician making home visits is marketing the services of the agency. Excellence in customer service is the agency's most effective strategy. The home health nurse who demonstrates courtesy, competence, and caring is fulfilling the most effective marketing strategy.

Some agencies provide health promotion and prevention services as a way to market the agency. Some examples include:

- providing annual flu and pneumonia vaccination clinics at a reduced fee or free of charge

- conducting blood pressure screenings at elderly housing complexes or local businesses

- offering community education programs about public health issues, such as Lyme disease and HIV transmission

- presenting at local philanthropic organizations such as a rotary club or Kiwanis about health-related issues, such as smoking cessation or domestic violence

- conducting hypo/hyperglycemia screenings at health fairs.

Participating in events such as these allows the agency to develop name recognition by potential or future recipients of the agency's services.

Additional marketing strategies include working with local media to highlight human interest stories or celebrating occasions, such as Nurses' Week, Home Health Care Week, and Rehabilitation and Hospice/Palliative Care Month.

Whatever marketing strategies are used by an agency, the responsibility for the development of positive relationships extends to every employee. Everyone has a role in marketing the agency as the best and easiest to work with – from the chief executive officer (CEO) who meets with insurance companies to negotiate contracts, to the receptionist answering the phone, to the medical records clerk.

The success of the marketing component directly affects every other component of the agency. The most immediate effects will be felt by the intake department.

INTAKE

The 3M National Expert Design Project identified the intake function as a key organizational component. *Intake* is the "component responsible for taking referrals, verifying their appropriateness, and collecting information needed by the clinical admissions staff" (Fazzi Associates, 2000, p. 11).

Depending on the size of the agency, there may be a single individual or an entire department dedicated to this function. Most agencies are organized in a manner that facilitates the acceptance of referrals 24 hours a day, 365 days per year. The intake department may be open and staffed to accept telephone referrals from morning until night. Some agencies have the capability to accept online referrals, whereas others only have an intake representative available by pager. Regardless of the method used to actually facilitate the intake process, agencies strive to have a streamlined, convenient process that promotes referral source satisfaction.

In addition to basic patient demographic data (name and age), the intake department collects information about where the patient is staying and the phone number at that address. Almost every home health nurse has had a patient who lives at one address but is staying at another. Sometimes the agency is unable to locate the patient until the physician or a family member calls in to complain about the lack of home care services. It is at this point that the agency realizes that the intake department did not get complete and accurate information at the time of the referral. Figure 5-1 provides an example of a form that might be used by the intake department.

The agency must also obtain physician-related information, such as the physician requesting the service and the physician who will be following the patient and signing the plan of care and other orders. The completed intake documents also

text continues on page 69

FIGURE 5-1: MY TOWN VNA REFERRAL FORM EXAMPLE (1 OF 3)

My Town Visiting Nurse Association	Request for Admission

DEMOGRAPHICS
Pg. 1 of 3

Patient Name: _____ Gender: ❑ M ❑ F ____ Medical Record #:_____

Address:_____ Phone #: _____

City: _____ State:_____ Zip Code: _____

DOB: _____ SS#: _____

Language: _____ Lives with:_____

Temporary Address: _____ Phone #: _____

CONTACT INFORMATION

Name: _____

Address:_____

City: _____ State:_____ Zip Code: _____

Phone #:_____

Relationship to patient:_____

SOURCE OF ADMISSION

❑ Transfer from another HHA   ❑ Transfer from a skilled nursing facility

❑ Readmission to same HHA   ❑ HMO referral

❑ Clinic referral   ❑ Emergency room

❑ Transfer from another health care facility   ❑ Court/Law enforcement

❑ Transfer from a hospital facility   ❑ Information not available

REFERRAL SOURCE

Referred by: _____ Phone #: _____

Primary Institution: _____ Admit Date: _____ D/C Date: _____

Prior Facility: _____ Admit Date: _____ D/C Date: _____

Referring Physician:_____ License Exp. Date: _____

   Address: _____

   Phone #: _____

Attending Physician: _____ License Exp. Date: _____

   Address: _____

   Phone #: _____

Consulting Physician: _____ License Exp. Date: _____

   Address: _____

   Phone #: _____

INSURANCE INFORMATION

Medicare #: _____ Managed by HMO ❑ Yes ❑ No

Medicaid #: _____ Managed by HMO ❑ Yes ❑ No

Insurance Company: _____ Subscriber's Name: _____

   Address: _____ Policy #: _____

   Phone #: _____ Group #: _____

Contact/Case Mgr.: _____ Type of Policy: ❑ Individual ❑ Family

Initial authorization needed? ❑ Yes ❑ No   Effective Date: _____

Person Contacted: _____ Termination Date:_____

Service Approved: _____ Signature & Date Referral Taken: _____

Authorization #: _____

FIGURE 5-1: MY TOWN VNA REFERRAL FORM EXAMPLE (2 OF 3)

MEDICAL INFORMATION
Pg. 2 of 3

Medical Diagnosis: _____ ICD9 Code: _____ Symptoms/Other Information Reported: _____

Surgical Intervention/Procedures: ____ ICD9 Code: ____ Symptoms/Other Information Reported: ____

Confirmed Infection: ❑ MRSA ❑ VRE ❑ C-Diff ❑ Other

SERVICE REQUESTED

❑ RN   To assess: ❑ C/P Status   ❑ Weight   ❑ Pain Control   ❑ Medication Compliance
❑ Other (specify) _____

To perform: ❑ Wound Care   Site ___   Frequency ___   Rx. ___
❑ Wound Care   Site ___   Frequency ___   Rx. ___
To teach: ❑ Medications   ❑ Diet   ❑ Other ___
❑ IV Care*   ❑ Pacemaker*   ❑ Tube feeding*   * SEE ATTACHED

❑ PT   Evaluation   Restricted Weight Bearing or ROM ?   ❑ Right   ❑ Left
❑ OT   Evaluation   Restricted ROM ?   ❑ Right   ❑ Left
❑ ST   Evaluation   Restrictions? (specify) ___
❑ MSW   Evaluation   ___
❑ HHA   Evaluation   ___

❑ Hospice Evaluation   ❑ Palliative Care   ❑ Cardiac Team   ❑ Telemonitor   ❑ Wound Team   ❑ EMD Visit   ❑ Psych Nurse

DIET, ALLERGIES, & MEDICATIONS

Diet: _____ Allergies: _____
Medications: ❑ Refer to hospital discharge information

1. _____ 6. _____
2. _____ 7. _____
3. _____ 8. _____
4. _____ 9. _____
5. _____ 10. _____

Special Instructions/Information: _____

*THIS PATIENT REQUIRES AUTHORIZATION. SEND EVALUATION & NOTES TO INTAKE ASAP.

FIGURE 5-1: MY TOWN VNA REFERRAL FORM EXAMPLE (3 OF 3)

IV, TUBE FEEDING, & PACEMAKER ORDERS   Pg. 3 of 3

❏ Peripheral Line   Flush with every infusion or daily if not in use

❏ Heparin Lock   3 cc of Normal Saline Solution

            3 cc of 10 units/ml Heparin

            Other per vendor (specify): _____

Catheter Length:_____ (inches/cm) Length Exposed:_____ (inches/cm)

❏ PICC   Flush with every infusion or daily for all ports not in use

❏ Midline   5 cc Normal Saline Solution

❏ CVP   3 cc of 100 units/ml Heparin

❏ Hickman   Other per vendor (specify): _____

❏ Groshong Catheter   Flush with every infusion or weekly if not in use

            5 cc Normal Saline Solution

            Other per vendor (specify): _____

Port-a-Cath   Flush with every infusion or weekly if not in use

❏ Single   5 cc Normal Saline Solution

❏ Double   5 cc of 100 units/ml Heparin

Flush Due (date):_____Other per vendor (specify): _____

Site: _____Date of insertions: _____

Dressing Change: ❏ Weekly ❏ 3x/week Other (specify): _____ Due: _____

Cap Change: ❏ Weekly   Other (specify): _____ Due: _____

Method of Infusion: ❏ Dial-a-Flow ❏ Gravity ❏ Push ❏ Pump _____

       Cassette Change ❏ q24hrs ❏ q48hrs

IV Solution: ❏ Hydration (specify) _____ ❏ TPN (specify) _____

    ❏ Additives/Medications (specify) _____

Vendor: _____ Phone #: _____ Delivery Time: _____

TUBE FEEDING

❏ PEG ❏ J-Tube ❏ G-Tube Size _____

❏ Clamped ❏ Bolus ❏ Gravity ❏ Pump ❏ Flush (specify) _____

Feeding Solution (specify):_____ Volume & Rate (specify): _____

Vender: _____ Phone #: _____ Delivery Time: _____

PACEMAKER/AICD

❏ AICD ❏ Pacemaker Type _____ Low Rate _____ High Rate _____

    Mode set at _____ Rate Responsiveness: _____

    Site:_____ Site Care (specify):_____

Name: _____Date: _____

include insurance information to identify any payment and eligibility issues.

During intake, clinical information such as the medical diagnoses and any surgical procedures is documented. Depending on the referral source, information related to medications, diet restrictions, equipment needs, and psychosocial issues may or may not be available.

The final piece of information required for a complete referral is the physician orders. Orders may be explicit and detailed, or they may be vague, requiring the home care nurse to make a visit and then call the physician with a report of the findings. In either case, the skilled home health nurse can take the information and conduct a thorough and efficient home visit.

A successful and efficient intake department must work closely with the marketing, clinical, and fiscal departments of the agency. Intake personnel must be fully aware of the agency's marketing strategy, clinical capacity, and competence of the visiting staff. They must be knowledgeable about the agency's admission policy and apply it consistently. The staff working in the intake department must be able to triage calls to assure that only appropriate referrals are accepted, while striving to maintain referral source satisfaction. Consider My Town VNA's admission policy, noted in Table 5-1.

Although My Town VNA is committed to providing care regardless of the patient's disease or disability, due to recent staffing issues, the agency lost the services of its psychiatric nurse. The intake department receives a referral for a patient whose primary diagnosis is schizophrenia. The referral is from a local psychiatric facility that is clearly looking for the skills of a psychiatric nurse. If you were the intake nurse on the phone with the referral source, what would your agency expect you to do to guarantee referral source satisfaction? Would they require you to:

• take the referral and forward it to the clinical

department to "figure out"

• inform the referral source that your agency can not accept the referral due to staffing issues

• take the referral information and notify the referral source that you will be forwarding it to another agency that can provide the necessary service?

It is important to explore the notion of appropriate referrals. Not every inquiry handled by the intake department does or should result in a referral for the clinical service department, particularly when referrals come from health and human service providers or other community organizations. It is not uncommon for the intake department to receive inquiries about types of and means to obtain other community-based services. For example, the intake department may receive calls to:

• identify where a family can arrange private duty services

• receive information related to Meals On Wheels or personal response systems

• receive requests for referrals to "good" doctors.

Some agencies use a liaison nurse to facilitate the referral process. The role of the liaison nurse differs from marketing in that the marketing component is responsible for developing new relationships, whereas the liaison nurse provides assistance to a referral source after contact has already been made. For example, a long-term care facility is planning the discharge of a patient to his home. The liaison nurse is called to participate in the discharge planning meeting to assist in identifying an agency and other community-based services that might be available to the patient.

In the hospital setting, patients are required to receive a list of all the home health providers in their geographic area. Once the patient chooses a home health agency, the liaison nurse may be called in to visit the patient and facilitate the discharge process and home health services.

TABLE 5-1: ACCEPTANCE/NONACCEPTANCE OF PATIENTS POLICY

My Town VNA will make decisions about admitting patients and providing care and services based on the following criteria:

- Patients shall be accepted for treatment without regard to age, race, religion, sex, mental or physical handicap, national origin, sexual preference, communicable disease, or payment source. Acceptance of a patient will be based on the reasonable expectation that their nursing, rehabilitative, and social service needs can be met adequately by My Town VNA, in conjunction with family and/or other community resources, in the patient's place of residence.

- Consideration for acceptance will be based on the adequacy and suitability of agency personnel within My Town VNA's scope of services. If the patient's needs exceed My Town VNA's serviceability, the patient will be referred to an appropriate source for care.

- There is the reasonable expectation that My Town VNA will receive reimbursement for services rendered. My Town VNA will assist families in exploring financial resources that may be available to eligible patients, including the patient care fund for indigent patients.

- Patients are expected to reside within the communities serviced by My Town VNA.

- When it is reasonably determined that unsafe conditions at a particular time and location place an employee in jeopardy, additional protocols may be implemented.

- Patients shall be accepted for care when the home situation is safe and beneficial to the patient – i.e., the patient has adequate or potential support services to be safely cared for in the community: support services can be defined as family, friends, substitute caregivers, or community organizations. The patient's home has adequate and safe physical facilities and equipment for the nurse, therapist, and homemaker, home health aide to provide safe care. The patient and/or family has made plans to meet medical emergencies.

- Unless otherwise specified or indicated at the time of referral, initial contact will be made with the patient/family within 24 hours of My Town VNA's receiving a request for service.

- When the home environment is assessed to be inadequate to safely meet the patient's needs or the care required by the patient is assessed to be beyond the scope of My Town VNA's services, the admitting clinician will review the findings with the clinical nurse manager. The patient/family will be notified at that time of My Town VNA's concerns. The patient/family and physician will be notified within 48 hours of My Town VNA's decision not to admit the patient and every attempt will be made by My Town VNA to find a suitable environment for the patient's care.

- Before patients are accepted for home care services from long-term care facilities (nursing homes, rehabilitation hospitals, etc.), a registered nurse may make an evaluation visit to the facility to determine whether My Town VNA can safely meet the patient's needs in the community.

- Before patients are accepted, a plan of care is initiated by the patient's physician. This plan of care is signed by the physician and forwarded to My Town VNA for the case to continue. *Exception:* An initial patient assessment may be made by a clinician without a physician's order to determine an individual's need for service or ongoing medical treatment.

- The patient or caregiver provides written consent for care.

- My Town VNA is committed to providing service to persons meeting admission criteria, inclusive of those whose primary language is not English.

- My Town VNA reserves the right not to accept those patients who do not meet the acceptance criteria stated above.

- Hospice patients must be certified as terminally ill. The patient's attending physician must attest that the patient has a medical prognosis of 6 months or less, and the hospice physician must concur.

CLINICAL SERVICE

Once the intake department completes the referral process, the patient information is forwarded to the clinical service department for admission. The 3M National Expert Design Project (Fazzi Associates, 2000) defines the clinical service component as the one responsible for admitting, servicing, and discharging patients.

Depending on the agency's size and scope of services, the clinical component can be highly complex or relatively simple. The structure of the clinical service component includes a clinical director, clinical manager, and direct care staff. In a small agency, the CEO commonly serves as the clinical director. In large agencies, the CEO role might be distinct, and one or more clinical directors may report to a CEO.

Regardless of an agency's size and structure, Medicare-certified agencies are required, by regulation, to have at least a bachelor's-prepared registered nurse providing clinical direction. In some hospital-based agencies, the home care department is managed by a director who is a registered nurse. The agency may also have additional managerial support from a nurse who is affiliated with the hospital, a medical director, or the hospital's chief nurse.

Chapters 2, 3, and 4 outlined the role and function of the home care nurse. The clinical service component of any agency encompasses additional disciplines, including but not limited to physical, occupational, speech-language, nutrition, and respiratory therapy. In addition, the services of the medical social worker and home health aide are crucial to the success of the entire home health team and plan. These disciplines may be generated from agency staff or contracted from an outside agency.

Although many nurses are exposed to these disciplines in facility-based settings, home care requires nurses to have a detailed understanding of the func-

tions, capabilities, and scope of practice for each discipline. The following sections contain descriptions of each of the disciplines, the populations they serve, and their basic educational preparation.

Physical Therapy

According to the U.S. Department of Labor (Bureau of Labor Statistics, 2009a), physical therapists (PTs) are required to have a minimum of a master's degree from an accredited physical therapy program. All PTs are required to take a national exam and then be licensed by the state in which they practice.

The PT's role is broad in scope and includes helping patients with orthopedic problems to regain optimal function and minimize pain. In any setting, PTs are experts in the diagnosis and treatment of musculoskeletal and neuromuscular problems that affect people's abilities to move and function in their daily lives (Bureau of Labor Statistics, 2009a). In home health, PT services are provided to patients who are recovering from surgery or trauma and chronically ill or deconditioned patients who require strength and endurance training.

Historically, the PT has also had a role in illness and injury prevention and in health promotion in a variety of settings. This role has also been extended to the home setting. Home health nurses and other referral sources request PT services for home safety evaluations, fall prevention plans, and evaluations to prevent further loss of functional ability.

PTs employ techniques such as joint mobilization and manipulation to extend a patient's range of motion, as well as massage, ultrasound, and hot or cold pack therapy. Some of the more progressive agencies utilize physical therapy staff to provide electrical stimulation to heal chronic wounds and have taken advantage of their skills by including them in incontinence management programs.

Like the relationship between the registered nurse and the licensed practical nurse (LPN) or licensed vocational nurse (LVN), the PT may work collaboratively with a physical therapy assistant (PTA) in the provision of patient care. A PTA is a licensed professional who must complete a 2-year educational program and work under the direct supervision of the PT. The PTA is limited by his or her scope of practice and is not allowed to complete patient assessments or establish a patient's plan of care and treatment. However, the PTA is qualified to carry out a plan of care that has been established and supervised by the PT.

Occupational Therapy

Occupational therapy is a skilled treatment that assists individuals achieve independence in all aspects of their lives (American Occupational Therapy Association, n.d.). A wide variety of conditions and deficits are treated by these skilled professionals. In home health, occupational therapy services may be requested to address such issues as limitations that result from chronic degenerative conditions like arthritis or neurological disorders; traumatic or sudden onset conditions such as stroke, heart attack, spinal cord injury, broken bones, or amputation; or children with birth injuries or developmental delays.

An occupational therapist (OT) develops and implements treatment plans that focus on improving the patient's ability to perform both activities of daily living (ADLs) and instrumental activities of daily living (IADLs). (See Tables 5-2 and 5-3.)

TABLE 5-2: LIST OF ACTIVITIES OF DAILY LIVING
• Grooming
• Dressing upper and lower body
• Bathing
• Toileting
• Transferring
• Ambulation/locomotion
• Feeding or eating

TABLE 5-3: LIST OF INSTRUMENTAL ACTIVITIES OF DAILY LIVING
• Transportation
• Planning and preparing light meals
• Laundry
• Housekeeping
• Ability to use the telephone
• Shopping

In addition to performing assessment and treatment, the OT has a wealth of knowledge related to the use and availability of adaptive equipment. Part of the OT's plan of care, includes teaching the patient and the patient's caregiver to utilize equipment in a manner that is safe, maximizes independence, and promotes a return to optimal function.

OTs may be prepared at the baccalaureate, masters or doctoral level. Regardless of the program, OTs must complete clinical internships in various supervised health settings. Like PTs, OTs must also pass a national certification exam and, in most states, are required to obtain licensure.

Many settings, including home health, employ certified occupational therapy assistants (COTA). COTAs typically graduate from associate degree programs and, like OTs, are trained in both the classroom and clinical setting. A COTA works under the direct supervision of an OT by following the treatment plans he or she establishes.

Speech-Language Pathologist

In home health, the speech-language pathologist (SLP) is consulted for patients who have difficulty swallowing (dysphagia), communicating, or maintaining adequate nutrition. The SLP must be proficient in addressing dysphagia in both adults and children (American Speech-Language-Hearing Association, n.d.).

An SLP completes a comprehensive medical history to evaluate the severity of the patient's symptoms and deficits. The assessment includes an evaluation of the strength and movement of the muscles involved in swallowing and communication.

The skills of an SLP may be requested to intervene with patients who have suffered birth defects, stroke, brain or spinal cord injury, or neurological disorders, such as multiple sclerosis, muscular dystrophy, and cerebral palsy. In addition, an SLP may be asked to treat patients with problems affecting the patient's head or neck, such as cancer, injury, surgery, or dental problems (American Speech-Language-Hearing Association, n.d.).

A certified SLP is a graduate of a master's degree program that includes a classroom and clinical component. An SLP is also required to pass a national certification exam and, in many states, must be licensed (American Speech-Language-Hearing Association, n.d.).

Respiratory Therapist

The registered respiratory therapist's (RRT's) expertise is in treating patients with breathing and oxygenation difficulties and deficits. Patients diagnosed with both acute and chronic lung problems, such as asthma, bronchitis, and emphysema are often referred to an RRT. An RRT's skills are also valuable in the treatment and management of heart attack patients, accident victims, premature infants, and patients with cystic fibrosis or lung cancer (Bureau of Labor Statistics, 2009c).

In home health, the RRT participates in the patient's plan of care by teaching the patient to maximize his or her respiratory function and capacity. The RRT may be an agency employee or, more likely, is available to the agency through working with a durable medical equipment company or by contract. The services of an RRT are not a directly reimburseable home health service under Medicare. The skills of the RRT may be required to teach the patient and caregiver to efficiently perform pulmonary toileting, chest physical therapy, or oxygen and equipment management.

An RRT is a graduate of an accredited respiratory therapy program that includes both a classroom and clinical component. RRTs typically hold at least an associate degree and, in most states, must be licensed to practice.

Registered Dietitian

The services of a registered dietitian (RD) have become an integral part of home health care. Through training and education, an RD assists patients to understand about the effects of nutrients on human life, health, and diseases, including dietary deficiency disease (Bureau of Labor Statistics, 2010).

In home health, the RD is responsible for assisting the patient and family in establishing and implementing prescribed therapeutic diets and goals. For the patient to achieve compliance, the RD must display a positive and motivating attitude and work well as part of the team. The RD must demonstrate an understanding of people of all ages, backgrounds, temperaments, and tastes (Bureau of Labor Statistics, 2010).

RDs usually have a Bachelor of Science degree and are required to complete graduate level education, resulting in a Master of Nutrition Science degree. Most states require an RD to obtain a license to practice.

In home health, the RD may be an agency employee or made available to patients by contract. As with RRT services, dietitian services are not a directly reimburseable home health service under Medicare. In addition to visiting patients with tube feedings or parenteral nutrition, some agencies screen patients for nutritional risk factors and refer those at risk to an RD for intervention. Over the last few years, home health clinicians have increased their use of RDs and frequently request their services for patients with wounds and respiratory, cardiac, developmental, and gastrointestinal disorders.

Medical Social Worker

Social work is a profession that is organized to assist people in improving their lives and circumstances. Medical social workers (MSWs) have specialized skills to help patients and their families cope with acute, chronic, and terminal illnesses. Through their counseling skills, MSWs help patients and their families to identify their concerns, consider effective solutions, and mobilize necessary resources to improve the situation or circumstance. MSWs follow through with patients to ensure that they make use of the available services.

In home health, the MSW is knowledgeable about the availability of supportive health and human services in each community as well as state and federal assistance programs. The MSW is essential to support the patient through almost any crisis or to facilitate the placement of a compromised elder in a long-term care facility. As an integral part of the home health team, the MSW helps other team members to identify strategies to manage issues that might limit the patient's return to optimal function and independence.

To practice as an MSW, an individual must be prepared at the graduate level and hold a master's degree. An MSW must complete at least 900 hours of supervised clinical experience before becoming qualified to practice independently (Bureau of Labor Statistics, 2009c).

Home Health Care Aide

The home health care aide (HCA) is usually the only paraprofessional that is part of the home health team. The HCA is assigned to assist patients who cannot meet their personal care needs independently or require assistance to follow a plan of care that has been established by a qualified therapist. The HCA works under the direct supervision of the registered nurse or PT, and, in a Medicare-certified agency, must be supervised at least every 2 weeks.

To a certain extent, each individual state regulates the tasks that may be delegated to an HCA.

For example, an HCA can assist a patient with a shower or the application of prosthetic devices, but in some states, cannot apply a prescription lotion or cream to a patient who has compromised skin integrity. Most agencies require the HCA to follow instructions on an individualized patient assignment list. The HCA should not perform duties he or she was not assigned.

Professional clinicians must always remember that it is not within the scope of HCA services to assess a patient. Instead, the HCA must be taught what patient-related issues should be observed and reported to the agency. For example, it is within the scope of the HCA's ability to observe a patient with an indwelling urinary catheter for signs and symptoms of a urinary tract infection; however, it is not appropriate for the HCA to notify the physician of such findings.

FISCAL

Prior to the federal law resulting in the Balanced Budget Act of 1997, the clinical and financial department, of many agencies functioned somewhat separately. The clinical service department performed the patient visits and the fiscal department billed the appropriate payer. Fiscal-clinical interaction was usually the result of billing problems that were created by clinical errors or omissions.

Since the Balanced Budget Act required the Centers for Medicare & Medicaid Services (CMS) to control home health expenditures, the CMS created an incentive for all agency departments to work more closely and efficiently than ever. Today, the financial health of an agency is directly related to the efficient management of agency operations, accurate patient assessment, and streamlined, efficient plans of care. More now than ever, agency staff members must access information related to patient acuity and the cost of providing care to Medicare patients. The fiscal department is largely responsible for generating this information in reports that are easily read and used to facilitate decision-making and strategic planning.

In addition to the billing function customarily associated with the fiscal department of an agency, many other roles and functions must be efficiently performed; yet, they are usually invisible to clinical staff. Some of the more common functions are outlined below.

Depending on the scope and size of the agency, there may be a single billing clerk or an entire department dedicated to this function. For the purposes of this course, *billing* is defined as the function of producing a bill (either electronically or on paper) that outlines the charges for agency services. In addition to bills for home visits, some agencies may generate bills for additional lines of business, such as adult day care, hospice, home infusion services, and medical supplies. An agency may generate hundreds or thousands of bills to 10, 20, or even 100 different payers in a month.

The accounts receivable function ensures that once the agency has billed for services, payment is actually received (either electronically or in cash) and recorded appropriately. In addition, accounts receivable tracks delinquent, unpaid, and partially paid claims. In some instances, accounts receivable must also substantiate and verify recoupments, payment adjustments, and process donations or charitable gifts.

The person who functions in the accounts payable role is responsible for paying all of the bills that are incurred by the agency in a timely manner. In addition to paying for necessities like the agency's rent, mortgage or utilities, the accounts payable function releases payment for other business expenses like equipment and office supplies.

In an effort to maintain tight control on spending, many agencies have developed a requisition or purchase order process by which designated signatures are required before items are ordered and paid for. The accounts payable clerk often has the responsibility to verify that the process has been followed and all required approvals have been obtained.

Depending on the size of the agency, there may be a single person in charge of making all agency purchases or an entire department may be necessary to expedite this function. The individual responsible for purchasing typically works very closely with the accounts payable clerk.

There are generally two categories of items purchased by the agency. The first is patient-related purchases. Patient-related purchases include items used directly in the provision of patient care, such as gloves, wound supplies, catheters, and intravenous supplies. The second type, agency-related supplies, are generally those supplies that the organization requires to function. Items such as furniture, computers, software, forms, and general office supplies fall into this category.

Payroll is a function that may be found in the finance component or the human resources component of the agency. For the purposes of this course, payroll will be described as a financial component of the organization. The primary responsibility of the payroll department is to ensure that all employees receive accurate payment for the hours they have worked. If the agency provides fringe benefits to its employees, the payroll department ensures that benefits are accrued accurately and timely.

Regardless of the size or structure of the agency, one person usually manages the fiscal component of the organization. Whether the manager is a chief financial officer, vice president or business manager, he or she ensures that the agency receives payment for the services it has rendered. This person may report directly to the CEO, the agency's board of directors or trustees, or to a vice president in a hospital system. Regardless of the reporting structure, the manager of the financial component is typically required to prepare monthly financial statements, negotiate rates with various contractors and vendors, and prepare or participate in financial audits.

QUALITY ASSURANCE/ PERFORMANCE IMPROVEMENT

The quality assurance/performance improvement (QA/PI) component of an agency is one that "works with other departments to develop, monitor, trend, and continually update meaningful performance measures and to implement processes that use the data to improve performance" (Fazzi Associates, 2000, p. 11).

Since the Balanced Budget Act and the mandatory use of the Outcome and Assessment Information Set (OASIS), this component of the organization has become highly organized and sophisticated. Although in many agencies the QA/PI functions have primarily impacted clinical and patient-related functions, the implementation of the Medicare prospective payment system has provided new incentives to develop performance measures for all departments. Examples of QA/PI

goals for each of the eight agency departments are outlined in Table 5-4.

In addition to the functions outlined above, the QA/PI component has a role in the management of the day-to-day operations of the agency. QA/PI functions may be centralized in a single department, disseminated among agency managers, or a combination of both. Some of the day-to-day activities of the QA/PI component include:

- review of admission documents, assessment paperwork, and plans of care

- evaluation of recertification of plans of care

- review of agency adverse event reports

- orientation of new staff to agency documents and expectations for documentation

- responding to Medicare and other payer's requests for additional documentation.

In many organizations, the QA/PI person is extremely knowledgeable about Medicare rules and regulations and is often used as a resource by all clinicians and staff.

TABLE 5-4: EXAMPLES OF QA/PI GOALS FOR EACH OF THE EIGHT AGENCY COMPONENTS	
Marketing	As a result of marketing efforts, the agency will receive three to five new patients from newly identified referral sources per week.
Intake	All referrals will be processed and forwarded to the clinical department for admission within 1 hour of receipt in the department.
Clinical	All patients will be screened for safety risk and referred to the rehabilitation department for evaluation.
Fiscal	All agency purchases will be accompanied by an authorized purchase order that includes the date and signature of the authorizing agent.
QA/PI	The agency will maintain a Medicare denial rate of less than 5%.
Medical Records	Filing will be placed in the medical record within 72 hours of receipt into the department.
Information Systems	All agency computers will have a screen saver password activated whenever the computer is unattended.
Human Resources	All new hires will receive a criminal background check before they are allowed to enter patient homes.

MEDICAL RECORDS

The medical records component is responsible to "safeguard complete and accurate information on the patient" (Fazzi Associates, 2000, p. 11). All Medicare-certified agencies are required to maintain complete and accurate patient-specific medical records. Therefore, the primary and overriding responsibility of the medical records department is to keep track of every patient record in a manner that protects confidentiality while making sure the information is readily accessible to the clinicians who need it. Although it is estimated that 50% of all agencies have made the transition to computerized or electronic medical records, that fact does not diminish the responsibility of this component.

Regardless of the type of medical record an agency uses, the medical records department is also responsible for the storage of completed or discharged records. Each state regulates the length of time that an agency has to keep a record available. Typically, agencies are required to maintain patient records for at least 7 years for adult patients and up to 30 years for pediatric patients.

Other functions of the medical records department might include tracking of physician orders to assure that they are returned, signed, and dated; managing and maintaining of agency forms and paperwork; and providing photocopies of medical records as necessary.

INFORMATION SYSTEMS

The 3M National Expert Design Project (Fazzi Associates, 2000) defines *information systems* as the component of the agency that "responds to needs of other departments for information systems support and data" (p. 11). Virtually all home health organizations are computerized to some degree. Whether the agency only has its billing component computerized or has a completely computerized electronic medical record, some-

body has to provide support to the staff using the hardware and the software.

As agencies become more and more sophisticated, the information systems (IS) component will become larger and larger. For example, the IS component may be supporting (implementing, troubleshooting, and maintaining) voice mail systems, answering systems, and OASIS and other electronic data submission requirements. If the agency has a web site or email, the IS department also supports these functions. If the agency uses software to track donations, maintain a telemonitoring program, or conduct a patient satisfaction program, information systems are essential to the success of these initiatives. All it takes is one day when the voice mail or email system does not function properly, and it quickly becomes clear how crucial the IS system is in the daily operations of the agency. The IS component may also play a role in the education of new staff to agency systems or updating the skills of current staff to software improvements and enhancement.

Regardless of the agency size, structure, and level of computerization, IS management exists somewhere. Although many field clinicians are not aware of whose responsibility it is to ensure that everything functions properly or what the IS component does, if this component of the agency is weak or nonfunctional, it will be felt by all agency departments.

One of the final responsibilities of the IS component is to utilize their skill in conducting research. In addition to seeking resources that might be available on the internet, the IS component is usually responsible for generating reports that reflect agency operations.

Although the generation of reports might not be considered research in the purest sense, creating reports that are useful requires the IS component to assist the agency in asking the "right" questions and developing a hypothesis. Once the hypothesis is clear, the IS component is skilled at assisting to identify all of the variables that might affect the results, such as age, referring physician, number of visits, and discharge disposition. Skilled IS personnel can assist agency staff to uncover the detailed agency data that are necessary for both clinical and organizational operations.

HUMAN RESOURCES

The function of the human resources (HR) component is "to meet the staffing needs of the organization" (Fazzi Associates, 2000, p. 11). The HR component may be part of the organization as a freestanding agency, or the organization may tap into the HR component of a larger organization, such as a hospital or facility-based organization. The human resources component of the agency has five major functions:

- compliance with laws designed to protect the rights of the employer and employee
- retention of current employees
- recruitment of new employees
- competency evaluation
- maintenance and fringe benefits administration.

Both the federal and state governments have enacted many laws that protect the rights of workers. The HR component ensures that the agency does not violate any of these laws. Violations of a worker's rights can result in heavy fines and penalties to the agency. For example, workers have a right to a lunch and break period after 6 hours of work; they also have the right to be paid for all hours worked and the right to work in a safe environment.

With the shortage of nurses and other healthcare workers, retention of current employees is one of the primary functions of the HR component. In addition to the lack of qualified employees, the expenses associated with recruitment of new employees can be staggering. The estimated cost associated with recruiting one new employee is $3000 to $5000. Clearly, it is more cost effective to retain the agency's current employees than to recruit new ones. Expenses that contribute to this cost include the cost of advertising, interviewing the candidate, verifying the health of the candidate, evaluating the candidate's competency, and ensuring that the new employee receives a thorough orientation to the duties of the job.

In some agencies, the HR department maintains the competency of the agency's staff. This may be accomplished through on-the-job training, in-servicing, continuing education programs, and self-learning modules. Depending on the size of the organization, this function is likely to be shared with the clinical department and other departments of the organization.

Finally, the HR department administers the agency's fringe benefits. Depending on the complexity of the agency's benefit package, this function is extremely important and detailed. HR ensures that all employees entitled to benefits receive them. Any change in an employee's status may have an effect on his or her benefits. For example, if a nurse increases or decreases the hours that they work, this may trigger a change in health insurance, life insurance, or vacation accruals. The HR component of the organization must track all these changes and make the necessary adjustments with absolute attention to detail and accuracy.

MEDICARE CERTIFICATION

"Medicare is the single largest purchaser of home care in the United States" (Medicare Payment Advisory Commission, 2009, p. 5). The privilege of participating in the Medicare program can mean the difference of existing or not for a home health agency.

Throughout this course, the phrases "Medicare certified" and "Medicare certification" have been used repeatedly. For an agency to receive reimbursement for services provided to Medicare beneficiaries, it must be certified to participate in the Medicare program. Certification requires the agency to meet and continuously adhere to the standards that are outlined in the Conditions of Participation (COPs). Once an agency "proves" that it meets the conditions, it is issued a Medicare provider number. The agency's provider number is unique and must be included in all billing and other correspondence with the CMS.

Not only is certification required to participate in the Medicare program, but other insurance companies that provide a home health benefit require the agencies that they contract with to meet the standards outlined in the home health COPs. Therefore, failure to achieve and maintain Medicare standards can effectively eliminate the agency from providing any home health services. Although numerous noncertified agencies also provide home health services, regulations usually limit them to the provision of nonskilled services, such as homemaking and personal care assistance. These services are paid out of pocket by the patient or his or her family, because traditional insurance plans do not usually cover nonskilled services.

Once an agency is certified, it is required to remain in compliance with the COPs at all times. The CMS conducts surveys (usually unannounced) of agencies to ensure compliance. If an agency fails to maintain compliance with the standards outlined in the Home Health Conditions of Participation, it may face fines, payment denials, or closure.

If an agency knowingly commits fraud or abuses the privilege of participating in the Medicare program, the consequences can be severe. Consequences may range from the owner or administration being subjected to criminal charges incarceration or revocation of the privilege of ever participating in any CMS-funded programs in the future. To date, over 25,000 individuals or entities have been excluded from participating in CMS programs (Office of Inspector General, 2007). Due to the serious nature of fraud and abuse violations,

Medicare-certified agencies cannot even employ an individual who has been excluded from the Medicare program. Therefore, HR departments commonly include an OIG as part of the prehiring screening.

Although a lifetime exclusion from participating in Medicare programs might sound severe, it is important to remember that the CMS uses public funds (collected through taxation) to purchase health services for Medicare beneficiaries. Because public funds are used, safeguards have been put in place to ensure that the funds are spent judiciously. As a certified provider, the agency is acting as a guardian of the Medicare trust fund, which is an asset of the American public. This responsibility is taken seriously by the CMS and the Office of Inspector General and should be taken seriously by all agencies and providers. For all intents and purposes, committing Medicare fraud or abuse is viewed as stealing money from the American taxpayers and is dealt with swiftly and severely.

CONDITIONS OF PARTICIPATION

The 15 Conditions of Participation (COPs) are found in the *Code of Federal Regulations* under Title 42: Public Health, Chapter IV: Centers for Medicare & Medicaid Services, Department of Health and Human Services, Part 484: Home Health Services (CMS, 2010). Although the COPs provide a very detailed and extensive explanation of the requirements for Medicare certification, this chapter will provide only a brief overview. In addition, Table 5-5 provides a summary list of the conditions to be discussed.

The COPs begin with an outline of the minimum qualifications of the administrative, managerial, and direct care staff. Condition 484.4 requires the administrator of the agency to be either a licensed physician, a registered nurse, or a person

TABLE 5-5: CONDITIONS OF PARTICIPATION FOR HOME HEALTH CARE AGENCIES
Section and Condition
484.1   Basis and scope
484.2   Definitions
484.4   Personnel qualifications
484.10   Condition of Participation: Patient rights
484.11   Condition of Participation: Release of patient-identifiable OASIS information
484.12   Condition of Participation: Compliance with federal, state, and local laws, standards, and principles
484.14   Condition of Participation: Organization, services, and administration
484.16   Condition of Participation: Group of professional personnel
484.18   Condition of Participation: Acceptance of patients, plan of care, and medical supervision
484.20   Condition of Participation: Reporting OASIS information
484.30   Condition of Participation: Skilled nursing services
484.32   Condition of Participation: Therapy services
484.34   Condition of Participation: Medical social services
484.36   Condition of Participation: Home health aide services
484.38   Condition of Participation: Qualifying to furnish outpatient physical therapy or speech pathology services
484.48   Condition of Participation: Clinical records
484.52   Condition of Participation: Evaluation of agency's program
484.55   Condition of Participation: Comprehensive assessment of patients
(CMS, 2010)

who has at least 1 year of training and experience in administration in home health or a related health field (CMS, 2010). In addition to outlining the experience and training requirements of the administrator, this section of the COPs details the minimum requirements for the following disciplines and services:

- audiologist
- HCA
- OT
- occupation therapy assistant
- PT
- PTA
- medical doctor
- public health nurse
- LVN or LPN
- registered nurse
- social work assistant
- social worker
- SLP.

The second COP provides a very detailed outline of the rights of home health patients. Chapter 3 of this course provided a detailed discussion of patient rights and, although the details will not be repeated here, they are extremely important. Both the state and federal regulating agencies treat violations of patient rights very seriously. Therefore, agencies should be judicious in the administration of these rights and ensure that violations are dealt with swiftly. Condition 484.10 includes requirements for:

- notifying the patient of his or her rights
- respecting property and person
- informing the patient about and allowing the patient to participate in the care planning process

- providing confidentiality

- explaining liability for payment

- Informing the patient of the home health state hotline to register complaints about care treatment or services.

(CMS, 2010)

As will be discussed in Chapter 6, the implementation of OASIS is highly regulated. Condition 484.11 outlines an agency's responsibility to maintain all patient-identifiable OASIS data with the strictest level of confidentiality (CMS, 2010). Condition 484.20 also outlines the federal requirements for the agency to encode, lock, and transmit the OASIS data in accordance with the time frames outlined in Chapter 6.

Agencies are also required to operate in compliance with all local, state, and federal laws. The staff is required to provide services that are in accordance with the state laws and standards of professional practice. Not every state requires home health agencies to be licensed to operate. However, if the agency is operating in a state that does require licensure, failure to obtain a license is considered a violation of a local and state law as well as a violation of this condition of participation.

The COPs outline the basic organizational and oversight structure required for a certified home health agency. Detailed in this section is the requirement that the agency have written policies and procedures that outline the administrative, supervisory, and direct care staff functions, including those functions that may be delegated and who is held accountable if issues arise.

The 10 standards that comprise Condition 484.14 begin with a description of the minimum services and disciplines that a Medicare-certified agency must provide. Although there is no limit to the number of services that an agency can provide, Medicare-certified agencies are required to provide skilled nursing and the services of at least one other discipline. The second discipline may be physical, speech, or occupational therapy; social work; or home health aide services. Once the agency meets the two discipline requirement, additional services may be purchased from other health care providers or staffing agencies.

All Medicare-certified agencies are required to have a governing body that assumes legal authority for the operations of the agency (CMS, 2010). In many agencies, the governing body is referred to as the "board of directors" or "board of trustees." The governing body is also responsible for overseeing the management and fiscal affairs of the agency. This is usually accomplished by the appointment of an agency administrator who reports directly to the governing body. As previously stated, the administrator may be a physician, nurse, or professional who possesses relevant experience and credentials.

Other responsibilities that the governing body may delegate to the administrator include the responsibility to ensure that the agency employs an adequate number of personnel and that the staff employed is qualified to meet patient care needs (CMS, 2010). The administrator is also responsible for the financial soundness of the agency and is held accountable for ensuring that the agency's system of accounting is reliable and accurate. In the absence of the administrator, written authorization of a qualified person to act in the administrator's absence must be provided.

Regardless of whether the administrator is a nurse or other health care professional, the COPs require Medicare-certified agencies to provide all services under the direction of a physician or registered nurse. Typically, this position is titled "clinical director" or "director of clinical services." The director is responsible for patient care services and must be available during all times that patient care is being delivered (CMS, 2010). If the director is not available to participate in all activities associated with professional services, the agency is required to identify a similarly qualified person who is.

The COPs also establish standards for HR management. Medicare-certified agencies are required to have written personnel policies and demonstrate practices that support the provision of patient care (CMS, 2010). Agencies are required to maintain a personnel record for all employees. At a minimum, the personnel record is required to identify the employee's qualifications and validate that the person is licensed to practice in the respective state.

Condition 484.16 requires each agency to establish a group of professional personnel (GPP). The role of the GPP is to act as a professional advisory committee and provide guidance in the areas of clinical practice and issues. The GPP must include at least one physician, one registered nurse (preferably with home health experience), and representation from other disciplines, such as physical therapy, social services, and nutrition. At least one member of the GPP must not be the agency owner or an employee (CMS, 2010). Some agencies also invite consumers to participate on their GPP. In a Medicare-certified agency, the GPP is required to review agency policies and procedures, and conduct an evaluation of the agency's services at least annually. In addition to the evaluation of clinical programs, the GPP has a responsibility to conduct a review of the administration's ability to promote patient care that is within the accepted standards of professional practice and ensure that this care is provided in a manner that is efficient and maximizes its patient outcomes.

As part of the agency evaluation, condition 484.48 requires the agency to conduct a clinical record review at least quarterly (CMS, 2010). The record review should include a sample of all disciplines and services provided by the agency and should include both active and discharged patients.

A Medicare-certified agency can only accept a patient if there is a reasonable expectation that the agency can meet the patient's medical, nursing, rehabilitation, social, and personal care needs. Condition 484.18 requires the agency to establish a written admission policy that outlines the agency's admission criteria and the services provided (CMS, 2010). In addition, condition 484.18 requires the agency to establish an individualized plan of care and provide all services under medical supervision. All changes and amendments to the plan must be obtained through the use of a physician order that is dated, signed, and maintained as part of the patient's medical record.

Conditions 484.30, 484.32, 484.34, and 484.36 outline the educational, licensure, and performance expectations for skilled nursing, therapy, social work, and home health aide services (CMS, 2010). Condition 484.30 outlines the expectations of the registered nurse in home health (CMS, 2010). The standards that comprise this condition are very similar to the Standards of Professional Performance discussed in earlier chapters. This COP requires the nurse to make an initial evaluation visit, regularly reevaluate the patient's nursing needs, initiate the plan of care and necessary revisions, furnish those services requiring substantial and specialized nursing skill, initiate appropriate preventative and rehabilitative nursing procedures, prepare clinical and progress notes, coordinate services, inform the physician and other personnel of changes in the patient's condition and needs, counsel the patient and family in meeting nursing and related needs, participate in in-service programs, and supervise and teach other nursing personnel (CMS, 2010).

Condition 484.32 requires a qualified therapist (either physical, occupational, or speech) to assist the physician in evaluating level of function, help develop the plan of care (revising it as necessary), prepare clinical and progress notes advise and consult with the family and other agency personnel, and participate in in-service programs (CMS, 2010). In addition, this condition includes a standard that states that it is the expectation of the PT or OT to supervise the care, treatment, and services provide by therapy assistants.

If an agency provides social work services, Condition 484.34 outlines the role as inclusive of assisting the physician and other team members in understanding the significant social and emotional factors related to the health problems, participating in the development of the plan of care, preparing clinical and progress notes, working with the family, using appropriate community resources, participating in discharge planning and in-service programs, and acting as a consultant to other agency personnel (CMS, 2010). If an agency utilizes a social work assistant, the agency is required by this standard to provide direct supervision by a qualified social worker.

In most instances, the HCA is considered the same as a certified nursing assistant found in other settings. However, the COPs recognize that the provision of personal care and support services to a patient in the home environment requires an additional set of skills. Condition 484.36 provides a detailed outline of the training that an HCA must complete before entering clinical practice.

Every HCA is required to complete 75 hours of classroom training, 16 of which must be in a clinical-like setting. The HCA must demonstrate competence in areas such as communication, recording of vital signs, infection control techniques as well as an understanding of basic bodily functions, maintenance of a clean and safe patient environment, and recognition of developmental and cultural needs of the patient. This COP also requires the agency to ensure that all HCAs receive 12 hours of in-service and training every year. Like the other services provided by "assistant" staff, the HCA must be supervised by a licensed professional. In fact, this condition requires the agency to ensure that the HCA is supervised in the patient's home at least every 2 weeks (CMS, 2010). Typically, these supervisory visits are completed by the registered nurse and must be documented in the patient's medical record.

The final condition to be discussed is the requirement for the agency to maintain a comprehensive medical record. Condition 484.48 requires the agency to maintain a medical record for every patient in accordance with professional standards and practices (CMS, 2010). In addition to requiring agencies to retain patient medical records for a specified number of years, this condition outlines the expectation for protection of the medical record from unauthorized use and safeguards it against loss.

SUMMARY

Millions of Americans receive home health services every year. It is important to remember that each of these patients is cared for in a unique setting: his or her home. The provision of patient care in the home setting requires a sophisticated, highly organized agency. The 3M National Expert Design Project identified eight components and departments that are common to all agencies, regardless of their size, structure, or location.

Changes in the industry have required agency departments to work together closely to ensure that operations are efficient and streamlined. Weakness in interdepartmental cooperation and collaboration has the potential to threaten the viability of the entire organization.

Although the home health COPs discussed in this chapter seem reasonable and straightforward, more than 1,171 home health agencies, owners, and administrators who have been excluded from participating in the Medicare program (Office of Inspector General, 2007). All agency employees have the responsibility to understand the COPs and work to ensure that all violations are avoided.

EXAM QUESTIONS

CHAPTER 5
Questions 43-52

Note: Choose the option that BEST answers each question.

43. An effective marketing strategy is one that

    a. increases the number of patient referrals to the agency.
    b. regularly advertises on the radio and television by highlighting human interest stories.
    c. participates in community-based health fairs and disease prevention and health promotion activities.
    d. strives to strengthen relationships with the physicians who customarily refer to the agency.

44. The intake department must work cooperatively with all agency components and

    a. take all referrals to ensure referral source satisfaction.
    b. consider the financial and insurance resources of every patient before accepting the referral.
    c. ensure that the agency only takes referrals that will be financially lucrative and decline referrals that might be complex or require large amounts of service.
    d. triage calls to ensure that only appropriate referrals are accepted, while striving to maintain referral source satisfaction.

45. The 3M National Expert Design Project defines the clinical service component as

    a. the largest of all agency components.
    b. one that is most often plagued with inefficiency and duplication.
    c. the most important of all agency components because it is the one responsible for direct patient care.
    d. one responsible for admitting, servicing, and discharging patients.

46. Depending on the agency's size and structure, the fiscal component of the agency is usually comprised of billing, accounts receivable, accounts payable, payroll, and

    a. marketing.
    b. HR.
    c. IS.
    d. purchasing.

47. The QA/PI component of an agency

    a. is to focus solely on the financial performance of the agency.
    b. is to focus solely on the clinical functions of the agency.
    c. is to assist in the development of performance measures for agency components.
    d. has been eliminated due to financial constraints.

48. The function of the medical records component of the agency

    a. will essentially be eliminated as agencies move to complete electronic medical records.

    b. is to safeguard complete and accurate information on the patient.

    c. is considered nonessential.

    d. will most likely be merged with another agency component to save time and money.

49. The IS component

    a. is only really important in agencies that have electronic medical records.

    b. is responsible to work primarily with the fiscal department to ensure timely billing.

    c. will most likely be eliminated due to the expense associated with it.

    d. may be responsible to support voice mail systems, telephone answering systems, and electronic data submission software.

50. Meeting the staffing needs of the agency is the primary function of

    a. QA/PI.

    b. HR.

    c. intake.

    d. marketing.

51. Medicare certification is important to a home health agency because

    a. it is required to provide a nonskilled level of care.

    b. physicians are not allowed to refer patients to noncertified agencies.

    c. it allows the agency to participate in Medicare and other insurance programs.

    d. it forces an agency to limit the number of patients it can have on service at any one time.

52. The COPs require the agency to establish a GPP, complete an annual evaluation of the agency's programs and services, and

    a. provide all nursing specialties, including pediatrics, psychiatric, and rehabilitation.

    b. provide free care to patients who are indigent but over the age of 50.

    c. conduct clinical record reviews at least quarterly.

    d. establish a relationship with a local hospital that will provide clinical oversight to the agency.

CHAPTER 6

OUTCOME AND ASSESSMENT INFORMATION SET

CHAPTER OBJECTIVE

After completing this chapter, the reader will be able to apply the Outcome and Assessment Information Set (OASIS) to patient scenarios.

LEARNING OBJECTIVES

After studying this chapter, the reader will be able to

1. identify the time frames allowed to complete the OASIS.

2. differentiate between the uses of each OASIS document.

3. list the rules that guide the completion of the OASIS documents.

4. describe the relationship between the OASIS and the plan of care.

INTRODUCTION

Like any "mature" industry, home health has had to evolve and expand to meet the changing needs and expectations of its customers. In any agency, nurses might be heard reminiscing about the "good old days." If a home health nurse was asked when the "good old days" were, he or she would likely say, "Before OASIS!"

If you have no home health experience, you might think it is odd that the word *oasis* represents something negative or overwhelming. In fact, an oasis is commonly defined as a "situation or place preserved from surrounding unpleasantness; a refuge" (American Heritage Dictionary, 2000). In home health, OASIS is an acronym for the Outcome and Assessment Information Set, a standardized patient assessment tool that must be completed for the majority of patients admitted to Medicare-certified home health agencies.

The OASIS document was developed by the Center for Health Care Policy and Research (CHCPR). The CHCPR was commissioned by the U.S. Department of Health and Human Services to develop a standardized patient data collection/assessment tool. The collection of a standardized information set was intended to provide the federal government a means to measure the quality of an agency's services. From the assessment, patient outcomes (results) of care could be calculated, and agencies could then be compared to identify the most effective service providers. As a result, the Centers for Medicare & Medicaid Services (CMS) would be able to identify agencies that demonstrated the "best" patient outcomes. Their "best practices" would then be shared with all other agencies, thereby improving the care of all home health patients. This sounds like a noble and worthwhile effort. How can one argue with initiatives aimed at improving the quality of patient care? Is it not our professional obligation to participate in initiatives to improve patient care?

In addition to the quality improvement applications, OASIS information also created the foundation to build the home health prospective payment system (PPS) of reimbursement, discussed in Chapter 8 of this book. These two factors were the impetus to require all Medicare-certified home health agencies to implement OASIS data collection in 1999. Since that time, changes have been made to OASIS with the most significant changes effective as of January 1, 2010. The latest set of OASIS measures include process driven measures, such as performing a pressure ulcer risk assessment, in addition to patient outcome measures. The current form of OASIS is called OASIS-C and all information in this chapter is in reference to this version. A detailed and specific set of implementation instructions is available at http://www.cms.hhs.gov/HomeHealthQualityInits/14_HHQIOASISUser Manual.asp. The implementation of OASIS required agencies to change many of their policies, procedures, and clinical documentation forms. The sections that follow provide a synopsis of the OASIS items, regulations and processes.

OASIS IMPLEMENTATION

To achieve the CMS's quality improvement goals, thousands of home health agencies were required to implement the OASIS system. To maximize the effectiveness of the quality initiative, all nurses working in home health were required to learn to correctly answer over 100 OASIS items/questions in a manner that was consistent with the intent of the questions. To facilitate the education and training of agency staff, the *Outcome and Assessment Information System User Manual* was published by the Health Care Financing Administration. The user manual provides agencies with hundreds of pages of instructions for the implementation of the OASIS system. As part of the implementation, agencies were required to:

• collect OASIS data for all eligible patients

• complete the patient assessment within the required time frames

• encode, lock, and electronically transmit the data within the required time frames.

Since the original publication of OASIS and the item-by-item tips found in the OASIS user manual, CMS has collated a comprehensive list of questions and answers (Q&As). The OASIS Q&As are the official responses of the CMS to clinician questions, and are released on a quarterly basis. They are designed to give OASIS users hints and details that should be considered when completing an item. The Q&As are arranged sequentially according to the item and can be found at http://www.oasisanswers.com/aboutoas_links.htm.

ELIGIBLE PATIENTS

The OASIS guidelines require agencies to complete the Start of Care (SOC) OASIS on all patients admitted to home health for the receipt of skilled nursing or therapy services. They also state that a nurse must complete the OASIS assessment unless therapy services are the only services requested at the time of admission; in this case, the therapist may complete the OASIS document. In multidisciplinary cases, the nurse is required to complete the OASIS assessment. This regulation has created a significant amount of confusion in the day-to-day operations of home health agencies.

Patients who are admitted to the agency for non-skilled services, such as homemaking, are excluded from the OASIS regulations. In addition, patients admitted with a maternity or postpartum diagnosis are excluded. Finally, it is important to note that the OASIS is not designed to be administered to the pediatric population; therefore, patients who are under 18 years of age are also excluded from the OASIS requirements. Although some home health agencies also provide hospice services, only home health patients are subject to the OASIS regulations and the collection of OASIS data.

TIME FRAMES

The OASIS regulations require agencies to pay attention to at least seven different time frames. The best way to illustrate the time frame requirements is to relate them to a patient example; therefore, consider the case of Mr. Hunt. Mr. Hunt was admitted to My Town Visiting Nurse Association (VNA) on November 1st. Since this is the date of the first skilled visit provided to Mr. Hunt, it is also his home health start of care (SOC) date.

48-Hour Start of Care

The first OASIS time frame that the agency must consider is the requirement to conduct a SOC visit within 48 hours of receiving a patient referral. If the agency is unable to accommodate the 48-hour requirement, the regulations require the agency to inform the referral source and provide them the option of referring the patient to an agency that can meet the patient's needs in a more timely fashion. If the agency does not or cannot make the visit within 48 hours, the patient's medical record should reflect the reason that the visit was not made and that the referral source, physician, and patient were notified.

In some instances, there are appropriate exceptions to this rule. For example, the physician may request that the agency visit the patient in 1 week to remove postoperative staples or in 1 month to administer a vitamin B12 injection or flush a venous access device. In any case, this instruction should be clearly documented in the patient's medical record.

5 Days to Complete the Start of Care OASIS

The completion of the SOC OASIS (see Appendix B) might be perceived as an overwhelming task by both the home health nurse and the patient. In deference to this perception, the OASIS regulations allow the agency up to 5 days to complete the

SOC OASIS, which seems like a reasonable consideration. However, because OASIS is designed to capture the patient's status at the beginning of the episode, most agencies require their staff to complete the SOC OASIS based on the condition of the patient at the first visit.

The reality of home health is that a patient may present very differently from one visit to the next. For example, after a hospitalization, a patient may "bounce back" once they are home for a few days. Therefore, most agencies consider the OASIS a snapshot and require that it be completed on the basis of one visit – not a video that can be viewed over a 5-day period. Typically, the SOC OASIS is completed within 24 to 48 hours of the SOC visit.

60-Day Episode

The second OASIS time frame is the 60-day episode. There is no limit to the number of 60-day episodes that a patient can have as long as the patient's condition meets payor criteria. However, the agency must be mindful that each 60-day episode is discrete and cannot overlap another episode in any way. In the case of Mr. Hunt, his 60-day episode runs from November 1st to December 30th. If Mr. Hunt receives a visit on December 31st, that visit would have occurred on the first day of his second episode of care.

30 Days to Transmit

As mentioned earlier, the intent of OASIS data collection is to provide a measure for patient outcomes and to compare one agency's performance to that of all other agencies. In order to accomplish this goal, OASIS regulations require agencies to encode and transmit all Medicare and Medicaid patient data to the federal government for analysis.

Simply stated, agencies are required to enter answers found on each patient OASIS assessment into a computer software program. In essence, the software packages the information in a way that protects confidentiality yet makes retrieval and analysis of the information possible. The process of computerizing and sending OASIS data is referred to as *encoding, locking* and *transmitting.*

In the case of Mr. Hunt, assume that My Town VNA requires its staff to complete the OASIS within 48 hours of the SOC visit (November 1st). If the agency utilizes a paper-based medical record, the nurse has to complete the initial OASIS paperwork, have it checked for errors and omissions, correct the errors or complete the omissions, and return the document to data entry for encoding and locking.

Once the agency encodes and locks the assessment, it then has 30 days to transmit the data to its respective state OASIS coordinator. The state OASIS coordinator acts as a facilitator for the federal government by electronically packaging the data received from all of the home health agencies in the state and then sending it along to the federal computer system. The state OASIS coordinator also provides technical support and assistance to agencies in relation to problems with encoding, locking, and transmitting data.

48 Hours to Complete a Transfer OASIS or Resumption of Care OASIS

From the OASIS perspective, a patient may experience three events that require the completion of an additional and specific assessment within a required time frame. Whenever a patient is transferred to an inpatient facility (e.g., hospital or rehab facility) for more than 24 hours, the agency is required to complete a Transfer to Inpatient Facility OASIS assessment (see Appendix C). This document must be completed within 48 hours of being notified that the patient was admitted. The detail to pay special attention to is the phrase "within 48 hours of being notified." It is not uncommon for the agency to be unaware that the patient was transferred to an inpatient facility. For some, the first notification that the patient was hospitalized occurs when the agency is notified that the patient will be retuning home and services should resume. When

this scenario occurs, the agency must still complete the Transfer OASIS within 48 hours so that it accurately reflects the sequence of events, even though the patient has already returned home.

The second event occurs whenever an agency resumes the care of a patient after an inpatient stay. The OASIS regulations require the agency to complete a Resumption of Care (ROC) OASIS. This document must be completed on the first visit after the patient returns home. The ROC OASIS is the same exact document as the SOC OASIS found in Appendix B.

5-Day Window

One of the most difficult OASIS time frames to track has been termed the "5-day window." The 5-day window only affects patients who receive home health services for subsequent 60-day episodes. The OASIS regulations require the agency to reassess the patient before the beginning of each subsequent episode of care. To operationalize this requirement, the CHCPR determined that the patient should be assessed any time after the 55th day of the episode but before the end of the 60th day.

To illustrate this point, once again consider the case of Mr. Hunt. Assume he was not discharged from My Town VNA by the end of the 60th day of the SOC episode, and his physician-ordered plan of care requires him to continue to receive care into a second episode. OASIS regulations mandate that the agency make a home visit, reassess his status, and document the findings using a Follow-Up (FU) OASIS assessment (see Appendix D). All of these steps must occur in the 5-day window of the current episode. When applied to the calendar, Mr. Hunt will have to receive a visit anytime from December 26th (day 56 of the episode) through December 30th (day 60 of the episode).

48 Hours to Complete a Discharge OASIS

The final time frame that the home health nurse must be aware of is the time allotted to complete, encode, and lock the Discharge (D/C) OASIS (see Appendix E). Most agencies require their staff to complete the Discharge OASIS within 48 hours of the last visit. OASIS regulations allow the agency 7 days to encode and lock the assessment. Table 6-1 provides a summary of the OASIS time frames using Mr. Hunt's schedule for illustration and clarification.

Now that a review of the OASIS time frames has been completed, it is necessary to review the actual OASIS documents that are provided in Appendices B through E and the rules that must be followed when completing them.

RULES FOR COMPLETION OF OASIS DOCUMENTS

It is imperative that, when completing the OASIS documents, the home health nurse is familiar with the rules as they are presented in the OASIS regulations. The five basic rules are outlined here.

Rule 1: OASIS questions are incorporated into the agency's comprehensive patient assessment. OASIS items are identified by the letter M followed by a number. Agencies are not allowed to take liberties with the wording or punctuation of any of the OASIS questions. If it suits the needs of the agency, the questions can be sequenced differently as long as the OASIS item number designations are not changed.

Rule 2: When completing the OASIS items, the nurse must pay careful attention to the directives that are included in each of the questions. Some questions direct the nurse to "Mark all that apply" or follow predetermined skip patterns. For example, if the home health nurse marks that the patient has not experienced an inpatient stay, the directives in the question instruct the nurse to skip all questions related to an inpatient stay.

TABLE 6-1: MR. HUNT'S OASIS TIME FRAMES AND SCHEDULES

Event #1: Referral received by agency on 10/31

	Time allowed to complete:	*To be completed by:*
SOC Visit	Within 48 hours of referral	11/2
SOC OASIS	5 days	11/7

Event #2: Agency notified of inpatient transfer on 12/1

	Time allowed to complete:	*To be completed by:*
Transfer OASIS completed	Within 48 hours of notification	12/3

Event #3: Patient re-referred on 12/5 to resume services 12/6

	Time allowed to complete:	*To be completed by:*
ROC Visit	Within 48 hours of referral	12/8
ROC OASIS completed	Within 48 hours of visit	12/10

Event #4: Patient requires services into a subsequent episode; 5-day window 12/26 through 12/30

	Time allowed to complete:	*To be completed by:*
Follow-Up OASIS completed	Within 48 hours of visit made on 12/26	12/28
Episode end	60 days from SOC	12/30

Event #5: Patient is discharged on 1/6

	Time allowed to complete:	*To be completed by:*
Discharge OASIS completed	Within 48 hours of discharge	1/8

Rule 3: Although many of the questions provide the option of choosing "Unknown" as an answer, this should be avoided as often as possible. Unknown responses eliminate the possibility of the agency measuring the patient's outcome on the question.

Rule 4: The OASIS assessments are not interview questionnaires. The nurse should use his or her assessment and observation skills to identify the answer that most accurately describes the patient's status or function.

Rule 5: The OASIS document is designed to capture the patient's usual status. However, it is not uncommon for a patient's functional abilities to vary from day to day. Therefore, the home health nurse is directed to answer the questions based on the patient's status most of the time on the day the patient assessment is being conducted.

(Centers for Medicare & Medicaid Services [CMS], 2009)

To clarify this point, consider a patient who receives outpatient chemotherapy. The home care nurse visits the patient the day after the treatment, when the patient is most debilitated. While the nurse is conducting the assessment, the patient reports that this will be the worst day of the week, and he is too fatigued and nauseous to participate in any activities of daily living (ADLs), such as showering and dressing. The patient also reports that as the week progresses, he expects he will feel progressively better and be able to get into the shower and dress. He reports that his usual routine is to get dressed every day after his morning shower. Following the instructions in the OASIS user's manual, the nurse must answer the questions based on the patient's status as he presents at the time of the assessment. In this case, the OASIS will reflect the patient's worst condition. If the assessment were conducted later in the week, a more positive presentation would be documented.

START OF CARE/ RESUMPTION OF CARE OASIS DOCUMENT

Any professional nurse who reviews the OASIS assessments provided in the appendices will quickly recognize that the OASIS questions are primarily functional in nature. In no way will the completion of the OASIS items provide the home health team with an adequate clinical picture of the patient. Despite the scope of the OASIS documents, they were never intended to replace the agency's documentation of the patient's clinical and physical status. In fact, they were designed as adjunctive documents to be incorporated into the agency's existing clinical assessments.

Outlined below is a review of each of the OASIS assessments, including points that require special attention from the home health nurse. The SOC OASIS basically collects 13 types of information (see Table 6-2).

Patient History and Diagnoses

There are 13 questions that capture patient data in this section of the assessment, of which 8 describe issues related to an inpatient stay. The remaining 5 questions primarily address the patient's prognosis and risk factors that have potential to impact the patient's ability to maximize his or her outcome. While reviewing OASIS questions, you will notice some instructions directing the nurse to either mark all that apply or skip ahead to other questions. Below, question M1000 exemplifies both of these instructions.

(M1000) From which of the following **Inpatient Facilities** was the patient discharged during the past 14 days? **(Mark all that apply).**

☐   1-   Long-term nursing facility (NF)

☐   2-   Skilled nursing facility (SNF/TCU)

☐   3-   Short-stay acute hospital (IPP S)

☐   4-   Long-term care hospital (LTCH)

TABLE 6-2: OASIS DATA INFORMATION TYPES	
• Demographics	• Elimination status
• Patient history and diagnoses	• Neuro/emotional/behavioral status
• Living arrangements	• ADLs/Instrumental activities of daily living (IADLs)
• Sensory status	• Medications
• Integumentary status	• Care Management
• Respiratory status	• Therapy need and plan of care

☐ 5- Inpatient rehabilitation hospital or unit (IRF)

☐ 6- Psychiatric hospital or unit

☐ 7- Other (specify) _____

☐ NA- Patient was not discharged from an inpatient facility (**If NA, go to M1016**)

If the patient was referred to the agency from a physician's office or a community referral was received, it is likely that the patient did not experience an inpatient facility discharge within the last 14 days. The home health nurse is then instructed to skip all of the questions related to an inpatient facility discharge (M1005, M1010, and M1012) and go ahead to the questions that address a change in the patient's medical condition and plan of treatment, beginning with question M1016.

If the patient was referred as a result of a hospitalization or other inpatient facility, all of the following questions must be answered.

(M1005) Inpatient Discharge Date (most recent):

_____/_____/_____

Month   Day   Year (4 digits)

☐ UK- Unknown

(M1010) List each Inpatient Diagnosis and ICD-9-CM code at the highest specificity for only those conditions treated <u>during an inpatient stay within the last 14 days</u> (no E-codes or V-codes)

<u>Inpatient Facility Diagnoses</u>   <u>ICD-9-CM</u>

a _____ (_ _ _._ _)

b _____ (_ _ _._ _)

(M1012) List each Inpatient Procedure and the associated ICD code categories (three digits required; five digits optional) <u>relevant to the plan of care.</u>

<u>Inpatient Procedure</u>   <u>ICD-9-CM</u>

a _____ (_ _ _._ _)

b _____ (_ _ _._ _)

Procedures that are relevant to the home health plan of care are listed here (for example, cardiac bypass surgery that requires post-operative wound care). Procedures that the patient received during an inpatient stay within the past 14 days can be included.

(M1016) Diagnoses Requiring Medical or Treatment Regimen Change Within Past 14 Days: List the patient's medical diagnoses and ICD-9-CM codes at the level of highest specificity for those conditions <u>requiring changed medical or treatment regimens</u> within the past 14 days (no surgical, E-codes or V-codes):

<u>Changed Medical Regimen Diagnosis</u> <u>ICD-9-CM</u>

a _____ (_ _ _._ _)

b _____ (_ _ _._ _)

c _____ (_ _ _._ _)

d _____ (_ _ _._ _)

e _____ (_ _ _._ _)

f _____ (_ _ _._ _)

☐ NA- Not applicable (no medical or treatment changes within the past 14 days)

The nurse must determine whether the patient experienced a change in the medical or treatment regimen within the past 14 days. Changes in a medical or treatment regimen might include something as simple as a new medication, or a change that is more complex such as the insertion of an indwelling urinary catheter for urinary retention. If the patient did not experience a change in medical regimen or an inpatient stay in the past 14 days, the nurse should mark option NA- and move on to question **M1018.**

(M1018) Conditions Prior to Medical or Treatment Regimen Change or Inpatient Stay Within Past 14 Days: If this patient experienced an inpatient facility discharge or a change in medical or treatment regimen within the past 14 days, indicate any conditions which existed prior to the inpatient stay or change in medical or treatment regimen. (Mark all that apply.)

- ☐   1-   Urinary Incontinence
- ☐   2-   Indwelling/suprapubic catheter
- ☐   3-   Intractable pain
- ☐   4-   Impaired decision-making
- ☐   5-   Disruptive or socially inappropriate behavior
- ☐   6-   Memory loss to the extent that supervision required
- ☐   7-   None of the above
- ☐   NA-   No inpatient facility discharge and no change in medical or treatment regimen in past 14 days
- ☐   UK-   Unknown

As mentioned earlier, some of the questions on the OASIS are very simple and straightforward, and others are more complex and require the nurse to pay close attention to the details that differentiate one category from the next. M1020 and M1022 are relatively complex and require the use of standardized definitions to classify the degree of symptom control for each diagnosis. Outlined below (following the M1020/1022/1024 instructions) are the definitions to facilitate rating in a consistent manner. The nurse must use these five definitions for all questions that require a symptom control rating. To simplify this section, only part of the M1020/1022/1024 OASIS-C chart is included below; refer to Appendix B for this chart in its entirety. Proper coding is essential to appropriate reimbursement under PPS. Most agencies employ individuals who are specifically trained in coding.

(M1020/1022/1024) Diagnoses, Symptom Control, and Payment Diagnoses: List each diagnosis for which the patient is receiving home care and enter the ICD-9-CM code at the level of highest specificity (no surgical/procedure codes). Diagnoses are listed in the order that best reflect the seriousness of each condition and that support the home care disciplines and services provided. Rate the degree of symptom control for each condition. Choose one value that represents the degree of symptom control appropriate for each diagnosis: V-codes (for M1020 or M1022) or E-codes (for M1022 only) may be used. ICD-9-CM sequencing requirements must be followed if multiple coding is indicated for any diagnoses. If a V-code is reported in place of a case mix diagnosis, then optional item M1024 Payment Diagnoses may be completed. A case mix diagnosis is a diagnosis that determines the Medicare PPS case mix group. Do not assign symptom control ratings for V- or E-codes.

0-   Asymptomatic, no treatment needed at this time

1-   Symptoms well controlled with current therapy

2-   Symptoms controlled with difficulty, affecting daily functioning; patient needs ongoing monitoring

3-   Symptoms poorly controlled, patient needs frequent adjustment in treatment and dose monitoring

4-   Symptoms poorly controlled, history of rehospitalizations

Using the guidance above, the home health nurse must identify the patient's home care diagnoses and rate the severity in questions M1020 and M1022.

(M1020) Primary Diagnosis	ICD-9-CM	Severity Rating
a _____	(_ _ _._ _)	□0 □1 □2 □3 □4

(M1022) Other Diagnosis	ICD-9-CM	Severity Rating
a _____	(_ _ _._ _)	□0 □1 □2 □3 □4
b _____	(_ _ _._ _)	□0 □1 □2 □3 □4
c _____	(_ _ _._ _)	□0 □1 □2 □3 □4
d _____	(_ _ _._ _)	□0 □1 □2 □3 □4
e _____	(_ _ _._ _)	□0 □1 □2 □3 □4
f _____	(_ _ _._ _)	□0 □1 □2 □3 □4

A case mix diagnosis is defined as a diagnosis that results in a patient score essential to determine the proper home health reimbursement. The CMS specifically defines secondary diagnoses as "all conditions that coexisted at the time the plan of care was established, or which developed subsequently, or affect the treatment of care (CMS, 2009). Due to the demographics of Medicare patients, it is likely that they will have several diagnoses for comorbid conditions. The CMS instructs the clinician to include conditions that are actively being addressed in the current plan of care or might be limiting the patient's responsiveness to treatment, but to also include any comorbidity affecting the patient's responsiveness to treatment and rehabilitative prognosis, even if the condition is not the focus of any home health treatment itself. For example, for a patient who requires wound care, his history of diabetes should be included. Although his blood glucose levels are stable, he is adherent to diet and activity, and the plan of care does not require a focus on diabetic education, diabetes may slow healing and should be listed in M1020/M1022.

(M1024) Payment Diagnoses (Optional): If a V code (e.g. surgical aftercare) is reported in M1022 in place of a case mix diagnosis that requires multiple diagnosis codes under ICD-9-CM coding guidelines, enter the diagnosis descriptions and the ICD-9-CM codes in the same row in Columns 3 and 4.

(M1024) Primary Diagnosis	ICD-9-CM
a _____	(_ _ _._ _)
(M1024) First Secondary Diagnosis	ICD-9-CM
b _____	(_ _ _._ _)

As part of the patient's medical plan of treatment, M1030 requires the nurse to indicate which nutrition and intravenous therapies a patient receives at home.

(M1030) Therapies the patient receives at home:
(Mark all that apply)

□   1-   Intravenous or infusion therapy (excludes TPN)

□   2-   Parenteral nutrition (TPN or lipids)

□   3-   Enteral nutrition (nasogastric, gastrostomy, jejunostomy, or any other artificial entry into the alimentary canal)

□   4-   None of the above

(M1030 Pointers)

- Response 1 should be selected even if the therapies are not administered by the home care nurse.

- Response 4 should be selected if the therapy is provided in an outpatient clinic.

- Response 4 should be selected if the therapy is for the treatment of a specific symptom that is not being treated on the day of the visit (i.e., if the patient has weight gain of more than 5 lbs, the family is to give intravenous fursomide).

• Flushing or using a nasogastric, gastrostomy, or jejunostomy tube solely for the administration of medications does not qualify as nutrition.

(M1032) Risk for Hospitalization: Which of the following signs or symptoms characterize this patient as at risk for hospitalization? (Mark all that apply)

☐   1-   Recent decline in mental, emotional, or behavioral status

☐   2-   Multiple hospitalizations (2 or more) in the past 12 months

☐   3-   History of falls (2 or more falls – or any fall with an injury – in the past year)

☐   4-   Taking five or more medications

☐   5-   Frailty indicators, e.g., weight loss, self-reported exhaustion

☐   6-   Other

☐   7-   None of the above

(M1034) Overall status: Which description best fits the patient's overall status? (Check one)

☐   0-   The patient is stable with no heightened risk(s) for serious complications and death (beyond those typical of the patient's age).

☐   1-   The patient is temporarily facing high health risk(s) but is likely to return to being stable without heightened risk(s) for serious complications and death (beyond those typical of the patient's age).

☐   2-   The patient is likely to remain in fragile health and have ongoing high risk(s) of serious complications and death.

☐   3-   The patient has serious progressive conditions that could lead to death within a year.

☐   UK-   The patient's situation is unknown or unclear.

(M1032 and M1034 Pointers)

These two questions – M1032 and M1034 – include both objective and subjective factors that must be answered based on the nurse's judgment. Reducing potentially avoidable hospitalizations for home care patients is of major concern to CMS. These items identify patients who are more frail or who have factors that place them at increased risk for hospitalizations, and should give the nurse direction in developing a plan of care and interventions to mitigate that risk. These items will be used in risk adjustment (addressed in Chapter 7).

(M1036) Risk Factors, either present or past, likely to affect current health status and/or outcome **(Mark all that apply.)**

☐   1-   Smoking

☐   2-   Obesity

☐   3-   Alcohol dependency

☐   4-   Drug dependency

☐   5-   None of the above

☐   UK-   Unknown

The OASIS User Manual suggests use of Body Mass Index guidelines for determining obesity. Amount and length of exposure to smoking, drugs or alcohol should be considered when answering this question. The intent is to identify factors that exert a substantial impact on the patient's health, response to treatment, and ability to recover from illnesses.

Living Arrangements

This section of the OASIS includes one question that requires the home health nurse to assess the patient's current living arrangements and the supportive assistance available to the patient.

(M1100) Patient Living Situation: Which of the following best describes the patient's residential circumstance and availability of assistance? (**Check one box only**)

Living Arrangement	*Availability of Assistance*				
	Around the clock	Regular daytime	Regular nighttime	Occasional/ Short-term	No assistance available
a) Patient lives alone	☐ 01	☐ 02	☐ 03	☐ 04	☐ 05
b) Patient lives with other person(s) in the home	☐ 06	☐ 07	☐ 08	☐ 09	☐ 10
c) Patient lives in congregate situation (e.g., assisted living)	☐ 11	☐ 12	☐ 13	☐ 14	☐ 15

(M1100 Pointers)

- Identify the frequency with which <u>in-person physical assistance</u> is provided; this includes assistance with ADLs and instrumental activities of daily living (IADLs), such as meal preparation and medication management.

- Use judgment in terms of ability/willingness of person to provide assistance if needed (cognitive, physical, emotional ability, availability).

- Paid help provided on an intermittent basis (a few hours a day, a few days per week) is not considered help that lives with the patient.

Sensory Status

The patient's ability to see, hear, experience pain, understand spoken language, and verbally express himself or herself are captured in the next set of questions as outlined below.

(M1200) Vision (with corrective lenses if the patient usually wears them)

☐   0-   Normal vision: sees adequately in most situations; can see medication labels, newsprint.

☐   1-   Partially impaired: cannot see medication labels or newsprint, but can see obstacles in path and the surrounding layout, can count fingers at arm's length.

☐   2-   Severely impaired: cannot locate objects without hearing or touching them or patient nonresponsive.

(M1200 Pointers)

- The patient's ability to read or understand written language should not be considered.

- A magnifying glass is not an example of a corrective lens.

- Nonprescription reading glasses (i.e., those bought at the local store) are considered corrective lenses.

(M1210) Ability to Hear (with hearing aids if the patient usually uses them):

☐   0-   Adequate: hears normal conversation without difficulty.

☐ 1- Mildly to moderately impaired: difficulty hearing in some environments or speaker may need to increase volume or speak distinctly.

☐ 2- Severely impaired: absence of useful hearing.

☐ UK- Unable to assess hearing.

(M1220) Understanding of Verbal Content (in patient's own language)

☐ 0- Understands: clear comprehension without cues or repetitions

☐ 1- Usually understands: understands most conversations, but misses some part/intent of message. Requires cues at times to understand.

☐ 2- Sometimes understands: understands only basic conversations or simple, direct phrases. Frequently requires cues to understand.

☐ 3- Rarely/Never understands

☐ UK- Unable to assess understanding

(M1230) Speech and Oral (Verbal) Expression of Language (in patient's own language)

☐ 0- Expresses complex ideas, feelings, and needs clearly, completely, and easily in all situations with no observable impairment.

☐ 1- Minimal difficulty in expressing ideas and needs (may take extra time; makes occasional errors in word choice, grammar or speech intelligibility; needs minimal prompting or assistance).

☐ 2- Expresses simple ideas or needs with moderate difficulty (needs prompting or assistance, errors in word choice, grammar organization or speech intelligibility). Speaks in phrases or short sentences.

☐ 3- Has severe difficulty expressing basic ideas or needs, and requires maximal assistance or guessing by listener. Speech is limited to single words or short phrases.

☐ 4- Unable to express basic needs even with maximal prompting or assistance but is not comatose or unresponsive (e.g., speech is nonsensical or unintelligible).

☐ 5- Patient nonresponsive or unable to speak.

(M1230 Pointers)

• Augmented speaking devices are considered verbal expression of language and should be considered when evaluating a patient's speech and verbal expression of language.

• For patients whose only means of communication is sign language, option 5 must be selected because the patient is not able to speak.

(M1240) Has this patient had a formal **Pain Assessment** using a standardized pain assessment tool (appropriate to the patient's ability to communicate the severity of pain)?

☐ 0- No standardized assessment conducted

☐ 1- Yes, and it does not indicate severe pain

☐ 2- Yes, and it indicates severe pain

• This item is one of the new process measures added to the OASIS-C version implemented in 2010. A standardized tool is defined by CMS (2009) as one that includes a standard response scale (e.g., 0-10 scale). The tool must be administered according to the tool's instructions. Severe pain would be defined according to the tool's scoring system.

(M1242) Frequency of Pain interfering with patient's activity or movement

- [ ] 0- Patient has no pain
- [ ] 1- Patient has pain that does not interfere with activity or movement
- [ ] 2- Less often than daily
- [ ] 3- Daily, but not constantly
- [ ] 4- All of the time

(M1242 Pointers)

- An accurate assessment of M1242 requires the nurse to integrate the patient's verbal response and nonverbal behavior as specifically determining what the patient might otherwise do if he or she did not have any pain. Would the patient walk to the mailbox every afternoon, attend church, go to the market, or sleep in the upstairs bedroom instead of on the living room sofa?

Item M1242 creates some confusion when nurses attempt to answer it. Some nurses report difficulty answering for patients who take medication to manage their pain. If a patient has daily pain but is able to control it with medication so that it does not interfere with activity or movement, how should this question be answered? Option 0 states the patient has no pain and Option 1 states that pain does not interfere with activity or movement. Once the patient takes medication, is option 0 the correct option for the patient? If the patient does not take his or her medications, option 1, 2, or 3 might be more appropriate. When answering this question, home health nurses might seek the assistance of a manager or the agency's OASIS coordinator to ensure that this question is interpreted in accordance with agency and OASIS policy.

Integumentary Status

With a few exceptions, the majority of the questions to this point have been relatively simply stated and easy to answer. The 16 questions that comprise the integumentary status portion of the OASIS assessment include questions that are detailed and more complex.

A review of questions M1300 to M1350 illustrates that, to complete an OASIS accurately, the home health nurse must be knowledgeable about the accepted definitions and descriptions of wounds and wound-related issues. The home health nurse has to learn to describe the status of wounds very rigidly. For example, these questions require the home health nurse to accurately differentiate between a pressure ulcer and a stasis ulcer.

(M1300) Pressure Ulcer Risk Assessment: Was this patient assessed for Risk of Developing Pressure Ulcers?

- [ ] 0- No assessment conducted (**Go to M1306**)
- [ ] 1- Yes, based on an evaluation of clinical factors, e.g. mobility, incontinence, nutrition, etc., without use of standardized tool
- [ ] 2- Yes, using a standardized tool, e.g., Braden, Norton, other

---

(M1302) Does this patient have a **Risk of Developing Pressure Ulcers?**

- [ ] 0- No
- [ ] 1- Yes

(M1300, M1302 Pointers)

- M1300 is another process measure
- A standardized tool is one that has been scientifically tested, includes a standard response scale, and has been evaluated with a population similar to the patient the nurse is assessing.

If a standardized tool was used in M1300, use the scoring parameters for the tool to answer M1302; if clinical factors were used to evaluate risk, the home care agency may define what comprises risk. Patients at greatest risk for developing pressure ulcers include those with limited mobility or patients who experience bowel or bladder incontinence. Patients with inadequate nutrition or sensory-perceptual deficits might also be at risk for developing pressure ulcers.

(M1306) Does this patient have at least one **Unhealed Pressure Ulcer at Stage II or Higher** or Designated as "Unstageable"?

☐   0-   No **(If No, go to M1322)**

☐   1-   Yes

(M1306 Pointers)

Stage III and IV pressure ulcers are not to be reverse-staged. That is, once a pressure ulcer is staged as a III or IV, it will always remain at that stage even once it is completely closed. However, according to an update announced by the National Pressure Ulcer Advisory Panel (NPUAP) in 2004, stage I and II pressure ulcers (partial thickness) can heal through the process of regeneration of epidermis across the wound surface which is also called epithelialization (Wound Ostomy and Continence Nurses Society, 2009).

The CMS has worked closely with the WOCN to provide home care nurses with a consistent set of guidelines for answering these questions. This document, which should be used as a foundational OASIS resource, can be found in Appendix F and is also available at http://www.wocn.org/pdfs/GuidanceOASIS-C.pdf.

Additionally:

- Debrided pressure ulcers remain pressure ulcers; they do not change to surgical wounds.

- Pressure ulcers closed with a muscle flap or skin graft are considered surgical wounds.

- A muscle flap or skin graft that fails as a result of pressure is considered a pressure ulcer.

Although most clinicians can readily identify the presence of a pressure ulcer, some difficulty might arise when answering M1306 and the following item M1308, which require the nurse to differentiate between the stages of the pressure ulcer(s). When responding to M1306 and M1308, it is important to read the detailed description of each stage and answer the questions as accurately as possible.

Note that this item appears in the Follow-Up (FU) and Transfer OASIS-C tools as discussed later in this chapter. This item contributes to an outcome measure that will make it evident if new pressure ulcers are occurring after the start of home care. It is clearly important to identify those patients at risk for developing pressure ulcers and developing a plan of care to reduce that risk. Plan of care interventions are captured later in the OASIS-C.

(M1308) Current Number of Unhealed (non-epithelialized) Pressure Ulcers at Each Stage: (Enter "0" if none; excludes Stage I pressure ulcers)

	Column 1 Complete at SOC/ROC/FU & D/C	Column 2 Complete at FU & D/C
Stage description – unhealed pressure ulcers	Number currently present	Number of those listed in Column 1 that were present on admission (most recent SOC/ROC)
a. Stage II: Partial thickness loss of dermis presenting as a shallow open ulcer with red pink wound bed, without slough. May also present as an intact or open/ruptured serum filled blister		
b. Stage III: Full thickness tissue loss. Subcutaneous fat may be visible but bone, tendon, or muscles are not exposed. Slough may be present but does not obscure the depth of tissue loss. May include undermining and tunneling.		
c. Stage IV: Full thickness tissue loss with visible bone, tendon, or muscle. Slough or eschar may be present on some parts of the wound bed. Often includes undermining and tunneling		
d.1. Unstageable: known or likely but not stageable due to non-removeable dressing or device		
d.2. Unstageable: known or likely but not stageable due to coverage of wound bed by slough and/or eschar		
d.3. Unstageable: Suspected deep tissue injury in evolution		

Directions for M1310, M1312, and M1314:
If the patient has one or more unhealed (non-epithelialized) Stage III or IV pressure ulcers, identify the Stage III or IV pressure ulcer with the largest surface dimension (length X width) and record in centimeters (cm). If no Stage III or Stage IV pressure ulcers, go to M1320.

(M1310) Pressure Ulcer Length: Longest length "head-to-toe"

__ __ . __ (cm)

(M1312) Pressure Ulcer Width: Width of the same pressure ulcer; greatest width perpendicular to the length

__ __ . __ (cm)

(M1314) Pressure Ulcer Depth: Depth of the same pressure ulcer; from visible surface to the deepest area

__ __ . __ (cm)

(M1310, M1312, M1314 Pointers)

- To determine the pressure ulcer with the largest surface dimension, the nurse must measure <u>every</u> existing non-epithelialized Stage III and IV pressure ulcer or unstageable pressure ulcer due to presence of slough/eschar.

- <u>Depth is not considered</u> in determining the largest ulcer.

- If all Stage III or IV pressure ulcers are either closed (completely re-epithelialized) or unstageable (because they can't be visualized due to dressings/casts), enter 00.0.

- Depth for a wound covered/filled with eschar can be entered as 00.0.

In addition to staging pressure ulcers and determining the ulcer with the largest surface dimension, the clinician must also identify which pressure ulcer is most problematic, both in status of wound healing (M1320) and by assignment of the stage (M1324). For instance, a patient may have more than one pressure ulcer at two different stages of healing. More specifically, the patient may have a Stage IV ulcer that demonstrates active and progressive healing in addition to a Stage III ulcer that is infected and filled with slough. Although a Stage IV ulcer results in more tissue destruction, it is less problematic than the infected Stage III ulcer. Therefore, it is important to pay close attention when answering M1320.

Refer to Appendix F for definitions related to the status of pressure ulcers.

(M1320) Status of Most Problematic (Observable) Pressure Ulcer:

☐   0-   Newly epithelialized

☐   1-   Fully granulating

☐   2-   Early/partial granulation

☐   3-   Not healing

☐   NA-   No observable pressure ulcer

(M1320 Pointers)

- An infected pressure ulcer at any stage is considered not healing.

- A pressure ulcer covered by eschar that can not be staged is classified as early/partial granulation (option 2) if necrotic or avascular tissue covers < 25% of the wound bed. If the wound has > 25% necrotic or avascular tissue, it is classified as non-healing (option 3) in M1320 in accordance with the WOCN guidelines (Appendix F).

- A pressure ulcer that is completely healed is option 0 (Newly epithelialized).

(M1322) Current Number of Stage I Pressure Ulcers: Intact skin with non-blanchable redness of a localized area usually over a bony prominence. The area may be painful, firm, soft, warmer or cooler as compared to adjacent tissue.

☐   0

☐   1

☐   2

☐   3

☐   4 or more

(M1324) Stage of Most Problematic Unhealed (Observable) Pressure Ulcer:

☐   1-   Stage I

☐   2-   Stage II

☐   3-   Stage III

☐   4-   Stage IV

☐   NA–   No observable pressure ulcer or unhealed pressure ulcer

For the purposes of responding to M1330, the clinician must determine the etiology of the wound. Stasis ulcers are typically located on the lower extremities and are the result of inadequate venous circulation. The development of stasis ulcers is often associated with stasis dermatitis. If the ulcer is arterial in nature or classified as a diabetic ulcer, M1330 should be marked option 0 (No).

The WOCN has produced a "Clinical Facts Sheet" that is intended to assist the home health nurse to differentiate between wounds (see Appendix G). However, if the etiology of the wound still cannot be ascertained from this reference, the referral documentation, or the nurse's assessment, OASIS guidelines direct the nurse to contact the physician for clarification (CMS, 2009, p. F-15).

(M1330) Does this patient have a Stasis Ulcer?

☐   0-   No **(Go to M1340)**

☐   1-   Yes, patient has BOTH observable and unobservable stasis ulcers

☐   2-   Yes, patient has observable stasis ulcers ONLY

☐   3-   Yes, patient has unobservable stasis ulcers ONLY (known but not observable due to non-removable dressing) **(Go to M1340)**

(M1332) Current Number of (Observable) Stasis Ulcer(s):

☐   1-   One

☐   2-   Two

☐   3-   Three

☐   4-   Four or more

(M1334) Status of Most Problematic (Observable) Stasis Ulcer:

☐   0-   Newly epithelialized

☐   1-   Fully granulating

☐   2-   Early/partial granulation

☐   3-   Not healing

In addition to documenting the presence of pressure and stasis ulcers, the home health nurse must also identify the status of any surgical wounds.

(M1340) Does this patient have a Surgical Wound?

☐   0-   No **(Go to M1350)**

☐   1-   Yes, patient has at least one (observable) surgical wound

☐   2-   Surgical wound known but not observable due to non-removable dressing **(Go to M1350)**

(M1340 Pointers)

•   For the purposes of OASIS, stapled or sutured incisions, orthopedic pin sites, central lines (except peripherally inserted central catheters), implanted infusion devices, and venous access devices are surgical wounds.

- Specific exclusions from this question are listed below. These may be reported in M1350 if they are receiving clinical assessment or intervention from the home care nurse.

  – suprapubic tube (cyctostomy)

  – ileal conduit (ileostomy)

  – PEG tube (gastrostomy)

  – cataracts

  – gynecological surgeries via a vaginal approach.

(M1342) Status of Most Problematic (Observable) Surgical Wound:

☐   0-   Newly epithelialized

☐   1-   Fully granulating

☐   2-   Early/partial granulation

☐   3-   Not healing

M1342 describes the stages of an actively healing surgical wound. A surgical wound that has completely healed, thus becoming a scar, is no longer identified as a surgical wound. For the purposes of OASIS documentation, a surgical site closed via primary intention (e.g. sutures, staples), is described as a surgical wound until re-epithelialization has been present for approximately 30 days (CMS, 2009, F-18). After that time period, it is considered a scar.

(M1350) Does this patient have a **Skin Lesion** or **Open Wound,** excluding bowel ostomy, other than those described above, that is receiving intervention by the home health agency?

☐   0-   No

☐   1-   Yes

(M1350 Pointers)

- Lesions are areas of pathologically altered tissue such as sores, skin tears, burns, rashes – anything except bowel ostomies

- The nurse should only consider lesions/wounds that are receiving clinical intervention from the

agency, such as a skin condition that is being clinically assessed on a regular basis

- PICC and peripheral IV sites are considered skin lesions/open wounds

- Ostomies (except bowel) are considered skin lesions/open wounds if clinical interventions (e.g. cleansing/dressing changes) are being provided

- Does not include cataract surgery, surgery to mucosal membranes, or gynecological surgical procedures via vaginal approach

Respiratory Status

The next two questions on the SOC OASIS direct the nurse to assess the patient's respiratory status.

(M1400) When is the patient dyspneic or noticeably **Short of Breath?**

☐   0-   Never, patient is not short of breath

☐   1-   When walking more than 20 feet, climbing stairs

☐   2-   With moderate exertion (e.g., while dressing, using commode or bedpan, walking distances less than 20 feet)

☐   3-   With minimal exertion (e.g., while eating, talking, or performing other ADLs) or with agitation

☐   4-   At rest (during day or night)

(M1400 Pointers)

- To assess the activity level of a chairfast patient that causes shortness of breath, assess the patient while he or she is performing ADLs.

- Since the chairfast patient cannot demonstrate the ability to ambulate 20 feet or climb stairs, the CMS has directed that the chairfast patient can be assessed when transferring or conducting demanding bed mobility activities (repositioning, rolling, or moving to the top of the bed).

(CMS, 2009, p. G-1)

Although the first question, M1400, does not direct the nurse how to answer if the patient utilizes oxygen, the *OASIS User Manual* does. The nurse must determine whether the patient uses oxygen, and if he or she does, the nurse must then identify whether the patient uses it intermittently or continuously.

If the patient uses oxygen intermittently, the nurse should answer M1400 after assessing the patient with the oxygen off. If the patient uses oxygen on a continuous basis, the nurse should assess the patient with the oxygen on (CMS, 2009, p. G-1).

(M1410) Respiratory Treatments utilized at home. **(Mark all that apply.)**

☐	1-	Oxygen (intermittent or continuous)
☐	2-	Ventilator (continually or at night)
☐	3-	Continuous/Bi-level positive airway pressure
☐	4-	None of the above

Elimination Status

The OASIS contains five questions intended to assess the patient's bowel and bladder function. These questions, M1600 through M1630, are relatively straightforward and require simple answers.

(M1600) Has this patient been treated for a **Urinary Tract Infection** in the past 14 days?

☐	0-	No
☐	1-	Yes
☐	NA-	Patient on prophylactic treatment
☐	UK-	Unknown

(M1610) Urinary Incontinence or Urinary Catheter Presence:

☐	0-	No incontinence or catheter (includes anuria or ostomy for urinary drainage) **(If No, go to M1620)**

☐	1-	Patient is incontinent
☐	2-	Patient requires a urinary catheter (i.e., external, indwelling, intermittent, suprapubic) **(Go to M1620)**

(M1610 Pointers)

• If the patient experiences stress incontinence only occasionally (such as when performing activities) the correct response is option 1, the patient is incontinent.

(M1615) When does **Urinary Incontinence** occur?

☐	0-	Timed-voiding defers incontinence
☐	1-	Occasional stress incontinence
☐	2-	During the night only
☐	3-	During the day only
☐	4-	During the day and night

(M1620) Bowel Incontinence Frequency:

☐	0-	Very rarely or never has bowel incontinence
☐	1-	Less than once weekly
☐	2-	One to three times weekly
☐	3-	Four to six times weekly
☐	4-	On a daily basis
☐	5-	More often than once daily
☐	NA-	Patient has ostomy for bowel elimination
☐	UK-	Unknown

(M1630) Ostomy for Bowel Elimination: Does this patient have an ostomy for bowel elimination that (within the last 14 days): a) was related to an inpatient facility stay, or b) necessitated a change in medical or treatment regimen?

☐	0-	Patient does not have an ostomy for bowel elimination.

☐   1-   Patient's ostomy was not related to an inpatient stay and did not necessitate change in medical or treatment regimen.

☐   2-   The ostomy was related to an inpatient stay or did necessitate change in medical or treatment regimen.

Neuro/Emotional/Behavioral Status

This section of the assessment is detailed and intended to uncover difficulties that might inhibit the patient from achieving an optimal level of function. This is the only section of the assessment that directs the nurse to answer questions based on what is "reported or observed" during the assessment process. The OASIS User Manual does not provide the nurse with any guidance about how to answer these questions if a conflict arises between the perceptions of the nurse and the behaviors reported by the patient or caregiver.

In the following questions, many of the responses are detailed and characterized by subtle variations. Ideally, when answering these questions, the nurse should read each of the options and pay careful attention to the subtle differences of each. Answering requires the nurse to use professional judgment to choose the option that best describes what he or she has observed. If there is inconsistency between the nurse, patient, or caregiver, the nurse should be sure to make a notation that describes the inconsistent views or conflicts in the patient's medical record.

(M1700) Cognitive Functioning: Patient's current (day of assessment) level of alertness, orientation, comprehension, concentration, and immediate memory for simple commands.

☐   0-   Alert/oriented, able to focus and shift attention, comprehends and recalls task directions independently.

☐   1-   Requires prompting (cueing, repetition, reminders) only under stressful or unfamiliar conditions.

☐   2-   Requires assistance and some direction in specific situations (e.g., on all tasks involving shifting of attention), or consistently requires low stimulus environment due to distractibility.

☐   3-   Requires considerable assistance in routine situations. Is not alert and oriented or is unable to shift attention and recall directions more than half of the time.

☐   4-   Totally dependent due to disturbances such as constant disorientation, coma, persistent vegetative state, or delirium.

(M1710) When Confused (Reported or Observed Within the Last 14 days):

☐   0-   Never

☐   1-   In new or complex situations only

☐   2-   On awakening or at night only

☐   3-   During the day and evening, but not constantly

☐   4-   Constantly

☐   NA-   Patient nonresponsive

(M1720) When Anxious (Reported or Observed Within the Last 14 Days):

☐   0-   None of the time

☐   1-   Less often than daily

☐   2-   Daily, but not constantly

☐   3-   All of the time

☐   NA-   Patient nonresponsive

(M1700, M1710, & M1720 Pointers)

- When considering the appropriate response for the patient, consider these questions all together. For instance if the patient's cognitive function in M1700 is assessed as other than option 0, alert and oriented, it would seem reasonable that this patient would have some level of confusion in new or complex situations, as questioned in M1710. Assuming both of the above statements are true, it would also seem reasonable that the patient would experience some level of anxiety, as questioned in M1720.

Depression is a prevalent condition affecting many home care patients and while it may not be a primary psychiatric diagnosis, it is a complicating factor for many common diagnoses affecting home care patients. Depression is associated with chronic illnesses or conditions such as heart failure, COPD, diabetes, and urinary incontinence and often results in poorer self-care management. For these reasons, screening for depression is one of the new 2010 OASIS-C measures.

(M1730) Depression Screening: Has the patient been screened for depression, using a standardized depression screening tool?

☐   0-   No

☐   1-   Yes, patient was screened using the PHQ-2©* scale. (Instructions for this two-question tool: Ask the patient: "Over the last two weeks, how often have you been bothered by any of the following problems")

PHQ-2©	Not at all 0-1 day	Several days 2-6 days	More than half of the days 7-11 days	Nearly every day 12-14 days	N/A Unable to respond
a) Little interest or pleasure in doing things	0	1	2	3	na
b) Feeling down, depressed, or hopeless?	0	1	2	3	na

*Copyright © Pfizer Inc. All rights reserved. Reproduced with permission.

☐   2-   Yes, with a different standardized assessment – and the patient meets the criteria for further evaluation for depression.

☐   3-   Yes, patient was screened with a different standardized assessment – and the patient does not meet the criteria for further evaluation for depression

(M1730 Pointers)

- While CMS does not require that depression screening be conducted, M1730 is a process item that will be used to measure home care agency best practices.
- A PHQ-2 score of 3 should trigger further evaluation such as notification of the physician and patient education.

(M1740) Cognitive, behavioral, and psychiatric symptoms that are demonstrated at least once a week **(Reported or Observed): (Mark all that apply.)**

☐ 1- Memory deficit: failure to recognize familiar persons/places, inability to recall events of past 24 hours, significant memory loss so that supervision is required

☐ 2- Impaired decision-making, failure to perform usual ADLs or IADLs, inability to appropriately stop activities, jeopardizes safety through actions

☐ 3- Verbal disruption: yelling, threatening, excessive profanity, sexual references, etc.

☐ 4- Physical aggression: aggressive or combative to self and others (e.g. hits self, throws objects, punches, dangerous maneuvers with wheelchair or other objects)

☐ 5- Disruptive, infantile, or socially inappropriate behaviors (excludes verbal actions)

☐ 6- Delusional, hallucinatory, or paranoid behavior

☐ 7- None of the above behaviors demonstrated

(M1745) Frequency of Disruptive Behavior Symptoms (Reported or Observed) Any physical, verbal, or other disruptive/dangerous symptoms that are injurious to self or others or jeopardize personal safety.

☐ 0- Never
☐ 1- Less than once a month
☐ 2- Once a month
☐ 3- Several times each month
☐ 4- Several times a week
☐ 5- At least daily

(M1750) Is this patient receiving **Psychiatric Nursing Services** at home provided by a qualified psychiatric nurse?

☐ 0- No
☐ 1- Yes

Activities of Daily Living and Instrumental Activities of Daily Living

The SOC OASIS assessment includes 13 questions that require the nurse to evaluate the patient's mental and physical ability to safely perform Activities of Daily Living (ADLs) and Instrumental Activities of Daily Living (IADLs). The guidelines provided in the *OASIS User Manual* instruct the home health nurse to differentiate between the patient's ability, **not** willingness, to perform ADLs and IADLs. To highlight the difference between ability and willingness, consider the following patient scenarios.

Mrs. Leger is a 68-year-old woman who tells the home health nurse that she has never taken a shower. She tells the nurse that she grew up only taking sponge baths and prefers not to get into the tub or shower. Does this mean she is unable?

Mr. Shoesmith is an elderly gentleman who has been recently widowed after being married all of his adult life. He reports to the nurse that he could not possibly perform grocery shopping because his wife had always performed this chore. Does that mean he is unable?

The OASIS regulations recognize that a patient may experience variation in ability on a day-to-day basis and instructs the nurse to "choose the response describing the ability more than 50 percent of the time" (CMS, 2009, p. K-1).

M1800 through M1890 require the clinician to consider what the patient is able to safely perform on the day of the assessment. If that patient's ability varies on that day, respond to these questions based on the patient's ability at least 51% (more than 12 hours) of the day.

(M1800) Grooming: Current ability to tend safely to personal hygiene needs (i.e., washing face and hands, hair care, shaving or make up, teeth or denture care, fingernail care).

☐ 0- Able to groom self unaided, with or without the use of assistive devices or adapted methods.

☐ 1- Grooming utensils must be placed within reach before able to complete grooming activities.

☐ 2- Someone must assist the patient to groom self.

☐ 3- Patient depends entirely upon someone else for grooming needs.

(M1810) Current **Ability to Dress Upper Body Safely** (with or without dressing aids) including undergarments, pullovers, front opening shirts and blouses, managing zippers, buttons and snaps.

☐ 0- Able to obtain clothes out of closets and drawers, put them on, and remove them from the upper body without assistance.

☐ 1- Able to dress upper body without assistance if clothing is laid out or handed to the patient.

☐ 2- Someone must help the patient put on upper body clothing.

☐ 3- Patient depends entirely upon another person to dress the upper body.

(M1820) Current Ability to Dress Lower Body Safely (with or without dressing aids) including undergarments, slacks, socks or nylons and shoes.

☐ 0- Able to obtain, put on, and remove clothing and shoes without assistance.

☐ 1- Able to dress lower body without assistance if clothing and shoes are laid out or handed to the patient.

☐ 2- Someone must help the patient put on undergarments, slacks, socks or nylons and shoes.

☐ 3- Patient depends entirely upon another person to dress the lower body.

(M1810 & M1820 Pointers)

• If the patient has to dress in stages but without any assistance, mark option 1.

• If the dressing occurs in stages because verbal cues or assistance is needed, option 1 or 2 would be appropriate, depending on the level of assistance.

• If the patient is wearing clothing that is not his or her customary manner of dress (e.g., pajamas, housecoat, or sweat pants) because they have difficulty managing buttons, hooks, or zippers, the nurse should assess the patient's ability to dress related to clothing that they wound have routinely worn.

(M1830) Bathing: Current ability to wash entire body safely. **Excludes grooming** (washing face and hands only).

☐ 0- Able to bathe self in shower or tub independently, including getting in and out of tub/shower.

☐ 1- With the use of devices, is able to bathe self in shower or tub independently, including getting in and out of tub/shower.

☐ 2- Able to bathe in shower or tub with the intermittent assistance of another person:

  (a) For intermittent supervision or encouragement or reminders, OR

(b) To get in and out of the shower or tub, OR

(c) For washing difficult to reach areas.

☐ 3- Able to participate in bathing self in shower or tub, but requires presence of another person throughout the bath for assistance or supervision.

☐ 4- Unable to use the shower or tub, but able to bathe self independently with or without use of devices at the sink, in chair, or on commode.

☐ 5- Unable to use the shower or tub, but able to participate in bathing self in bed, at the sink, in bedside chair, or on commode with the assistance of another person throughout the bath.

☐ 6- Unable to participate in effectively bathing and is totally bathed by another person.

(M1830 Pointers)

• If the patient's shower or tub is nonfunctioning, option 4 or 5 would apply.

• If the patient is medically restricted from bathing in the shower or tub, option 4 or 5 would apply.

• If the patient is afraid to shower or get in the tub, option 4 or 5 would apply.

• If the patient chooses not to use the shower or tub, the nurse should use skilled assessment of the patient's ability to perform other activities, such as transferring or ambulating, to answer this question. The clinician must differentiate between the patient's choice and ability.

(M1840) Toilet Transferring: Current ability to get to and from the toilet or bedside commode safely and transfer on and off toilet/commode.

☐ 0- Able to get to and from the toilet and transfer independently with or without a device.

☐ 1- When reminded, assisted, or supervised by another person, able to get to and from the toilet and transfer.

☐ 2- Unable to get to and from the toilet but is able to use a bedside commode (with or without assistance).

☐ 3- Unable to get to and from the toilet or bedside commode but is able to use a bedpan/urinal independently.

☐ 4- Is totally dependent in toileting.

(M1840 Pointers)

• If the patient uses the toilet during the day but uses a commode for convenience during the night, the correct response is option 0 (CMS, 2009, p. K-8).

(M1845) Toileting Hygiene: Current ability to maintain perineal hygiene safely, adjust clothes and/or incontinence pads before and after using toilet, commode, bedpan, urinal. If managing ostomy, includes cleaning area around stoma, but not managing equipment.

☐ 0- Able to manage toileting hygiene and clothing management without assistance.

☐ 1- Able to manage toileting hygiene and clothing management without assistance if supplies/implements are laid out for the patient.

☐ 2- Someone must help the patient to maitain toileting hygiene and/or adjust clothing.

☐ 3- Patient depends entirely upon another person to maintain toileting hygiene.

(M1845 Pointers)

- Toileting hygiene includes pulling clothes up or down as well as adequately cleaning the perineal area.

(M1850) Transferring: Current ability to move safely from bed to chair, or ability to turn and position self in bed if patient is bedfast.

- ☐   0-   Able to independently transfer.
- ☐   1-   Able to transfer with minimal human assistance or with use of an assistive device.
- ☐   2-   Able to bear weight and pivot during the transfer process but unable to transfer self.
- ☐   3-   Unable to transfer self and is unable to bear weight or pivot when transferred by another person.
- ☐   4-   Bedfast, unable to transfer but is able to turn and position self in bed.
- ☐   5-   Bedfast, unable to transfer and is unable to turn and position self.

(M1850 Pointers)

- Requiring extra time or using the arms of the chair to push up does not constitute dependence in transfer ability (CMS, 2009, p. K-13).

- Medical restrictions should be taken into consideration when evaluating the patient's ability to safely transfer (CMS, 2009, p. K-13).

(M1860) Ambulation/Locomotion: Current ability to walk safely, once in a standing position, or use a wheelchair, once in a seated position, on a variety of surfaces.

- ☐   0-   Able to independently walk on even and uneven surfaces and climb stairs with or without railings (e.g., needs no human assistance or assistive device).
- ☐   1-   With the use of a one-handed device (e.g., cane, single crutch, hemi-walker), able to independently walk on even or uneven surfaces and negotiate stairs without railings.
- ☐   2-   Requires use of a two-handed device (e.g. walker or crutches) to walk alone on a level surface and/or requires human supervision or assistance to negotiate stairs or steps or uneven surfaces.
- ☐   3-   Able to walk only with supervision or assistance of another person at all times.
- ☐   4-   Chairfast, unable to ambulate but is able to wheel self independently.
- ☐   5-   Chairfast, unable to ambulate and is unable to wheel self.
- ☐   6-   Bedfast, unable to ambulate or be up in a chair.

(M1870) Feeding or Eating: Current ability to feed self meals and snacks safely. *Note:* **This refers only to the process of** *eating, chewing,* **and** *swallowing, not preparing* **the food to be eaten.**

- ☐   0-   Able to independently feed self.
- ☐   1-   Able to feed self independently but requires:
  - (a)   meal set-up; <u>OR</u>
  - (b)   intermittent assistance or supervision from another person; <u>OR</u>
  - (c)   a liquid, pureed or ground meat diet.
- ☐   2-   Unable to feed self and must be assisted or supervised throughout the meal/snack.
- ☐   3-   Able to take in nutrients orally and receives supplemental nutrients through a nasogastric tube or gastrostomy.

☐ 4- Unable to take in nutrients orally and is fed nutrients through a naso-gastric tube or gastrostomy.

☐ 5- Unable to take in nutrients orally or by tube feeding.

(M1870 Pointers)

• The CMS has clarified "meal set-up" to include activities such as "mashing a potato, cutting up meat/vegetables when served, pouring milk on cereal, opening milk carton, adding sugar to coffee or tea, arranging the food on the plate for ease of access, etc., all of which are special adaptations of the meal for the patient" (CMS, 2009, p. K-16).

• When responding to M1870, differentiate between the assistance needed or required and the assistance offered or provided that is not necessarily needed or required.

(M1880) Current Ability to Plan and Prepare Light Meals (e.g., cereal, sandwich) or reheat delivered meals safely:

☐ 0- (a) Able to independently plan and prepare all light meals for self or reheat delivered meals: OR

 (b) Is physically, cognitively, and mentally able to prepare light meals on a regular basis but has not routinely performed light meal preparation in the past (i.e., prior to this home care admission).

☐ 1- Unable to prepare light meals on a regular basis due to physical, cognitive, or mental limitations.

☐ 2- Unable to prepare any light meals or reheat any delivered meals.

(M1890) Ability to Use Telephone: Current ability to answer the phone safely, including dialing numbers, and effectively using the telephone to communicate.

☐ 0- Able to dial numbers and answer calls appropriately and as desired.

☐ 1- Able to use a specially adapted telephone (i.e., large numbers on the dial, teletype phone for the deaf) and call essential numbers.

☐ 2- Able to answer the telephone and carry on a normal conversation but has difficulty with placing calls.

☐ 3- Able to answer the telephone only some of the time or is able to carry on only a limited conversation.

☐ 4- Unable to answer the telephone at all but can listen if assisted with equipment.

☐ 5- Totally unable to use the telephone.

☐ NA- Patient does not have a telephone.

(M1900) Prior Functioning ADL/IADL: Indicate the patient's usual ability with everyday activities prior to this current illness, exacerbation, or injury. Check only one box in each row.

Functional Area	Independent	Needed Some Help	Dependent
a. Self-care (e.g., grooming, dressing, and bathing)	☐ 0	☐ 1	☐ 2
b. Ambulation	☐ 0	☐ 1	☐ 2
c. Transfer	☐ 0	☐ 1	☐ 2
d. Household tasks (e.g., light meal preparation, laundry, shopping)	☐ 0	☐ 1	☐ 2

- Note that self-care excludes medication management.

- Transfer includes tub, shower, commode, and bed to chair transfer.

- If previously independent in some self-care tasks (or some transfers, or some household tasks) but needed help or completely dependent in others, pick the response that best describes ability to perform <u>the majority</u> of the tasks.

(M1910) Has this patient had a multi-factor **Fall Risk Assessment** (such as falls history, use of multiple medications, mental impairment, toileting frequency, general mobility/transferring impairment, environmental hazards)?

☐	0-	No multi-factor falls risk assessment conducted
☐	1-	Yes, and it does not indicate a risk for falls
☐	2-	Yes, and it indicates a risk for falls

This final question in this section is another process measure that was added to the 2010 OASIS-C revisions. Again, as with all of the process measures, CMS does not require that agencies conduct fall risk assessment for all patients. However, this is an important clinical concern. Falls are prevalent among older patients and contribute to injury and unplanned hospitalizations. If patients at risk are identified, planned interventions to mitigate the risk can be implemented.

Medications

The next six OASIS questions include a combination of process and outcomes measures. Medication management is extremely important in terms of patient outcomes. Complex drug regimens are common among the chronically ill and contribute to potential problems such as drug interactions, difficulty in adherence, and financial problems. Careful assessment of the medication regimen, medication

reconciliation as patients transfer from one setting to another, and patient education are essential. Patient education and prompt communication of medication related problems or issues to the physician must be timely. The questions related to oral and injectable medication management require the nurse to consider what the patient is able to safely perform on the day of the assessment. If the patient's ability varies on that day, respond to these questions based on the patient's ability at least 51% (more than 12 hours) of the day.

(M2000) Drug Regimen Review: Does a complete drug regimen review indicate potentially clinically significant medication issues, e.g., drug reactions, ineffective drug therapy, side effects, drug interactions, duplicate therapy, omissions, dosage errors, or noncompliance?

☐	0-	Not assessed/reviewed **(Go to M2010)**
☐	1-	No problems found during review **(Go to M2010)**
☐	2-	Problems found during review
☐	NA-	Patient is not taking any medications **(Go to M2040)**

- The Conditions of Participation for Home Health Agencies require a drug regimen review so option 0 would not meet the regulatory requirements.

- Some guidance in answering this question is found in the Guidance Manual. For example, no problems found during review (option 1) would be selected if all of the following are present:

  – List of medications from inpatient facility discharge matches medications shown to home care clinician at SOC/ROC visit. (This includes all medications – both prescription and over the counter medications)

– Diagnoses/symptoms for which patient is taking medications are adequately controlled (as able to be assessed)

– Patient has ALL medications

– Patient has a plan for taking medications safely at the right time

– Patient is not showing signs or symptoms that could be adverse reactions from medications

– No significant drug interactions

(CMS, 2009, p. L-2).

(M2002) Medication Follow-up: Was a physician or the physician-designee contacted within one calendar day to resolve clinically significant medication issues, including reconciliation?

☐   0-   No

☐   1-   Yes

(M2002 Pointers)

• CMS (2009) defines clinically significant medication issues as "those that, in the care provider's judgment, pose an actual or potential threat to patient health & safety, such as drug reactions, ineffective drug therapy, side effects, drug interactions, duplicate therapy, medication omissions, dosage errors, or nonadherence to prescribed medication" (p. L-3).

• The physician may be contacted by phone, voicemail, fax, or other means to convey the clinical medication issues; however, the clinician can only answer yes if there is acknowledgement by the physician regarding the information within one calendar day.

(M2010) Patient/Caregiver High Risk Drug Education: Has the patient/caregiver received instruction on special precautions for all high-risk medications (such as hypoglycemics, anticoagulants, etc.) and how and when to report problems that may occur?

☐   0-   No

☐   1-   Yes

☐   NA-   Patient not taking any high risk drugs OR patient/caregiver fully knowledgeable about special precautions associated with all high-risk medications

(M2010 Pointers)

• This item addresses the process of patient education upon admission and targets high risk medications that may have potentially negative impacts on health and safety.

• A listing of high risk medications can be found from a number of sources including the Institute for Safe Medication Practices (http://ismp.org/Tools/highalertmedications.pdf).

• Examples include: anticoagulants, opioids, hypoglycemics, chemotherapy.

(M2020) Management of Oral Medications: <u>Patient's current ability</u> to prepare and take <u>all</u> prescribed oral medications reliably and safely, including administration of the correct dosage at the appropriate times/intervals. **Excludes injectable and IV medications. (*Note:* this refers to ability, not compliance or willingness.)**

☐   0-   Able to independently take the correct oral medication(s) and proper dosage(s) at the correct times.

☐   1-   Able to take medication(s) at the correct times if:

    (a)   individual dosages are prepared in advance by another person; <u>OR</u>

    (b)   another person develops a drug diary or chart.

☐   2-   Able to take medication(s) at the correct times if given reminders by another person at the appropriate times.

☐ 3 - <u>Unable</u> to take medications unless administered by someone else.

☐ NA- No oral medications prescribed.

(M2020 Pointers)

- A patient who fills his or her own medication box for convenience is independent in ability to take oral medications. If someone else fills the patient's pill box for convenience, the nurse must further investigate to determine the **patient's** ability.

- Even though this question directs the clinician to consider the patient's ability to take **all** medications, the CMS instructs the clinician to consider the patient's ability to take the majority of his or her medications.

- Patient knowledge related to side effects should not be considered when responding to the question, however, should be considered as part of the patient's overall plan of care.

(M2030) Management of Injectable

Medications: <u>Patient's current ability</u> to prepare and take <u>all</u> prescribed injectable medications reliably and safely, including administration of the correct dosage at the appropriate times/intervals. **<u>Excludes</u> IV medications.**

☐ 0- Able to independently take the correct medication(s) and proper dosage(s) at the correct times.

☐ 1- Able to take injectable medication(s) at the correct times if:

    (a) individual syringes are prepared in advance by another person; <u>OR</u>

    (b) another person develops a drug diary or chart.

☐ 2- Able to take medication(s) at the correct times if given reminders by another person based on the frequency of the injection.

☐ 3- <u>Unable</u> to take injectable medications unless administered by another person.

☐ NA- No injectable medications prescribed.

When answering the medication management questions, the nurse must assess and document the patient's ability to perform, not willingness or compliance with, medication management activities. When answering these questions, the nurse should use his or her best judgment related to the patient's cognitive and physical ability. When completing the OASIS, the nurse should disregard whether the patient has demonstrated compliance, but should document any compliance issues in the patient's medical record.

(M2040) Prior Medication Management:

Indicate the patient's usual ability with managing oral and injectable medications prior to this current illness, exacerbation, or injury. Check only one box in each row.

Functional Area	Independent	Needed Some Help	Dependent	Not applicable
a. Oral medications	☐ 0	☐ 1	☐ 2	☐ NA
b. Injectable medications	☐ 0	☐ 1	☐ 2	☐ NA

(M2040 Pointers)

- If patient's ability to manage oral or injectable medications varied from medication to medication, CMS directs the clinician to consider the medication for which the most assistance was needed (CMS, 2009, L-12).

Care Management

(M2100) Types and Sources of Assistance: Determine the level of caregiver ability and willingness to provide assistance for the following activities, if assistance is needed. **Check only one box in each row.**

Type of assistance	No assistance needed in this area	Caregiver(s) currently provide assistance	Caregiver(s) need training/ supportive services to provide assistance	Caregiver(s) not likely to provide assistance	Unclear if Caregiver(s) will provide assistance	Assistance needed, but no Caregiver(s) available
a. ADL assistance (e.g., transfer, ambulation, bathing, dressing, toileting, eating, feeding)	☐ 0	☐ 1	☐ 2	☐ 3	☐ 4	☐ 5
b. IADL assistance (e.g., meals, housekeeping, laundry, telephone, shopping, finances)	☐ 0	☐ 1	☐ 2	☐ 3	☐ 4	☐ 5
c. Medication administration (e.g., oral, inhaled, or injectable)	☐ 0	☐ 1	☐ 2	☐ 3	☐ 4	☐ 5
d. Medical procedures or treatments (e.g., changing wound dressing)	☐ 0	☐ 1	☐ 2	☐ 3	☐ 4	☐ 5
e. Management of equipment (includes oxygen, IV/infusion equipment, enteral/parenteral nutrition, ventilator therapy equipment or supplies)	☐ 0	☐ 1	☐ 2	☐ 3	☐ 4	☐ 5
f. Supervision and safety (e.g. due to cognitive impairment)	☐ 0	☐ 1	☐ 2	☐ 3	☐ 4	☐ 5

M2100 continued on next page

Type of assistance	No assistance needed in this area	Caregiver(s) currently provide assistance	Caregiver(s) need training/ supportive services to provide assistance	Caregiver(s) not likely to provide assistance	Unclear if Caregiver(s) will provide assistance	Assistance needed, but no Caregiver(s) available
g. Advocacy or facilitation of patient's participation in appropriate medical care (includes transportation to and from appointments)	☐ 0	☐ 1	☐ 2	☐ 3	☐ 4	☐ 5

(M2100 Pointers)

- Select "caregiver not likely to provide" if the caregiver has indicated that they are unwilling to help or if the assessment indicated the caregiver may have physical and/or cognitive limitations that preclude ability to provide assistance.

- Examples of medical treatments include wound care, intermittent urinary catheterization, range of motion exercises.

- Examples of medical equipment include intravenous pumps/equipment, oxygen, wheelchair, hoyer lift.

(M2110) How often does the patient receive ADL or IADL assistance from any caregiver(s) (other than home health agency staff)?

☐ 1- At least daily.
☐ 2- Three or more times per week.
☐ 3- One to two times per week.
☐ 4- Received, but less often than weekly.
☐ 5- No assistance received
☐ UK- Unknown

Therapy Need and Plan of Care

This section of the SOC/ROC OASIS has two questions. In the first question (M2200), the clinician completing the OASIS is required to identify the total number of therapy visits – physical, speech, or occupational – planned for the payment episode. This question is only important for Medicare payment purposes. If the home health patient has a payer other than Medicare, for example, a managed care organization, the correct answer is "NA - Not Applicable."

The second question (M2250) requires the clinician to answer questions regarding whether the physician-ordered plan of care includes specific best practices. In addition to earlier process questions including formal pain assessment, pressure ulcer risk assessment, depression screening, falls risk assessment and medication process items, these questions follow up to ask, if those problems are present, were specific interventions included in collaboration with the physician. In addition, care coordination through establishment of patient-specific reporting parameters, diabetic foot care, and moist wound healing for pressure ulcers are addressed in M2250. As stated earlier, the care processes included in the OASIS-C are not mandated by CMS, however, some of these items will support publicly reported measures and if the care processes are not addressed by the agency, it will be reflected in their Home Health Compare scores (CMS, 2009).

(M2200) Therapy Need: In the home health plan of care for the Medicare payment episode for which this assessment will define a case mix group, what is the indicated need for therapy visits

(total number of reasonable and necessary physical, occupational, and speech-language pathology visits combined)? **(Enter zero ["000"] if no therapy visits indicated.)**

(__ __ __)   Number of therapy visits indicated (total of physical, occupational, and speech-language pathology combined.

☐   NA-   Not applicable: No case mix group defined by this assessment.

Because this question has significant financial implications, agencies typically implement systems and processes to ensure that this question is answered accurately. Some of the systems require a physical therapist to visit the patient before this question is answered or may require the nurse to conduct a case conference with a member of the rehabilitation department to ensure accuracy.

(M2250) Plan of Care Synopsis: (Check only <u>one</u> box in each row.) Does the physician-ordered plan of care include the following:

Plan/Intervention	No	Yes	Not applicable	
a. Patient-specific parameters for notifying physician of changes in vital signs or other clinical findings	☐ 0	☐ 1	☐ n/a	Physician has chosen not to establish patient-specific parameters for this patient. Agency will use standardized clinical guidelines accessible for all care providers to reference.
b. Diabetic foot care including monitoring for the presence of skin lesions on the lower extremities and patient/caregiver education on proper foot care	☐ 0	☐ 1	☐ n/a	Patient is not diabetic or is bilateral amputee.
c. Falls prevention interventions	☐ 0	☐ 1	☐ n/a	Patient is not assessed to be at risk for falls
d. Depression intervention(s) such as medication, referral for other treatment, or a monitoring plan for current treatment	☐ 0	☐ 1	☐ n/a	Patient has no diagnosis or symptoms of depression
e. Intervention(s) to monitor and mitigate pain	☐ 0	☐ 1	☐ n/a	No pain defined
f. Intervention(s) to prevent pressure ulcers	☐ 0	☐ 1	☐ n/a	Patient is not assessed to be at risk for pressure ulcers
g. Pressure ulcer treatment based on principles of moist wound healing OR order for treatment based on moist wound healing has been requested from physician	☐ 0	☐ 1	☐ n/a	Patient has no pressure ulcers with need for moist wound healing

(M2250 Pointers)

- Patient-specific parameters might include ranges for acceptable blood pressure, temperature, or weight; anything outside of those parameters would be reported to the physician.

- Interventions for depression may include new medications, referrals to agency resources (such as social workers), and patient education.

- Interventions for pain must include both monitoring and interventions. Examples are medications and thermal applications.

- Wet-to-dry dressings are not an example of moist wound healing as they allow the wound to dry out between wound treatments. An example of a moist wound healing product is a hydrogel dressing.

To this point, a review of the SOC OASIS data set has been completed. The SOC/ROC assessment is the most extensive of the OASIS assessments. The Follow-Up/Significant Change in Condition OASIS assessment is comprised of a selected sample of the questions found on the SOC assessment as well as additional questions related to clinical processes. The financial implication of these assessments will be discussed in Chapter 8.

TRANSFER OASIS DOCUMENT

As discussed earlier, essentially all home health occurs in 60-day episodes of care. A patient may be admitted to a home health agency and be discharged with his or her goals met, or experience a transfer to an inpatient facility for acute or rehabilitative care. Because there are several different discharge options for home health patients, the OASIS regulations require the agency to "track" what has happened to the patient by completing the appropriate OASIS document. A Transfer OASIS should be completed when a patient is transferred to an inpatient facility for more than 24 hours. *(Note:*

There are a few exceptions to this rule, but they are beyond the scope of this course.) In the 2010 OASIS-C version, the number of Transfer OASIS items increased from 11 to 19. This is because hospitalization rates are a priority for CMS; completion of the OASIS-C items at transfer will help to identify the reason for hospitalizations. Many of the items address care processes. Some of the items are seen for the first time when completing a Transfer OASIS, such as the questions about vaccinations and heart failure follow-up.

Completion of the Transfer OASIS is complex because it requires evaluation of the care throughout the episode of care, such as review of clinical notes and physician orders. To avoid a review of every clinical note from every home visit, agencies are developing strategies to follow information related to the care processes measured, such as manual tracking tools of events (e.g. check off tools completed by the clinician when signs of heart failure occur and what interventions were completed), or electronic tools that pull information from visit notes into a report.

The first items of the Transfer OASIS-C ask about vaccinations. The basic focus of these questions are, was the vaccine given during the episode, and if not, why. It is well known that patients are at high risk for complications from influenza as well as pneumococcal disease and that vaccinations protect patients and prevent hospitalizations and deaths.

M1040 Influenza Vaccine: Did the patient receive the influenza vaccine from your agency for this year's influenza season (October 1 through March 31) during this episode of care?

☐   0-   No

☐   1-   Yes **(Go to M1050)**

☐   NA-   Does not apply because entire episode of care (SOC/ROC to Transfer/Discharge) is outside this influenza season **(Go to M1050)**

M1045 Reason Influenza Vaccine not received:
If the patient did not receive the influenza vaccine from your agency during this episode of care, state reason:

☐ 1- Received from another health care provider (e.g., physician)

☐ 2- Received from your agency previously during this year's flu season

☐ 3- Offered and declined

☐ 4- Assessed and determined to have medical contraindication(s)

☐ 5- Not indicated; patient does not meet age/condition guidelines for influenza vaccine

☐ 6- Inability to obtain vaccine due to declared shortage

☐ 7- None of the above

M1050 Pneumococcal Vaccine: Did the patient receive pneumococcal polysaccharide vaccine (PPV) from your agency during this episode of care?

☐ 0- No

☐ 1- Yes **(Go to M1500)**

M1055 Reason PPV not received: If the patient did not receive the pneumococcal polysaccharide vaccine (PPV) from your agency during this episode of care (SOC/ROC to Transfer/Discharge), state reason:

☐ 1- Patient has received PPV in the past

☐ 2- Offered and declined

☐ 3- Assessed and determined to have medical contraindication(s)

☐ 4- Not indicated; patient does not meet age/condition guidelines for PPV

☐ 5- None of the above

(M1040, M1045, M1050, M1055 Pointers)

• Information about timeframes, indications, and contraindications for administration of influenza vaccine can be obtained from the Centers for Disease Control and Prevention (CDC) at the CDC's Website (www.cdc.gov). For example, some of the 2009 indications for PPV vaccination are: all adults 65 years of age and older (at least once in lifetime), all who live in long term care facilities, and all aged 2-64 years who have high risk conditions such as diabetes, nephrotic syndrome, ESRD, heart failure, COPD, HIV, and asplenia.

The next focus of the Transfer OASIS-C is heart failure. Heart failure is one of the most prevalent diagnoses among home care patients and is a leading reason for hospitalizations among home care patients.

M1500 Symptoms in Heart Failure Patients: If a patient has been diagnosed with **heart failure,** did the patient exhibit symptoms indicated by clinical **heart failure** guidelines (including dyspnea, orthopnea, edema, weight gain) at any point since the previous OASIS assessment?

☐ 0- No **(Go to M2004)**

☐ 1- Yes

☐ 2- Not assessed **(Go to M2004)**

☐ NA- Patient does not have a diagnosis of heart failure **(Go to M2004)**

M1510 Heart Failure Follow-Up: If a patient has been diagnosed with heart failure and has exhibited symptoms indicative of heart failure since the previous OASIS assessment, what action(s) has (have) been taken to respond? **(Mark all that apply)**

☐ 0- No action taken

☐ 1- Patient's physician (or other primary care practitioner) contacted the same day

☐ 2- Patient advised to get emergency treatment (e.g. call 911 or go to emergency room)

☐ 3- Implement physician-ordered patient-specific established parameters for treatment

☐ 4- Patient education or other clinical interventions

☐ 5- Obtained change in care plan orders (e.g. increased monitoring by agency, change in visit frequency, telehealth, etc.)

(M1510 Pointers)

- Option 1 is appropriate only if the physician responds to the communication acknowledging receipt of information and/or further orders or instructions. If the physician does not respond to the communication, Option 1 cannot be selected, even though the physician was contacted with information about the patient's condition.

- Option 3 includes interventions such as reminding a patient to implement existing orders for treatment. For example, taking an extra dose of furosemide for 2 days if the patient's weight goes up 3 pounds.

(M2004) Medication Intervention: If there were any clinically significant medication issues since the previous OASIS assessment, was a physician or the physician-designee contacted within one calendar day of the assessment to resolve clinically significant medication issues, including reconciliation?

☐ 0- No

☐ 1- Yes

☐ NA- No clinically significant medication issues identified since the previous OASIS assessment

(M2004 Pointers)

- Clinically significant medication issues are those that pose an actual or potential threat to patient health and safety, such as drug reactions, ineffective drug therapy, side effects, drug interactions, duplicate therapy, medication omissions, dosage errors, or non-adherence to prescribed medication regimen.

- Contact with physician must include not only reporting by the nurse, but an acknowledgement by the physician that the information was received.

(M2015) Patient/Caregiver Drug Education Intervention: Since the previous OASIS assessment, was the patient/caregiver instructed by agency staff or other health care provider to monitor the effectiveness of drug therapy, drug reactions, and side effects, and how and when to report problems that may occur?

☐ 0- No

☐ 1- Yes

☐ NA- Patient not taking any drugs

(M2300) Emergent Care: Since the last OASIS data were collected, has the patient utilized a hospital emergency department (includes holding/observation)?

☐ 0- No **(Go to M2400)**

☐ 1- Yes, used hospital emergency department WITHOUT hospital admission

☐ 2- Yes, used hospital emergency department WITH hospital admission

☐ NA- Unknown **(Go to M2400)**

(M2300 Pointers)

- For the purposes of OASIS, an inpatient admission is different than a patient who has a trip to the emergency room and remains in a holding unit or bed and is then discharged home. This distinction is sometimes difficult for the home care clinician to determine. Often, the patient is not aware of the difference and cannot provide any assistance to the nurse attempting to answer these questions. It is not uncommon for the representative of the home health agency to call the hospital to try to determine whether the patient meets the definition of an inpatient facility admission.

(M2310) Reason for Emergent Care: For what reason(s) did the patient receive emergent care (with or without hospitalization)? **(Mark all that apply.)**

☐ 1- Improper medication administration, medication side effects, toxicity, anaphylaxis

☐ 2- Injury caused by fall

☐ 3- Respiratory infection (e.g. pneumonia, bronchitis)

☐ 4- Other respiratory problem

☐ 5- Heart failure (e.g. fluid overload)

☐ 6- Cardiac dysrhythmia (irregular heartbeat)

☐ 7- Myocardial infarction or chest pain

☐ 8- Other heart disease

☐ 9- Stroke (CVA) or TIA

☐ 10- Hypo/Hyperglycemia, diabetes out of control

☐ 11- GI bleeding, obstruction, constipation, impaction

☐ 12- Dehydration, malnutrition

☐ 13- Urinary tract infection

☐ 14- IV catheter-related infection

☐ 15- Wound infection or deterioration

☐ 16- Uncontrolled pain

☐ 17- Acute mental/behavioral health problem

☐ 18- Deep vein thrombosis, pulmonary embolus

☐ 19- Other than above reasons

☐ UK- Reason unknown

The Intervention Synopsis follows from the Plan of Care Synopsis (M2250) completed at the start or resumption of care. This process measure evaluates whether a physician ordered plan of care was in place and at the time of transfer or discharge, and were the interventions specified actually implemented.

(M2400) Intervention Synopsis: (Check only <u>one</u> box in each row.) Since the previous OASIS assessment, were the following interventions BOTH included in the physician-ordered plan of care AND implemented?

Plan/Intervention	No	Yes	Not applicable	
a. Diabetic foot care including monitoring for the presence of skin lesions on the lower extremities and patient/caregiver education on proper foot care	☐ 0	☐ 1	☐ n/a	Patient is not diabetic or is bilateral amputee
b. Falls prevention interventions	☐ 0	☐ 1	☐ n/a	Formal multi-factor Fall Risk Assessment indicates the patient was not at risk for falls since the last OASIS assessment

M2400 continued on next page

Plan/Intervention	No	Yes	Not applicable	
c. Depression intervention(s) such as medication, referral for other treatment, or a monitoring plan for current treatment	☐ 0	☐ 1	☐ n/a	Formal assessment indicates the patient did not meet criteria for depression AND patient did not have diagnosis of depression since the last OASIS assessment
d. Intervention(s) to monitor and mitigate	☐ 0	☐ 1	☐ n/a	Formal assessment did not indicate pain since the last OASIS assessment
e. Intervention(s) to prevent pressure ulcers	☐ 0	☐ 1	☐ n/a	Formal assessment indicates the patient was not at risk of pressure ulcers since the last OASIS assessment
f. Pressure ulcer treatment based on principles of moist wound healing OR order for treatment based on moist wound healing has been requested from physician	☐ 0	☐ 1	☐ n/a	Dressings that support principles of moist wound healing not indicated for this patient's pressure ulcers OR patient has no pressure ulcers with need for moist wound healing

(M2410) To which **Inpatient Facility** has the patient been admitted?

☐ 1- Hospital **(Go to M2430)**

☐ 2- Rehabilitation facility **(Go to M0903)**

☐ 3- Nursing home **(Go to M2440)**

☐ 4- Hospice **(Go to M0903)**

(M2430) Reason for Hospitalization: For what reason(s) did the patient require hospitalization)?

(Mark all that apply.)

☐ 1- Improper medication administration, medication side effects, toxicity, anaphylaxis

☐ 2- Injury caused by fall

☐ 3- Respiratory infection (e.g. pneumonia, bronchitis)

☐ 4- Other respiratory problem

☐ 5- Heart failure (e.g. fluid overload)

☐ 6- Cardiac dysrhythmia (irregular heartbeat)

☐ 7- Myocardial infarction or chest pain

☐ 8- Other heart disease

☐ 9- Stroke (CVA) or TIA

☐ 10- Hypo/Hyperglycemia, diabetes out of control

☐ 11- GI bleeding, obstruction, constipation, impaction

☐ 12- Dehydration, malnutrition

☐ 13- Urinary tract infection

☐ 14- IV catheter-related infection or complication

☐ 15- Wound infection or deterioration

☐ 16- Uncontrolled pain

☐ 17- Acute mental/behavioral health problem

☐ 18- Deep vein thrombosis, pulmonary embolus

☐ 19- Scheduled treatment or procedure

☐ 20- Other than above reasons

☐ UK- Reason unknown **(Go to M0903)**

(M2440) For what Reason(s) was the patient Admitted to a Nursing Home? (Mark all that apply.)

☐   1-   Therapy services

☐   2-   Respite care

☐   3-   Hospice care

☐   4-   Permanent placement

☐   5-   Unsafe for care at home

☐   6-   Other

☐   UK-   Unknown **(Go to M0903)**

In addition to the questions noted above, the Transfer OASIS document includes two specific questions related to date of transfer and date of last visit.

DISCHARGE OASIS DOCUMENT

The Discharge OASIS document is intended to measure the change in the patient's health status at the completion of the home health plan of treatment. In order to identify the change in health status, a comparison of the information on the SOC OASIS and the Discharge OASIS must be completed. For that reason, many of the questions found on the previous OASIS documents discussed are repeated on the Discharge OASIS, including the process measures of vaccines, heart failure, medication processes, and the intervention synopsis. For the purpose of this course, only the questions that are unique to the Discharge OASIS will be reviewed.

(M1307) The **Oldest Non-epithelialized Stage II Pressure Ulcer** that is present at discharge

☐   1-   Was present at the most recent SOC/ROC assessment

☐   2-   Developed since the most recent SOC/ROC assessment: record date pressure ulcer first identified

     __ /__ /__
     month/date/year

☐   NA-   No non-epithelialized Stage II pressure ulcers are present at discharge

(M1307 Pointers)

• Note that this item applies only to Stage II ulcers

• Never reverse the stage of pressure ulcers to describe the healing process (e.g., Stage III down to Stage II)

(M2420) Discharge Disposition: Where is the patient after discharge from your agency? **(Choose only one answer.)**

☐   1-   Patient remained in the community (without formal assistive services)

☐   2-   Patient remained in the community (with formal assistive services)

☐   3-   Patient transferred to a non-institutional hospice

☐   4-   Unknown because patient moved to a geographic location not served by this agency

☐   UK-   Other unknown **(Go to M0903)**

(M0903) Date of Last (Most Recent) Home Visit:

    _____/_____/_____
    Month   Day   Year (4 digits)

(M0906) Discharge/Transfer/Death Date: Enter the date of the discharge, transfer, or death (at home) of the patient.

    _____/_____/_____
    Month   Day   Year (4 digits)

NOTICE OF PRIVACY

A complete OASIS assessment obviously provides a very detailed description of the patient's status and functional abilities in many areas. For these reasons, the CMS has very strict expectations for the security and confidentiality of the patient's OASIS data.

To demonstrate their commitment, the CMS requires agencies to inform patients of their rights specifically in relation to this information. Appendix H provides a copy of the federally mandated "Home Health Agency OASIS Statement of Patient Privacy Rights" for review. Although this privacy statement is comprehensive, it is not a consent form. Most agencies require a patient to sign a separate consent form that states that the patient has been given the privacy statement, understands the information, and agrees to the release of his or her medical information.

OASIS AND THE PLAN OF CARE

Although a significant amount of time has been spent reviewing details of the OASIS questions, it is important to understand that the OASIS is only part of the patient's medical record. It is not a document that is intended to "stand alone." It has to be incorporated into the agency's comprehensive patient assessment and the patient's overall plan of treatment or plan of care. The plan of care includes diagnoses, types of services and equipment required, frequency of visits, prognosis, rehabilitation potential, functional limitations, activities permitted, nutritional requirements, medications and treatments, safety measures, and instructions for timely discharge or referral. Historically, a form called the Medicare 485 was required for use. Some agencies still use this form but it is not required.

Although this duplication seems benign, it can create difficulties if the nurse does not pay close attention to what he or she is documenting. If the nurse is not careful, this duplication can lead to inconsistent and contradictory documentation in the medical record. From the agency's perspective, these errors can lead to payment denials, poor patient outcomes, and medical records that would not stand up well if scrutinized in a court of law. For these reasons, it is always a good idea to closely review and compare the answers on the OASIS with those on the plan of care and follow the agency's policy for making any necessary corrections or additions.

SUMMARY

Since the inception of the OASIS, most agencies have worked diligently to follow the instructions and interpret the individual assessment questions consistently. The implementation regulations clearly stated that the OASIS was not to be completed as "extra" pieces of paper, and required agencies to incorporate the OASIS questions into existing documents. After reviewing the examples of the OASIS items provided in this chapter, one can appreciate the potential for misinterpretations and inaccuracies in the patient descriptors.

As stated in the beginning of this chapter, the intent of the OASIS was to provide agencies with a mechanism to measure the quality of their services. Although the system is not perfect, it has provided the first set of objective measures that can be applied to almost all patients admitted to home health. As the OASIS assessments evolve, the questions will be "fine tuned," and agencies will be able to increase the ability of their staff to answer the questions consistently. The goal of identifying "best practices" will come to fruition, and all home health patients will benefit.

EXAM QUESTIONS

CHAPTER 6
Questions 53-77

Note: Choose the one option that BEST answers each question.

53. Collecting, encoding, locking, and transmitting OASIS data are

    a. required to comply with the requirements outlined in the *OASIS User Manual.*

    b. required only of agencies with more than 60 patients.

    c. voluntary until the revised Conditions of Participation are finalized.

    d. necessary to obtain a certificate of compliance.

54. OASIS regulations mandate that agencies adhere to many different time frames and schedules. Which of the following statements is true?

    a. Agencies must complete the SOC visit within 72 hours of receiving the referral. F
    48

    b. All episodes are limited to 60 days.

    c. Agencies must complete the SOC OASIS within 7 days of the visit. F
    5

    d. All OASIS documents must be encoded and locked within 5 days. F
    7

55. The electronic packaging and transmission of the entire state's OASIS database to the federal government is the responsibility of the

    a. state OASIS coordinator.

    b. nurse or therapist who collected the data.

    c. Department of Information Systems and Data Quality.

    d. Department of Public Health.

56. If a patient experiences a transfer to an inpatient facility or returns from an inpatient stay, OASIS regulations mandate that the agency

    a. complete an additional and specific assessment within the required time frame.

    b. notify the physician.

    c. discharge the patient from agency services.

    d. amend the physician-ordered plan of care.

57. Clinicians should minimize choosing the "Unknown" option found in some OASIS questions because

    a. the assessment does not meet the definition of a comprehensive assessment if too many areas are not thoroughly assessed.

    b. marking this option is associated with poor clinical practice.

    c. the agency might be penalized for failing to take the OASIS mandate seriously.

    d. it eliminates the possibility of measuring the patient's outcome.

58. A referral from a physician to evaluate a patient's technique when self-administering insulin, insert an indwelling urinary catheter to treat urinary retention, or evaluate a patient's tolerance to a new antidepressant medication

 a. exemplifies changes in the patient's plan of treatment.

 b. represents tasks that do not require the skills of a registered nurse and therefore do not represent a change in the patient's plan of treatment.

 c. are tasks that should be delegated to a home care aide.

 d. are tasks that should be delegated to a licensed practical or vocational nurse.

To view the OASIS items referred to in some of the following questions, please see Appendix B.

59. Pain assessment is a care process that agencies may incorporate into their expectations for best practices. An example of a formal pain assessment in relation to completion of M1240 is:

 a. asking the patient to use their words to best describe their pain.

 b. asking the caregiver of a patient with limited cognitive abilities to rate their perception of the patient's pain using a 0-10 scale.

 c. using the 0-10 pain scale.

 d. using an agency developed tool that the nurses prefer for pain assessment.

Question 60 refers to the case of Mrs. Jones.

Mrs. Jones has been deaf since childhood. While conducting her assessment, she gives you a written note that asks you to look directly at her and speak slowly to facilitate her ability to read your lips. She is able to respond to your questions using a combination of signals and written responses.

60. The OASIS assessment requires you to answer M1230, which relates to the speech and oral expression of language (in patient's own language). M1230

 a. should always be answered with an interpreter present.

 b. should only be answered for a patient who does not have an obvious hearing deficit.

 c. should only be answered if the patient has an obvious hearing deficit.

 d. should be answered "patient nonresponsive or unable to speak."

Questions 61 through 64 refer to the case of Mrs. McMillan.

After a prolonged hospitalization, Mrs. McMillan is admitted to your home health care agency for services. She complains of bilateral heel pain whenever she is in a standing position. Inspection of her heels reveals bilateral necrotic blackened areas of eschar that are approximately the size of a quarter.

61. The best description of the sores on Mrs. McMillan's heels is

 a. pressure ulcers, because they are blackened areas over a bony prominence.

 b. stasis ulcers, because they have occurred on her lower extremities.

 c. not pressure ulcers, because they must be open to be classified as such.

 d. not pressure ulcers, because they must be open, draining, and painful to be classified as such.

62. When answering M1308, Mrs. McMillan's heels would be classified as

    a. Stage 1: Nonblanchable erythema of intact skin; the heralding of skin ulceration. In darker-pigmented skin, warmth, edema, hardness, or discolored skin may be indicators.

    b. Stage 3: Full-thickness skin loss involving damage or necrosis of subcutaneous tissue, which may extend down to, but not through, underlying fascia. The ulcer presents clinically as a deep crater with or without undermining of adjacent tissue.

    c. Stage 4: Full-thickness skin loss with extensive destruction, tissue necrosis, or damage to muscle, bone, or supporting structures (e.g., tendon, joint capsule, etc.).

    d. Unstageable due to coverage of wound bed by slough and/or eschar.

63. M1324 asks the clinician to stage the most problematic (observable) pressure ulcer. When answering this question for Mrs. McMillan, the correct response would be

    a. Stage 1: Nonblanchable erythema of intact skin; the heralding of skin ulceration. In darker-pigmented skin, warmth, edema, hardness, or discolored skin may be indicators.

    b. Stage 3: Full-thickness skin loss involving damage or necrosis of subcutaneous tissue, which may extend down to, but not through, underlying fascia. The ulcer presents clinically as a deep crater with or without undermining of adjacent tissue.

    c. Stage 4: Full-thickness skin loss with extensive destruction, tissue necrosis, or damage to muscle, bone, or supporting structures (e.g., tendon, joint capsule, etc.).

    d. no observable pressure ulcer or unhealed pressure ulcer.

64. After identifying and staging Mrs. McMillan's heels, item M1320 requires the nurse to describe the status of the most problematic wound. Due to the presence of eschar that fills the wound bed with blackened, dead tissue, the correct response would be

    a. wounds are healing and filled with granulation tissue.

    b. wounds are partially healed, and granulation tissue must be present even though it is not easily observed.

    c. wounds are nonhealing due to the presence of eschar.

    d. this determination can only be made by a certified wound, ostomy, and continence nurse.

65. When answering M1330, the clinician must identify whether the patient has a stasis ulcer. Stasis ulcers are typically

    a. described as an ulceration caused by inadequate venous circulation in the affected area and often associated with stasis dermatitis.

    b. described as an ulceration caused by inadequate arterial circulation in the affected area and typically occur on the trunk.

    c. the result of skin inflammation, sores, or ulcers resulting from tissue hypoxia due to prolonged pressure most often occurring over bony prominences.

    d. only diagnosed by nurses who are certified in wound, ostomy, and continence nursing.

66. Which of the following would be considered skin lesions or open wounds according to M1350?

    a. The surgical wound from a laporoscopic hysterectomy.

    b. A urostomy which the patient manages completely independently.

    c. A peripherally inserted central catheter (PICC).

    d. A stage I pressure ulcer.

67. If a patient uses oxygen, prior to answering M1400, the OASIS guidelines instruct the nurse to first

    a. determine whether the patient uses oxygen intermittently or continuously.

    b. assess the patient without the oxygen in place.

    c. assess the patient with the oxygen in place.

    d. skip this question, and only answer M1410 because the patient has an obvious deficit.

68. The Neuro/Emotional/Behavioral Status section of the OASIS (questions M1700 through M1750) instructs the nurse to answer the questions based on behaviors reported or observed. If a conflict arises between the nurse's observations and what the patient or caregiver report, the nurse should

    a. answer the questions to the best of his or her ability.

    b. use professional judgment to choose the option that best describes the patient and make a notation that clarifies the inconsistency between the observed and reported behaviors.

    c. discuss the correct response with the patient's physician.

    d. request the services of a psychiatric clinical nurse specialist to complete this portion of the assessment.

Question 69 refers to the case of Mrs. Leger.

Mrs. Leger is a 68-year-old woman who tells the home health care nurse that she has never taken a shower. She tells the nurse that she grew up only taking sponge baths and prefers not to get into the tub or shower. The nurse observes that her gait is steady, and she is able to easily rise out of a soft cushioned chair or couch.

69. M1830 requires the nurse to describe the patient's ability to wash her entire body. The choice that best describes Mrs. Leger's ability is that she is

    a. able to bathe herself in the shower or tub independently.

    b. able to bathe herself in the shower or tub with the use of an assistive device.

    c. able to bathe herself in the shower or tub with the assistance of another person.

    d. unable to bathe in the shower or tub.

Question 70 refers to the case of Mr. Shoesmith.

Mr. Shoesmith is an elderly gentleman who has been recently widowed after being married all of his adult life. He is being admitted to your agency after suffering a mild stroke. He has no residual deficits. The physician has ordered skilled nursing assessments of his cardiovascular and neurological status and teaching about his new medications. From your assessment, it is clear that he has no cognitive limitations. He reports to you that he is unwilling to perform any tasks associated with meal preparation because his wife has always performed that chore. (In answering OASIS questions related to ADLs and IADLs, the nurse must answer considering only the patient's cognitive and physical ability, not their willingness.)

70. Even though Mr. Shoesmith has not had to complete the tasks associated with meal preparation, from your assessment, it appears that he

    a. is physically and cognitively able to perform the tasks associated with meal preparation despite his unwillingness.

    b. able to select the foods he would like to eat but needs some assistance in preparing them.

    c. unable to make his own meals.

    d. in need of someone to do all of the meal preparation.

71. A complete drug regimen review is required according to M2000. In order to answer that there were "no problems" found during the review of the patient's medication regimen, the following should be in place:

    a. the patient has all of his medications in the home except for two which are in the pharmacy ready to be picked up.

    b. the patient has a plan for taking his medications safely at the right time.

    c. the patient takes his diuretic every day as his doctor has ordered but his lower extremity edema has increased.

    d. all prescription medications listed from the hospital match, except the patient occasionally also takes extra strength acetaminophen at home for a headache.

Question 72 refers to the case of Ms. Maury.

You are the home health care nurse conducting the SOC OASIS assessment of Ms. Maury. She is a 79-year-old woman who has a history of cardiac disease and insulin-dependent diabetes. As you evaluate her ability to manage her medication regimen, you note that she is taking all medications correctly except her insulin. As she demonstrates her technique, you note that there is a significant air bubble in the syringe. Ms. Maury does not seem to notice this detail. When you ask her about the presence of the air bubble, she states, "Oh dear, I have been taking insulin so long that I don't worry about such things anymore, but if it makes you happy, I will do it without a bubble." She demonstrates the filling of a second syringe without difficulty.

72. Although Ms. Maury is not always careful when prefilling her syringes, she is

    a. able to independently take the correct medication and proper dosages at the correct times.

    b. able to take medications at the correct times, if individual syringes are prepared in advance by another person.

    c. able to take medications at the correct times, if given daily reminders.

    d. unable to take injectable medications, unless administered by someone else.

73. Unlike a patient on medicare, the correct response to M2200 for a patient on an HMO who requires five physical therapy visits and one speech therapy visit is

    a. _ _5.

    b. _ _6.

    c. NA-not applicable.

    d. Unknown.

74. You are completing a Transfer OASIS for a patient who has been admitted to the hospital with an exacerbation of heart failure. You notified the physician two days earlier when you assessed that the patient's lower extremity edema was increasing and he was feeling more fatigued. The physician never called you back. You told the patient that his heart failure could be getting worse and that he should continue to monitor his condition and report any increased edema. Based on your actions, which of the following options could you document on M1510 Heart Failure Follow-Up?

    a. Patient's physician (or other primary care practitioner) contacted the same day.
    b. Patient advised to get emergency treatment (e.g. call 911 or go to emergency room).
    c. Patient education or other clinical interventions.
    d. Obtained change in care plan orders (e.g. increased monitoring by agency, change in visit frequency, telehealth, etc.).

75. The agency must ensure that a Transfer OASIS is completed when the patient is

    a. transferred to the emergency room.
    b. held in a holding unit.
    c. transferred to hospice services.
    d. transferred to an inpatient facility for more than 24 hours.

76. Informing the patient of his or her right to the confidentiality of OASIS data

    a. is optional.
    b. is unnecessary, because everybody knows that health care data is kept confidential.
    c. should only be done if the patient requests the information.
    d. is mandated by federal regulations.

77. The OASIS and the plan of care should

    a. be separate, standalone documents.
    b. never be completed at the same time by the same clinician.
    c. remain separate, because one is for assessment and the other is for payment purposes.
    d. be reviewed for inconsistency and contradiction.

CHAPTER 7

MEASURING QUALITY OUTCOMES

CHAPTER OBJECTIVE

After completing this chapter, the reader will be able to describe how Outcome and Assessment Information Set (OASIS) data can be used to measure patient outcomes.

LEARNING OBJECTIVES

After studying this chapter, the reader will be able to

1. describe how OASIS and performance improvement are related.

2. differentiate between three possible patient outcomes.

3. identify the value of determining statistical significance.

4. recall the importance of risk adjusting.

5. describe how an agency utilizes best clinical practices to improve patient outcomes.

INTRODUCTION

Medicare-certified home health agencies have always had performance improvement programs. Until the implementation of OASIS, most initiatives were aimed at improving the process of care (the way care is delivered). Depending on the size of the organization, agencies may have had a person or an entire department dedicated to eval-uating compliance with policies and procedures. One example of a process that was (and still is) frequently measured is the level of compliance with conducting home health aide supervision visits every 14 days.

Agencies that were interested in measuring patient outcomes usually did not have an objective measure that could be used. Attainment of the care plan goals was often the only measure of patient outcomes available to staff. For instance, a patient's goal might be to verbalize three signs or symptoms of exacerbation to be reported to the physician. Although this information might be helpful for discharge planning, it did not capture a change in the patient's clinical or functional status.

The implementation of OASIS enabled agencies to measure the clinical outcomes of the care provided to an individual patient or to an entire group of patients. Before the types of outcomes that can be measured are discussed, it is important to define exactly what is meant by "outcome." For the purpose of this course, a patient outcome is defined as a change in the patient's clinical or functional status between two points in time. With the advent of OASIS-C, new items were added to measure not only specific patient outcomes, but also processes of care. These refer to the "use of assessment tools or the planning and delivery of specific clinical interventions" (CMS, 2009, 1-5).

TYPES OF PATIENT OUTCOMES

To measure an outcome, an agency must be able to compare a patient at two different points in time. OASIS regulations require agencies to collect patient data:

- at the start of care
- whenever the patient is transferred to an inpatient facility
- at the resumption of care
- with every recertification
- at discharge.

The collection of data at these time points provides opportunities to compare the patient's response to the same question at different times.

Three general types of patient outcomes can be measured using OASIS data. The first and most obvious outcome is an improvement. An improvement in status or functional ability occurs whenever a patient moves from a less functional status to a more functional status.

Using M1242 as an example, consider a patient who reports that he has pain daily (but not constantly) when first admitted to home health care. By the time the patient is discharged, he reports that his pain occurs less often than daily. The change from daily to less than daily pain is a positive change, which represents an improved outcome.

(M1242) Frequency of Pain interfering with patient's activity or movement

☐	0-	Patient has no pain
☐	1-	Patient has pain that does not interfere with activity or movement
☐	2-	Less often than daily
☐	3-	Daily, but not constantly
☐	4-	All of the time

Conversely, a patient who denies pain at the time of admission and reports any level of pain at the time of discharge would have experienced a decline, which represents the second type of general outcome: a negative patient outcome.

The final outcome that can be measured is one in which the patient has stabilized; the outcome is said to be "null." Stabilization means that the patient's condition did not improve or decline; it was unchanged.

One question that agencies must answer in relation to stabilization outcomes is: "Are stabilized outcomes a reasonable expectation for some patients, or does it illustrate that an agency's services were inadequate?" Would it not be reasonable to expect that after receiving the services of a skilled nurse or therapist that the patient's status would be improved? Consider the case of Mrs. Huff.

Mrs. Huff

Mrs. Huff is a 46-year-old woman who is a quadriplegic. Her caregiver uses a Hoyer lift to transfer her from her bed to a specially equipped wheelchair. When in bed or the chair, she is unable to change her position or move any part of her body without the assistance of a caregiver. Is it reasonable to expect, even with intense home health care services, that she will demonstrate an improvement in areas such as M1850, which measures her ability to transfer?

(M1850) Transferring: Current ability to move safely from bed to chair, or ability to turn and position self in bed if patient is bedfast.

☐	0-	Able to independently transfer.
☐	1-	Able to transfer with minimal human assistance or with use of an assistive device.
☐	2-	Able to bear weight and pivot during the transfer process but unable to transfer self.

☐   3-   Unable to transfer self and is
         unable to bear weight or pivot
         when transferred by another person.

☐   4-   Bedfast, unable to transfer but is
         able to turn and position self in
         bed.

☐   5-   Bedfast, unable to transfer and is
         unable to turn and position self.

Although most patients have the opportunity to achieve outcomes mentioned above, some do not have the ability to get better and others could possibly get worse.

To clarify, consider the patient who denies any pain at the start of care. This patient is already at the most functional state and could not possibly get better. On M1242 there are only two possible outcomes for this patient: to stabilize (remain pain free) or destabilize (develop a pain issue) and experience a negative outcome.

The same thinking can also be applied to patients who are in the most dependent functional state. Reconsider the case of Mrs. Huff in light of M1850. She is a quadriplegic and in the most dependent functional state. The only two potential outcomes that she can experience are to stabilize (remain unchanged) or improve by moving to a less dependent state. In reality, it is unlikely that she will demonstrate much improvement in her ability to transfer, so the most likely outcome for her will be to remain stable.

CARE PROCESS MEASUREMENTS

If an agency improves its processes of care through the use of evidence-based guidelines, it should be anticipated that better patient outcomes will follow. Referring back to Chapter 6, care process measures were added to the OASIS C tool and include the following:

- Patient specific parameters for notifying the physician (M2250)

- Administration of influenza and pneumoccocal vaccines (M1040-M1055)

- Standardized pain assessment (M1240) and interventions to monitor and mitigate pain (M2250, M2400)

- Pressure ulcer risk assessment (M1300) and interventions to prevent pressure ulcers (M2250, M2400)

- Diabetic foot care including monitoring for lesions and patient education (M2250, M2400)

- Heart failure symptoms and actions taken (M1500, M1510)

- Depression screening (M1730) and interventions (M2250, M2400)

- Falls risk assessment (M1910) and interventions to reduce risk (M2250, M2400)

- Medication adverse events, reconciliation and follow-up and patient education (M2002, M2010, M2004, M2015)

Consider the process measure of pressure ulcer risk assessment (M1300). A methodical assessment for patient risk factors, such as moisture problems, nutrition, and/or mobility, allows the nurse to develop an appropriate plan of care. For example, if the patient has mobility problems, teaching the patient and family about frequent position changes and developing a turning schedule should reduce the risk of the patient developing new pressure ulcers or worsening of existing pressure ulcers as measured in OASIS items M1306, M1308, M1310/1312/1314, M1320, M1322, and M1324.

As noted in Chapter 6, CMS does not require or mandate that the home health care agency implement the care processes, as they are not required under the Conditions of Participation. However, some of the OASIS-C process measures will support the publicly reported measures.

AGGREGATE REPORTS

Not only has the OASIS provided agencies with a mechanism for measuring individual patient outcomes, the system also enables an agency to compare its performance to all other agencies that provide care for Medicare and Medicaid patients. These aggregate reports provide outcome measures for all of the patients cared for in a specified time period.

The ability to compare an agency's performance (benchmark) with the performance of other agencies makes it possible to set realistic patient outcome goals. Although one would hope that patients who receive home health care services would experience improvements in their clinical and functional status, one must question whether that expectation is realistic. Do you think that it is reasonable to expect 100% of patients who report pain at the start of care to experience an improvement by discharge? If a 100% rate of improvement is expected and not achieved, does that mean that an agency's care is inadequate, or does it mean that it is not a realistic goal?

If benchmarking against other agencies reveals that approximately 70% of all home care patients experience an improvement in outcome, would you still consider the 100% expectation realistic? When looking at your agency's performance, is it important to compare it to a large sample of other agencies? You might question:

- If an agency's performance is better than others, how much better is it? Is it significantly better?

- Can the agency's performance in this area be attributed to a commitment to improve pain management?

- Has the agency conducted educational programs for the staff to improve their ability to manage pain?

- If an agency consistently performs better than all other agencies in the area of improvement in

pain management, has it identified a "best practice" that should be shared with other agencies?

To help answer some of these questions, the Centers for Medicare & Medicaid Services (CMS) has facilitated the development of the Outcome-Based Quality Improvement (OBQI) and Outcome-Based Quality Monitoring (OBQM) Reports. These reports are created by analyzing all of the OASIS data that is encoded and transmitted to the state and federal OASIS computers.

Once the statistical analysis is complete, the information is presented in three agency-specific reports. The Adverse Event Outcome Report (Figure 7-1), the Patient Outcome Report (Figure 7-2), and the Case Mix Report (Figure 7-3) all provide the agency with information on how its patient outcome results compared with all other agencies who contributed their OASIS data. Through the use of a secure web site, agencies are able to download their individual reports at will.

Outcome-Based Quality Monitoring

Despite an agency's best effort, it is not uncommon for a patient to experience a decline in condition or an adverse event. The OBQM Report provides the agency with a means to compare its incidence of adverse event outcomes during a specified time period with all other agencies that contributed data during the same period.

Figure 7-1 provides a sample of one agency's Adverse Event Outcome Report. A preliminary review of the report reveals a list of patients who received emergent care for an injury caused by a fall or accident at home. An agency's incidence is calculated by dividing the number of patients who experienced the adverse event (9) by the total number of patients in the same time period (572). For this agency, the incidence is 1.6%.

Like one blood pressure reading, one adverse event report does not tell the agency much about its overall performance until it is benchmarked (compared). The agency may choose to benchmark its

FIGURE 7-1: ADVERSE EVENT OUTCOME REPORT

Agency Name: Faircare Home Health Services
Agency ID: HHA01
Location: Anytown, USA
Medicare Number: 007001
Medicaid Number: 999888001

Requested Current Period: 09/1999-08/2000
Actual Current Period: 09/1999-08/2000
Number of Cases in Current Period: 601
Number of Cases in Reference Sample: 29983
Date Report Printed: 11/30/2000

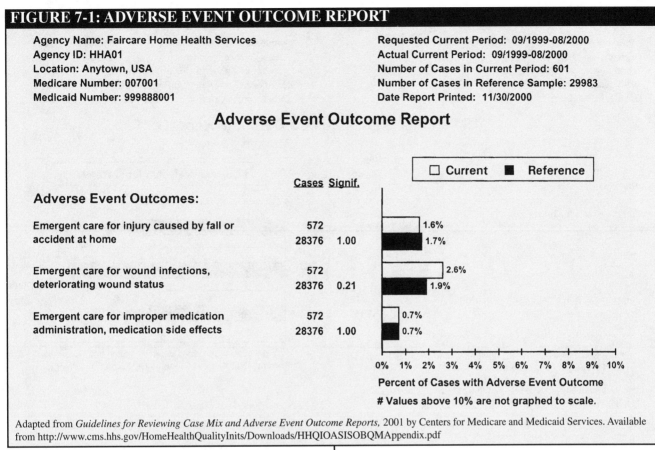

Adapted from *Guidelines for Reviewing Case Mix and Adverse Event Outcome Reports,* 2001 by Centers for Medicare and Medicaid Services. Available from http://www.cms.hhs.gov/HomeHealthQualityInits/Downloads/HHQIOASISOBQMAppendix.pdf

performance from month to month or may choose to benchmark against the performance of all other agencies, commonly referred to as the "reference group." Whichever option the agency chooses, paying close attention to the adverse events that agency patients experience might provide the agency with some insight into areas of weakness in its clinical services.

When looking at this report, it would not be uncommon for agency staff to become defensive and list a number of reasons why they feel these adverse outcomes occurred. It is important to listen to the staff's theory about why these events occurred, but it is even more important to attempt to identify the actual reason for occurrence. If a lot of time is spent trying to undermine the credibility of the report, the opportunity to avoid future adverse events could be lost. For this reason, many agencies review the medical records of the patients who experienced an adverse event. The review of these records might reveal trends in diagnoses, cli-

nicians, or services. If a trend is identified, the agency can then work to identify strategies that might be beneficial in decreasing the occurrence of the adverse event.

When reviewing any of these outcome reports, a column titled "Signif." will be found. The level of significance is a statistical value that identifies the probability that the difference between your agency and the reference group is due to chance. Levels of significance are usually presented as numbers that are less than 1.0. The smaller the number, the more likely (or the higher the probability) that the difference in performance is the result of something that the agency is (or is not) doing. In general, levels of less than 0.5 are accepted as clinically significant. This means that less than 5% of the time, the results would be attributed to chance.

The significance value is an important part of the report because it helps the agency to determine if the difference in its performance when compared with the reference group is a random variation or

FIGURE 7-2: PATIENT OUTCOME REPORT

Agency Name: FAIRCARE HOME HEALTH SERVICES
Agency ID: HHA01
Location: ANYTOWN, USA
Medicare Number: 007001
Medicaid Number: 999888001

Requested Current Period: 01/2001 - 12/2001
Actual Current Period: 01/2001 - 12/2001
Number of Cases in Current Period: 374
Number of Cases in Natl Ref Sample: 357978
Date Report Printed: 02/28/2002

All Patients' Risk Adjusted Outcome Report

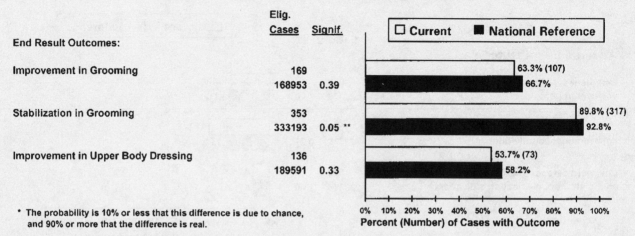

End Result Outcomes:	Elig. Cases	Signif.	
Improvement in Grooming	169		63.3% (107)
	168953	0.39	66.7%
Stabilization in Grooming	353		89.8% (317)
	333193	0.05 **	92.8%
Improvement in Upper Body Dressing	136		53.7% (73)
	189591	0.33	58.2%

Percent (Number) of Cases with Outcome

* The probability is 10% or less that this difference is due to chance, and 90% or more that the difference is real.

** The probability is 5% or less that this difference is due to chance, and 95% or more that the difference is real.

Adapted from *Guidelines for Reviewing Case Mix and Adverse Event Outcome Reports,* 2001 by Centers for Medicare and Medicaid Services. Available from http://www.cms.hhs.gov/HomeHealthQualityInits/Downloads/HHQIOASISOBQMAppendix.pdf

FIGURE 7-3: CASE MIX REPORT

Agency Name: Faircare Home Health Services
Agency ID: HHA01
Location: Anytown, USA
Medicare Number: 007001
Medicaid Number: 999888001

Requested Current Period: 09/1999-08/2000
Actual Current Period: 09/1999-08/2000
Number of Cases in Current Period: 601
Number of Cases in Reference Sample: 29983
Date Report Printed: 11/30/2000

All Patients' Case Mix Profile at Start/Resumption of Care

	Current Mean	Reference Mean	Sig.
Demographics			
Age (average in years)	70.75	72.78	**
Gender: Female (%)	69.4%	62.9%	**
Race: Black (%)	1.7%	10.7%	**
Race: White (%)	97.5%	85.5%	**
Race: Other (%)	0.8%	3.8%	**

Adapted from *Guidelines for Reviewing Case Mix and Adverse Event Outcome Reports,* 2001 by Centers for Medicare and Medicaid Services. Available from http://www.cms.hhs.gov/HomeHealthQualityInits/Downloads/HHQIOASISOBQMAppendix.pdf

representative of a true difference in performance. In Figure 7-1, the level of significance was calculated at 1.0, which means the difference between the performance of the agency and the reference group is likely to be the result of random variation and not the result of the agency's performance.

Outcome-Based Quality Improvement

The second report available to agencies is the Risk Adjusted Outcome Report. This report provides a graphical depiction of an agency's end-result and utilization outcomes.

As previously discussed, an *end-result outcome* is defined as the patient's change in health status between two points in time. Although patient outcomes are primarily measured as improvements, it is also possible for a patient to stabilize (experience no change) or to experience a decline in functional or clinical status.

There are 41 patient outcomes that can be measured (see Table 7-1). Because the acuity of patients can vary from one agency to the next, the Center for Healthcare Policy and Research applies statistical techniques to the data to minimize the influence of factors that might impact the agency's outcomes. The application of these techniques is commonly known as "risk adjusting." Twenty-six of the outcomes on the report are risk-adjusted.

For example, assume that My Town Visiting Nurse Association (VNA) receives a large number of its referrals from a post-acute rehabilitation stroke unit, and the majority of these patients demonstrate a high level of functional dependence. When completing the OASIS, My Town VNA will have low scores in the ADL and IADL sections of the assessment. The outcome report for My Town VNA may demonstrate a large number of stabilized outcomes and fewer improved outcomes.

Across town, Global Home Health Care accepts the majority of its referrals from an acute care hospital that is renowned for its care of cardiac patients. Global's patients are usually referred to home care after experiencing a 3- to 4-day hospitalization. The typical patient admitted by this agency receives six or seven home health care visits and is then discharged to outpatient cardiac rehabilitation. In terms of the OASIS, the majority of Global's patients demonstrate a high level of functional independence and return to complete independence by the time they are discharged. The Risk Adjusted Outcome Report for Global Home Health Care

---

TABLE 7-1: END-RESULT PATIENT OUTCOMES*

• Improvement in Grooming	• Stabilization in Housekeeping
• Improvement in Dressing Upper Body	• Stabilization in Shopping
• Improvement in Dressing Lower Body	• Stabilization in Phone Use
• Improvement in Bathing	• Stabilization in Management of Oral Medications
• Improvement in Toileting	• Improvement in Speech or Language
• Improvement in Transferring	• Improvement in Pain Interfering with Activity
• Improvement in Ambulation/Locomotion	• Improvement in Number of Surgical Wounds
• Improvement in Eating	• Improvement in Status of Surgical Wounds
• Improvement in Light Meal Preparation	• Improvement in Dyspnea
• Improvement in Laundry	• Improvement in Urinary Tract Infection
• Improvement in Housekeeping	• Improvement in Urinary Incontinence
• Improvement in Shopping	• Improvement in Bowel Incontinence
• Improvement in Phone Use	• Improvement in Behavior Problem Frequency
• Improvement in Management of Oral Medications	• Improvement in Cognitive Functioning
• Stabilization in Grooming	• Improvement in Confusion Frequency
• Stabilization in Bathing	• Improvement in Anxiety Level
• Stabilization in Transferring	• Stabilization in Speech or Language
• Stabilization in Light Meal Preparation	• Stabilization in Cognitive Functioning
• Stabilization in Laundry	• Stabilization in Anxiety Level

* End-result outcomes are health status outcomes.

Note. From "OASIS-C Guidance Manual" by Centers for Medicare & Medicaid Services, 2009, *OASIS User Manual*. Washington, DC: U.S. Government Printing Office. Available online from http://www.cms.gov/HomeHealthQualityInits/14_HHQIOASISUserManual.asp

reveals a large number of improved outcomes and few that only stabilized.

From the examples above, it is clear that the type of patients an agency admits to its caseload can have an impact on its Patient Outcome Report. The process of risk adjusting allows a statistical comparison of the factors that result from the characteristics of the patients. Risk adjusting is necessary to ensure that the outcomes reported are the result of patient care and not underlying characteristics of the patients. In essence, risk adjusting allows agencies to compare apples to apples and not apples to oranges.

The utilization outcomes provided in Table 7-2 provide the agency with the type of services its patients used while they were active or the services its patients required at the time of discharge. As stated above, utilization outcomes can be greatly influenced by the characteristics of the agency's patient population.

Case Mix Report

The third and final report is the Case Mix Report (see Figure 7-3). Like the two previous reports, this report provides the agency with notations when its results are statistically significant. The Case Mix Report provides the agency with a description of all of the patients who have been included in the two reports previously outlined. The description includes patient demographics, such as age, living situation, and presence of a primary caregiver. In addition, the Case Mix Report provides a summary of some of the OASIS data collected. The report allows the agency to identify trends in diagnosis, medical condition, and clinical and functional status of patients in the sample.

Finally, the Case Mix Report provides the agency with information related to discharge disposition and length of stay.

This report helps the agency to identify in detail the characteristics of the patients it serves and may influence the agency's decisions related to resource utilization and allocation. Differences like those between My Town VNA and Global Home Health Care become obvious.

OBQM OR OBQI?

Now that the three reports available to agencies have been reviewed, it is important to differentiate between OBQM and OBQI. Although these acronyms are often used interchangeably, they do represent different approaches to quality management.

In short, the monitoring of data does not impact the delivery of patient care. For instance, the Adverse Event Outcome Report lists the patients who experienced a negative outcome. The disadvantage to using only this report is that it can only identify variations in an agency's performance after they have occurred. Although the agency can then review patient medical records to identify what happened, it is too late to change the negative effects it had on the patients.

The OBQI Report provides the agency with an opportunity to analyze current performance and make the changes in the care delivery process necessary to ensure that the patient does not experience a negative or adverse outcome. The use of this report provides an opportunity to identify areas of weakness, implement measures to improve identified

TABLE 7-2: UTILIZATION OUTCOMES	
• Any Emergent Care Provided • Acute Care Hospitalization	• Discharged to the Community

* Utilization outcomes suggest but do not unequivocally reflect health status changes (and, as a result, can be regarded as proxy or surrogate outcomes).

Note. From "OASIS-C Guidance Manual" by Centers for Medicare & Medicaid Services, 2009, *OASIS User Manual*. Washington, DC: U.S. Government Printing Office. Available online from http://www.cms.gov/HomeHealthQualityInits/14_HHQIOASISUserManual.asp

weaknesses, and evaluate the effectiveness of the changes made.

The CMS makes agency performance on 12 outcomes available to the public on the Medicare website (www.medicare.gov). Providing agency-specific information to consumers is intended to allow them to choose the agency with the "best" performance in their area of need. For example, if you are seeking a home health agency to assist you or a family member to deal with issues of incontinence, you can now identify each home health agency's outcome score in this area.

Searching the CMS website by zip code even provides a consumer with the opportunity to compare the outcome scores of several different agencies in the same geographic area and choose the "best" performer. Over the last several years, CMS has changed the outcomes that have publicly reported scores. Table 7-3 provides a listing of current agency-specific outcomes as of January 2010. The CMS has converted the OASIS M0 item language to a more consumer-friendly statement and has provided a feature that allows consumers to print a graphical comparison of agencies.

As a field nurse, you might be thinking "So what? Why do I care about this information? All I want to do is take care of my patients." Remember, all of this information begins with one nurse and one patient. How the nurse assesses that patient and answers the OASIS items not only impacts the agency's financial health (as will be described in Chapter 8) but also its publicly reported outcomes.

BEST CLINICAL PRACTICES

The CMS continues to raise the quality expectations and standards for all certified home health agencies across the country. Recognizing that changing and standardizing clinical practice will ultimately improve patient outcomes requires a significant amount of scarce agency resources. The CMS has historically provided support through each state's Quality Improvement Organization (QIO). While the current scope of work by the QIOs is not specific to home care, quality improvement interventions and associated tools, toolkits, presentations, and links to resources, including clin-

TABLE 7-3: CURRENT AGENCY-SPECIFIC OUTCOMES AS OF APRIL 2010

- Three measures related to improvement in getting around:
  - Percentage of patients who get better at walking or moving around
  - Percentage of patients who get better at getting in and out of bed
  - Percentage of patients who have less pain when moving around

- Four measures related to meeting the patient's activities of daily living:
  - Percentage of patients whose bladder control improves
  - Percentage of patients who get better at bathing
  - Percentage of patients who get better at taking their medicines correctly (by mouth)
  - Percentage of patients who are short of breath less often

- Two measures about how home health care ends:
  - Percentage of patients who stay at home after an episode of home health care ends
  - NEW! Percentage of patients whose wounds improved or healed after an operation

- Three measures related to patient medical emergencies:
  - Percentage of patients who had to be admitted to the hospital
  - Percentage of patients who need urgent, unplanned medical care
  - NEW! Percentage of patients who need unplanned medical care related to a wound that is new, is worse, or has become infected

Note. From *Home Health Compare,* by U.S. Department of Health & Human Services, 2008. Retrieved June 23, 2010, from http://www.medicare.gov/HH Compare/Home.asp?version=default&browser=IE%7C7%7CWinXP&language=English&defaultstatus=0&pagelist=Home&CookiesEnabledStatus=True

ical tools, continue to be available on the Medicare Quality Improvement Community (MedQIC) Web site at http://www.qualitynet.org/dcs/ContentServer?c=MQParents&pagename=Medqic%2FContent%2FParentShellTemplate&cid=1089990236808&parentName=Setting.

The Home Health Quality Improvement (HHQI) National Campaign is a grassroots movement designed to unite home health stakeholders and multiple health care settings under a shared vision of reducing avoidable hospitalizations and improving medication management. Home care agencies can join HHQI by registering online. Access to agency data reports and tools to set outcome targets are available. The first Best Practice Intervention Package (BPIP) was released in January 2010, addressing reduction of acute care hospitalizations. A schedule of future BPIPs can be found on the Home Health Quality Improvement web page at http://www.homehealthquality.org/hh/default.aspx.

Before an agency selects a tool to use in the development of its best practice standard, it should complete an extensive record review to determine its exact area of clinical weakness. If this step is skipped, the agency might find that it has implemented what it thought was a best clinical practice standard that did not result in an improvement of its publicly reported outcomes. How? Without knowing exactly what the specific area of weakness is, the agency might have implemented a tool that is not necessary.

For example, if the agency's clinicians already complete a thorough and accurate patient assessment but do not implement interventions to address the problems found on the assessment, it will do the agency no good to change the assessment. What the agency needs to do is to determine that it is not the assessment that is the weakness, but that the staff could use assistance with planning interventions. Completing such a "process of care" investigation is a laborious process that the agency cannot afford to skip. Each agency must develop a best clinical practice based on its unique patient population and areas of weakness.

To consistently improve patient outcomes, the agency has to reduce the clinician-to-clinician variability of care provision. Clinician-to-clinician variability occurs when similar patients receive differing levels of care. The differing levels of care may be the result of a clinician's experience, education, or skill. The development of a best clinical practice guideline is an effective means to accomplish this task. You might be asked (or volunteer) to participate in a quality improvement team to help develop your agency's best clinical practice to improve one of the publicly reported outcomes.

Consider an improvement effort to improve the outcome score for urinary incontinence. A process of care investigation has determined that:

Clinical Weakness #1: The assessment of a patient's continence status is inadequate and varies from clinician to clinician.

The agency's first best clinical practice statement might be:

Best Clinical Practice #1: All patients who score other than a 0 on M1610 will receive a comprehensive continence assessment identifying the type of incontinence that best describes the patient's clinical situation.

A review of the literature would provide guidance in assessing the types and characteristics associated with different types of chronic urinary incontinence (Dowling-Castronovo & Bradway, 2008):

- *Stress incontinence:* involuntary loss of urine associated with activities that increase intra-abdominal pressure such as coughing or sneezing.

- *Urge incontinence:* involuntary loss of urine associated with a strong urge to void; patients may have leaking on the way to the bathroom. The patient may have frequency, nocturia and enuresis. Causes may include changes in the bladder associated with aging.

- *Overflow incontinence:* involuntary loss of urine associated with bladder over-distention; causes include under-active detrusor muscle or outlet obstruction causing over-distention. The patient may complain of urine leakage, dribbling, retention, hesitancy, sensation of bladder fullness or pressure.

- *Functional incontinence:* inability to be independent in voiding, most often from cognitive or physical impairments that limit the patient's ability to get to the bathroom/remember to go rather than urological or genital causes.

An assessment will act as your foundational urinary incontinence improvement tool. In addition, you might determine that the staff needs additional education and resources to improve their competence and skills in this area. You might search the literature for educational tools. The implementation of this best practice standard provides a measurable standard that the agency can use in its compliance monitoring.

Depending on other areas of weakness in the agency, additional best clinical practice standards might include:

Clinical Weakness #2: Not all patients experiencing urinary incontinence have strategies to improve incontinence consistently addressed in the plan of care.

Best Clinical Practice #2: All patients experiencing urinary incontinence will have the interventions found in the Managing Urinary Incontinence – Patient Self-Care Workbook (Appendix I) included in their plans of care, or barriers to intervention will be documented.

A review of the resource package reveals that before a urinary incontinence care plan can be established, the clinician must determine a patient's bladder habits. Understanding when incontinence occurs is crucial to the development of appropriate and effective interventions. Determining trends in urinary incontinence occurrences (e.g., during the

night, only in the morning, or after taking diuretics) is important information for care plan development; therefore, a bladder diary is a best clinical practice.

Clinical Weakness #3: Clinical staff are not consistently identifying bladder habits for all patients who score other than a 0 (on incontinence or catheter) on M1610.

Best Clinical Practice #3: For all patients experiencing urinary incontinence, identification of bladder habits will be documented using the Bladder Diary (in Appendix I).

A review of the literature in the resource package reveals that pelvic floor (Kegel) exercises are an important intervention for improving urinary incontinence. However, to be effective, they must be practiced on a consistent basis. As a result, patient compliance with this intervention is often problematic. Therefore, to change clinical practice and ensure an improvement in patient outcomes, the following best clinical practices should be considered.

Clinical Weakness #4: All patients experiencing urinary incontinence are not consistently taught to perform pelvic muscle floor exercises.

Best Clinical Practice #4: All patients experiencing urinary incontinence will be taught to perform pelvic muscle floor exercises utilizing the techniques found in the Managing Urinary Incontinence – Patient Self-Care Workbook (Appendix I).

Clinical Weakness #5: Patients do not consistently follow-through with pelvic muscle floor exercises.

Best Clinical Practice #5: Patients will be given the Pelvic Floor Exercise Log found in Managing Urinary Incontinence – Patient Self-Care Workbook and instructed in its use (Appendix I).

Although this is a brief example of the development of a best clinical practice, the process can be quite long. Once staff is educated and their skill levels enhanced, interventions can be implemented. Monitoring of compliance with the new best clinical practice standard is crucial to ensure that clinician-to-clinician variability is eliminated. New staff will need to be taught the information and best practice standard during their orientation period. Remember, the actual publicly reported improvement scores may take several months to change. Therefore, it is necessary for the agency's internal quality monitoring process to be implemented to ensure the improvement efforts will be reflected in the agency's future score.

SUMMARY

Through the use of Adverse Event Outcome Reports, OBQI Reports, and the Case Mix Report, agencies have data that describe their performance as it compares with reference groups. The identification of statistically significant variations allows the agency to focus its performance improvement efforts on areas that will not only effect care of the individual patient but also put the agency in a position to flourish in a highly competitive and regulated environment.

Through the use of home health report cards, consumers, physicians, and other community providers are able to compare the performance of all of the agencies in their geographic location. This comparison is intended to assist the consumer with choosing the agency that meets their needs and provides the "best" clinical and functional outcomes.

EXAM QUESTIONS

CHAPTER 7
Questions 78-85

Note: Choose the one option that BEST answers each question.

78. Prior to the implementation of OASIS, an agency's performance improvement initiatives were

    a. nonexistent.

    b. subjective in nature.

    c. most often aimed at improving the process of care delivery.

    d. complex and ineffective.

79. An outcome can be determined

    a. at the completion of the OASIS Start of Care assessment.

    b. whenever the patient achieves the goals on the physician-certified plan of care.

    c. when the agency is able to compare the same patient at two points in time.

    d. when the patient returns the post-discharge satisfaction survey.

80. Using the OASIS assessment data that follows, compare the patient's status at the start of care and at discharge. When reviewing these results, one can determine that the patient experienced

    a. a stabilized outcome.

    b. an improved outcome.

    c. a declined outcome.

    d. an indeterminable outcome.

Start of Care OASIS Assessment

(M1400) When is the patient dyspneic or noticeably Short of Breath?

☐	0-	Never, patient is not short of breath
■	1-	When walking more than 20 feet, climbing stairs
☐	2-	With moderate exertion (e.g., while dressing, using commode or bedpan, walking distances less than 20 feet)
☐	3-	With minimal exertion (e.g., while eating, talking, or performing other ADLs) or with agitation
☐	4-	At rest (during day or night)

Discharge OASIS Assessment

(M1400) When is the patient dyspneic or noticeably Short of Breath?

☐	0-	Never, patient is not short of breath
■	1-	When walking more than 20 feet, climbing stairs
☐	2-	With moderate exertion (e.g., while dressing, using commode or bedpan, walking distances less than 20 feet)
☐	3-	With minimal exertion (e.g., while eating, talking, or performing other ADLs) or with agitation
☐	4-	At rest (during day or night)

81. Care processes as measured by OASIS-C

    a. are required by CMS for implementation.

    b. are only included in the Discharge OASIS.

    c. include the use of assessment tools in the planning of specific clinical interventions.

    d. will not be publicly reported.

82. OBQM

    a. does not provide the agency with useful data.

    b. should only be used as a quality measure when the agency has identified the existence of a problem.

    c. provides the agency with a means to compare its incidence of adverse event outcomes to those of other agencies.

    d. provides a graphical depiction of end-result and utilization outcomes.

83. The level of significance

    a. is only important in validating that the agency's performance is better than all others in the reference group.

    b. is only important in validating that the agency's performance is worse than all others in the reference group.

    c. assists the agency to determine if the difference in its performance compared with the reference group is a random variation or representative of a true difference in performance.

    d. is too complex for most agencies to effectively evaluate.

84. The process of risk adjustment

    a. is only important in validating that the agency's performance is better than all others in the reference group.

    b. is only important in validating that the agency's performance is worse than all others in the reference group.

    c. ensures that the outcomes are the result of patient care and not the characteristics of the patient.

    d. is too complex for most agencies to engage in.

85. A best clinical practice standard is intended to

    a. have no impact on the agency's outcome scores.

    b. reduce clinician-to-clinician variations in the delivery of patient care.

    c. prevent staff from having to make clinical judgments.

    d. use anecdotal information and apply it to all similar patients.

CHAPTER 8

REIMBURSEMENT OF HOME HEALTH SERVICES

CHAPTER OBJECTIVE

After completing this chapter, the reader will be able to discuss payment mechanisms for home health care reimbursement.

LEARNING OBJECTIVES

After studying this chapter, the reader will be able to

1. state how case mix management can significantly improve the financial performance of a home health care agency.

2. differentiate between a full episode and a low utilization payment.

3. specify which services are bundled into the Medicare episodic payment.

INTRODUCTION

Most of us did not choose nursing as a profession because it is glamorous. We are not usually excited to work every other weekend and holiday. Most of us do not enjoy rotating shifts and being subjected to mandatory overtime. There is no thrill in working short staffed and being required to complete volumes of paperwork to validate our contribution to patient care. We are nurses because of a desire to care for people.

The Code of Ethics for Nurses dictates that all patients should receive care regardless of race, religion, sexual orientation, age, or ability to pay (American Nurses Association, 2001). However, the reality is that very few nurses volunteer their time, knowledge, and skills to their employers. Nurses expect to be fairly compensated for the skills and services they provide. In fact, by exercising the right to participate in collective bargaining, some nurses have picketed to improve working conditions and wages. At the same time, it is naïve not to acknowledge the nursing role in the financial health of the organizations where nurses are employed.

Now, more than ever, home health nurses are being held accountable for providing patients with a clinically appropriate level of service. It is imperative that home health nurses differentiate between the "wants" and "needs" of patients. Surely, there are hundreds (maybe even thousands) of patients who want a daily visit from a home health care nurse. The question that must be answered is: Does the patient *need* that level of intensive service? Since the implementation of the Medicare prospective payment system (PPS), unnecessary visits can quickly jeopardize the financial health of an entire organization.

In theory, home health reimbursement is simple. There are generally two payment mechanisms for home health care: fee-for-service and prospective payment. Because Medicare is the largest purchaser of home health care services, the PPS will be presented first, followed by a description of fee-for-service payment systems.

MEDICARE PROSPECTIVE PAYMENT SYSTEM

Simply stated, in the PPS, Medicare provides one lump sum to an agency to provide all of the beneficiary's home care required for a 60-day period. This lump sum is adjusted up or down based on the patient's acuity as it is documented on selected OASIS assessment questions. The Medicare PPS, originally implemented in 2000, became effective January 2008. The necessity for accuracy in scoring OASIS items has become even greater since then to ensure that the agency receives optimal reimbursement for each patient. In addition to the primary diagnosis, the first five secondary diagnoses contribute to the scoring that determines reimbursement. Certain diagnoses, along with OASIS item coding, may interact together to increase payment. Accurate diagnosis coding is also essential to ensure payment for medical supplies, a significant agency cost. The 2008 PPS changes are complicated and, most often, agencies depend on certified or coding experts to ensure that diagnoses are listed and coded correctly.

As with all things, the "devil is in the detail," and Medicare PPS is no exception. The principles of case mix, episodic payment, low utilization payment adjustments, bundling of supplies and outpatient services, therapy add-ons, and outlier payments will be fully explained in the remainder of this chapter.

Principle One: Case Mix

PPS reimbursement to the agency is based on averages. With some patients, the agency may achieve a profitable episode, and with others, the agency may experience a financial loss. Fiscal viability requires agencies to closely balance profitable and losing episodes. If the agency experiences too many losing episodes, it will quickly find its financial soundness in jeopardy. The mechanism by which this balance of profit and loss is achieved is called "case mix adjusting" or "case mix management."

Case mix management requires the agency to understand exactly what types of patients are referred and the amount of service and visits these patients typically receive. In a small agency, one patient who requires twice-daily home health care aide (HCA) and nursing can lead to financial instability or ruin. How can one patient have such an impact? Consider the detailed case of Mr. Bailey outlined below.

Mr. Bailey

Mr. Bailey is an 84-year-old patient who is known to My Town VNA. Mr. Bailey's physician prescribed nursing visits once a month for the injection of vitamin B12 to treat his pernicious anemia. As a result of a surgery to remove Mr. Bailey's ruptured gallbladder, the intake department received a referral from the local hospital requesting an increase in agency services. Mr. Bailey experienced a postoperative complication resulting in an opening of his surgical wound. The opening is currently infected and requires daily dressing changes. In addition, the hospital is requesting HCA services and physical therapy (PT).

Although Mr. Bailey is able to ambulate short distances with a walker, the hospital's discharge planner has already requested home-delivered meals and homemaking services. Mr. Bailey is a Medicare beneficiary, and the patient assessment reveals the scored questions from the OASIS profile outlined in Figures 8-1, 8-2, and 8-3.

Note: For the purposes of this chapter, all points assigned in Chapter 8 figures are based on a first episode from Table 4 in Appendix J. With the advent of OASIS-C in 2010 the OASIS item numbering system changed, though there was no change in the actual items used to determine payment. The nurse must recognize that reimburse-

FIGURE 8-1: MR. BAILEY'S OASIS CLINICAL SCORING DETAIL

	Question	Response	Point Value
M0110	Is the Medicare home health payment episode for which this assessment will define a case mix group an "early" or "later" episode in the patient's current or first or sequence of adjacent Medicare home health payment episodes?	1-Early (the only episode or first or second episode in a sequence of adjacent episodes)	NA
M1020	Primary diagnosis: Disruption of external surgical wound 998.32		2
M1022	Other diagnosis: Weakness, generalized		0
M1022	Other diagnosis: Pernicious anemia		2
M1022	Other diagnosis: Aftercare following GI		0
M1024	Payment diagnosis: cholelithiases		2
M1030	Therapies the patient receives at home	4 – none of the above	0
M1200	Vision with corrective lenses if the patient usually wears them	0-normal vision	0
M1242	Frequency of pain interfering with activity	3 – Daily but not constantly	1
M1308	Current number of unhealed (non-epithelialized) pressure ulcers at each stage	0-none	0
M1322	Current number of Stage I pressure ulcers	0 – none	0
M1330	Does this patient have a stasis ulcer?	No stasis ulcer	0
M1342	Status most problematic (observable) surgical wound	3 – Not healing	4
M1400	When is patient dyspneic or noticeably short of breath?	2-With moderate exertion	2
M1610	Urinary incontinence or urinary catheter present	0 – No incontinence or catheter	0
M1620	Bowel incontinence frequency	0 – Very rarely or never	0
M1630	Ostomy for bowel elimination	0 – None	0
M2030	Management of injectable medications	2 – Unable to take injectable medications unless administered by another person.	1
TOTAL CLINICAL POINTS			**14**

(Home Health Resource Grouper [HHRG], 2010)

FIGURE 8-2: MR. BAILEY'S OASIS FUNCTIONAL SCORING DETAIL

Question	Response	Point Value
M1810 Ability to dress upper body (with or without dressing aids)	0-Able upper body without assistance	0
M1820 Ability to dress lower body (with or without dressing aids)	2-Someone must help patient dress lower body	0
M1830 Bathing: Ability to wash entire body	2-Able to bathe with the assistance of another person	3
M1840 Toileting: Ability to get to and from the toilet or bedside commode and safely transfer on and off the toilet or commode	0-Able to get to and from the toilet or commode and transfer independently	0
M1850 Transferring: Ability to move from bed to chair, and ability to turn and position self in bed if patient is bedfast	1-Transfers with minimal assistance or with use of an assistive device	0
M1860 Ambulation/locomotion: Ability to safely walk once in a standing position, or use a wheelchair once in a seated position, on a variety of surfaces	1-Requires/uses a one-handed device	1
TOTAL FUNCTIONAL POINTS		4

(HHRG, 2010)

FIGURE 8-3: MR. BAILEY'S OASIS SERVICE UTILIZATION SCORING DETAIL

Question	Response
M2200 Therapy need: In the home health plan of care for the Medicare payment episode for which this assessment will define a case mix group, what is the indicated need for therapy visits (total number of reasonable and necessary physical, occupational, and speech-language pathology visits combined?)	12
Based on the completion of the OASIS for Mr. Bailey, his severity levels in the Clinical (C), Functional (F), and Service Utilization (S – based on number of therapy visits) in a first episode of care is C3F1S5, with an expected episode reimbursement of $4016.13 (Calculated from CMS, 2007, Table 5: Case-Mix Groups, Average Cost, and Case-Mix Weight)	

(HHRG, 2010)

ment rates fluctuate and change. The purpose of the case examples in this chapter is to demonstrate how OASIS items are used in payment and the importance of OASIS accuracy in determination of payment. See Appendix J.

From Mr. Bailey's OASIS assessment, it is evident that he has many deficits. Based on the combination of the OASIS answers, the agency will receive $4016.13 to provide all of Mr. Bailey's care. Additionally, based on diagnostic coding, including a nonhealing surgical wound (M1342),

the agency can also bill for nonroutine dressing supplies at $207.76 (CMS, 2007).

At Mr. Bailey's start of care (SOC), the physician orders for the plan of care are found in Figure 8-4. At the SOC, the plan of treatment established for Mr. Bailey appears to be clinically appropriate. Now consider the cost of providing this same level of service to him for the next 60-day period. Assume that My Town VNA's average costs per visit are approximately:

FIGURE 8-4: MR. BAILEY'S PHYSICIAN-ORDERED PLAN OF CARE

Orders for Discipline and Treatments (Specify Amount/Frequency/Duration)

- *Skilled Nursing* 1 visit/day x 60 days to perform dressing change to abdominal wound. Wound care – lightly pack wound with hydrogel impregnated gauze; cover with ABD. Skilled nursing p.r.n. x 4 visits for excessive drainage, dislodged dressing, or complaints of pain. Skilled nursing to perform the administration of vitamin B$_{12}$. Skilled nursing to assess vital signs, wound healing, pain, hydration, nutrition, mobility, safety, and bowel function. Instruct in pain management including use of analgesics and monitor response. Notify MD if fever > 101° F or if signs of wound infection including purulent drainage.

- *Physical Therapy* 3 times/week for up to 4 weeks to perform home safety evaluation, strengthening, and gait training. Patient to progress from walker to cane.

- *Home Health Care Aide* 1 visit/day x 60 days under the direct supervision of skilled nurse or therapist to assist the patient with ADLs, including transfer to shower.

- Registered nurse visits = $100/visit

- PT visit = $100/visit

- HCA visit = $25/visit.

By simply performing the math, the cost of Mr. Bailey's plan of treatment is estimated to be $8,687 (see Figure 8-5). The agency can expect to be reimbursed from Medicare $4,224. If this plan of treatment does not change, that is, if services are not reduced as Mr. Bailey's condition improves, the agency will lose $4,463 on this one case.

FIGURE 8-5: COSTS ASSOCIATED WITH MR. BAILEY'S PLAN OF CARE

Skilled Nursing
1 visit/day x $100/visit = $100/day x 60 days
= $6,000

Physical Therapy
3 visits/week x $100/visit = $300/week x 4
weeks = $1,200

Home Health Care Aide
7 visits/week x $25/visit = $175/week x
8.5 weeks = $1,487

Cost of Care = $8,687
Anticipated Medicare PPS Payment = $4,016
Anticipated Nonroutine Supply Payment = $208
Agency Profit/(Loss) = ($4,463)

As stated earlier, the Medicare PPS is based on averages. The case of Mr. Bailey illustrates why it is imperative to have a detailed understanding of the patients an agency serves, the expectations of the referring community, and the skills of the agency's clinicians. For every patient that represents a significant loss to the agency, there must be patients for whom the agency is able to generate a substantial profit. Mr. Dean represents such a case.

Mr. Dean

Mr. Dean is a 65-year-old patient who was referred to My Town VNA after a myocardial infarction (MI) and pacemaker insertion. His hospital course was also complicated by an occurrence of pulmonary edema. Until this MI, Mr. Dean has had a benign medical history.

Mr. Dean lives with his wife, who is supportive and is a recently retired certified nurse's aide. He was referred to My Town VNA for medication and diet teaching. Mr. Dean's physician has prescribed a titrating warfarin regimen, atenolol, and sublingual nitroglycerin tablets. He has also ordered a skilled nursing assessment of the pacemaker insertion site. Once the home health care nurse completes Mr. Dean's OASIS document, his Medicare PPS score is calculated (see Figures 8-6, 8-7, and 8-8).

Mr. Dean's plan of treatment is illustrated in Figure 8-9. Like Mr. Bailey's plan of treatment, the cost of providing this level of care to Mr. Dean can easily be calculated. The physician has ordered seven nursing visits for the entire 60-day period. We

FIGURE 8-6: MR. DEAN'S OASIS CLINICAL SCORING DETAIL

	Question	Response	Point Value
M0110	Is the Medicare home health payment episode for which this assessment will define a case mix group an "early" or "later" episode in the patient's current or first or sequence of adjacent Medicare home health payment episodes?	1-Early (the only episode or first or second episode in a sequence of adjacent episodes)	NA
M1020	Primary diagnosis: MI 410.42		2
M1022	Other diagnosis: pulmonary edema		0
M1022	Other diagnosis: Aftercare following surgery of the circulatory system		0
M1030	Therapies the patient receives at home	4 – none of the above	0
M1200	Vision with corrective lenses if the patient usually wears them	0-normal vision	0
M1242	Frequency of pain interfering with activity	3 – Daily but not constantly	1
M1308	Current number of unhealed (non-epithelialized) pressure ulcers at each stage	0-none	0
M1322	Current number of Stage I pressure ulcers	0 – none	0
M1330	Does this patient have a stasis ulcer?	No stasis ulcer	0
M1342	Status most problematic (observable) surgical wound	2-Early/partial granulation	0
M1400	When is patient dyspneic or noticeably short of breath?	2-With moderate exertion	2
M1610	Urinary incontinence or urinary catheter present	0 – No incontinence or catheter	0
M1620	Bowel incontinence frequency	0 – Very rarely or never	0
M1630	Ostomy for bowel elimination	0 – None	0
M2030	Management of injectable medications	NA – No injectable medications prescribed	0
	TOTAL CLINICAL POINTS		**5**

(HHRG, 2010)

already know that the cost of a nursing visit at My Town VNA is approximately $100; therefore, the anticipated cost for Mr. Dean's care will be $700. From the OASIS scoring, the agency anticipates a Medicare PPS payment of $1665, which leaves the agency with a profit of $965 (see Figure 8-10).

These two examples are realistic examples of patients found in home care, and they represent both extremes of care and the associated profit and loss. From a financial perspective, agencies would clearly prefer to care for patients who are similar to Mr. Dean as opposed to Mr. Bailey. In reality, the

FIGURE 8-7: MR. DEAN'S OASIS FUNCTIONAL SCORING DETAIL

Question	Response	Point Value
M1810 Ability to dress upper body (with or without dressing aids)	2-Someone must help patient dress upper body	2
M1820 Ability to dress lower body (with or without dressing aids)	0-Able to dress lower body without assistance	0
M1830 Bathing: Ability to wash entire body	0-Able to bathe in shower or tub independently	0
M1840 Toilet transferring: Ability to get to and from the toilet or bedside commode and safely transfer on and off the toilet or commode	0-Able to get to and from the toilet or commode and transfer independently	0
M1850 Transferring: Ability to move from bed to chair, and ability to turn and position self in bed if patient is bedfast	0-Able to independently transfer	0
M1860 Ambulation/locomotion: Ability to walk safely once in a standing position, or use a wheelchair once in a seated position, on a variety of surfaces	0-Able to walk independently on even and uneven surfaces and climb stairs with or without railings	0
TOTAL FUNCTIONAL POINTS		2

(HHRG, 2010)

FIGURE 8-8: MR. DEAN'S OASIS SERVICE UTILIZATION SCORING DETAIL

Question	Response
M2200 Therapy Need: In the home health plan of care for the Medicare payment episode for which this assessment will define a case mix group, what is the indicated need for therapy visits (total number of reasonable and necessary physical, occupational, and speech-language pathology visits combined?)	0

Based upon the completion of the OASIS for Mr. Dean, his severity levels in the Clinical (C), Functional (F), and Service Utilization (S – based on number of therapy visits) in a first episode of care is C2F1S1 with an expected episode reimbursement of $1665.19 (Calculated from CMS, 2007, Table 5: Case-Mix Groups, Average Cost, and Case-Mix Weight)

(HHRG, 2010)

FIGURE 8-9: MR. DEAN'S PHYSICIAN-ORDERED PLAN OF TREATMENT

Orders for Discipline and Treatments (Specify Amount/Frequency/Duration)

- *Skilled Nursing* 2 visits/week x 1 week, then 1 visit/week x 2 weeks, then 1 visit every other week x 3 weeks and p.r.n. x 2 visits for symptom management and complications related to medications or cardiac status. Skilled nurse to teach patient medication regimen, Coumadin titration, and diet restrictions. Skilled nursing to assess vital signs, medication and diet compliance, cardiac status, hydration, nutrition, and emergency plan. Instruct patient in pain management including analgesic use and monitor response. Report any signs of wound infection including temperature >101° F.

FIGURE 8-10: COSTS ASSOCIATED WITH MR. DEAN'S PLAN OF CARE

Skilled Nursing

7 visits/60 days x $100/visit = $ 700

Anticipated Medicare PPS Payment = $1,665

Agency Profit/(Loss) = $ 965

most common home health patient falls somewhere between the extreme loss associated with Mr. Bailey and the profit associated with Mr. Dean. It is important to remember that for every patient like Mr. Bailey, the agency needs approximately 11 patients as profitable as Mr. Dean to cover the cost.

From these examples, it is clear that the agency and its clinicians have to manage patients efficiently to minimize financial losses and maximize agency profits. Case mix management requires agencies to know which patients and diagnoses are most profitable to the agency and market to referral sources for these types of patients. Most agencies would not turn a case like Mr. Bailey away, but they certainly would not compete with other agencies to gets lots of referrals like his.

To further illustrate this point, consider the example of Happy Home Health Care (HHHC). HHHC is the largest provider of home health care services in their geographic location. Diabetes is one of the top three diagnoses that this agency admits to service. HHHC has a highly developed diabetes team, which includes:

- a certified diabetes educator (CDE)

- a certified ostomy, wound, continence nurse (CWOCN)

- a team of staff nurses who have participated in intensive training and demonstrated competence in diabetes management

- collaborative relationships with the local diabetic clinics and endocrinology physician practices.

For every Medicare PPS diabetes episode, HHHC averages a profit of $325; however, the agency is also aware that, although psychiatric diagnoses are also one of the top ten diagnoses that it receives, it does not have a highly specialized psychiatric care management team. In fact, they no longer have a psychiatric clinical nurse specialist, and their patient outcomes are not as positive as the agency would like.

HHHC also finds that its clinicians are providing a large number of nursing and HCA visits to the psychiatric patient population. As a group, the OASIS scoring profile for the psychiatric patients tends to be very low, translating into a low clinical and function acuity. For every Medicare beneficiary with a psychiatric diagnosis that HHHC admits to service, the agency loses approximately $250 per 60-day episode.

The Medicare PPS reimbursement system forces the management team at HHHC to face a very important decision. Should the agency continue to admit a category of patients that represent financial losses and inadequate patient outcomes? Figure 8-11 numerically outlines the simple problem that the agency must consider.

The profit generated by the expert and efficient management of the diabetes patients was lost to the agency through the inefficient management of the psychiatric patients. Based on this simplified example,

FIGURE 8-11: PROFITABILITY OF PATIENTS WITH DIABETES VERSUS PSYCHIATRIC DIAGNOSES

# Patients	Primary Diagnosis	Average P/(L) per episode*	Aggregate P/(L)*	Patient Outcomes
17	Diabetes	$325	$5565	Excellent
23	Psychiatric	($250)	($5750)	Marginal
			($185)	

* P-profit * (L)-loss

what do you think the management of HHHC should do? Here are some options:

- manage the agency's case mix by no longer accepting psychiatric cases

- increase the agency's marketing efforts to increase the number of diabetic patients and off-set the losses incurred from psychiatric patients

- reallocate agency resources to increase the skills of the agency's staff and develop a specialty team for psychiatric patients

- develop a partnership or collaborative relationship with other community-based providers of psychiatric services to improve the agency's patient and financial outcomes.

Although there is no "right" answer that is applicable to every agency, the decision to discontinue admitting psychiatric patients is a serious one and will not be taken lightly by the agency's administrator and board of directors.

The same principles of case mix management can also be applied to physicians or agency staff. Consider the comparison of Dr. Kolb and Dr. Stritter. Both of these physicians have internal medicine practices that provide a large number of referrals to your agency. Historically, Dr. Kolb aggressively manages her patients and makes frequent adjustments to her patient's medication regimen based on the patient's response as it is reported by the home health care nurse. Dr. Kolb usually implements the heart failure guidelines recommended by the Center for Health Care Policy and Research (CHCPR), and all of her patients are placed on angiotensin-converting enzyme (ACE) inhibitors.

Dr. Stritter also refers a significant number of heart failure patients to your agency; however, he manages his patients very differently than Dr. Kolb. He typically places his patients on digoxin and furosemide and tends to avoid the medications recommended by the CHCPR, stating, "Those drugs

are too expensive and have too many side effects." Although this statement has some level of truth, your agency has also noticed that Dr. Stritter's patients have a significantly longer length of stay and require many more skilled nursing visits than do Dr. Kolb's patients. Despite phone calls from the home health care nurse, Dr. Stritter rarely changes a home health plan of care without first seeing the patient or recommending that the patient return to the local emergency department instead of attempting to manage the patient's condition at home. Figure 8-12 depicts a side-by-side comparison of Dr. Kolb and Dr. Stritter during a 3-month period.

FIGURE 8-12: EFFECTS OF PHYSICIAN PRACTICE ON AGENCY PROFITABILITY		
	Dr. Kolb	**Dr. Stritter**
Number of heart failure patients referred	25	27
Average age	83	83
Average acuity	0.8703	0.8700
Changes in drug regimen	85%	15%
Patients rehospitalized in 60-day period	20%	48%
Average number of registered nurse visits per 60-day period	9	15
Discharge due to goals met	93%	79%
Average profit/(loss) per 60-day episode	$776	$176

Case mix management requires the agency's management team to evaluate whether it can afford to continue to take referrals from Dr. Stritter. The agency has clearly identified some differences between the practices of these two physicians and must decide if it is willing to continue to take risk for both financial and patient outcomes.

The same comparative analysis can be applied to agency clinicians. If a nurse or therapist tends to provide "extra" or unnecessary visits to a Medicare beneficiary, this will likely impact the agency's financial situation. As discussed in Chapter 6, the OASIS scoring provides a mechanism to clinically compare patients, and it is reasonable to expect that patients with similar acuity levels will require a similar number of home visits. If large variations in practice occur, it is likely that the agency will investigate the variations, assist clinicians with understanding the financial impact of their decisions, and assist them to develop more reasonable plans of care.

Principle Two: Episodic Payment

The implementation of the Medicare PPS on October 1, 2000, changed reimbursement to home health care agencies from a per-visit system to one that was episodic. In general, episodic payment is designed to make one payment for all of the home health care services that are provided to a beneficiary for a 60-day period.

Medicare PPS reimbursement begins and ends with the completion of a patient assessment. As discussed in Chapter 6, assessment data are collected and documented on the OASIS-C, which consists of approximately 100 federally mandated questions.

Selected OASIS questions are categorized into clinical severity (C), functional status (F), and service utilization (S). The CFS score determines the home health resource group (HHRG). The HHRG converts the OASIS score into a number that is similar to an acuity number. This determines the Medicare payment that the agency will receive to provide 60 days of home health services to a patient with that level of acuity. This was demonstrated in the cases of Mr. Bailey and Mr. Dean.

Acuity ranges from low, for a patient who has minimal clinical severity, functional status, or service utilization points (C1F1S1), to a patient who is in a completely dependent state and receives a maximum score of C3F4S5. With the 2008 changes in the PPS, the number of acuity categories increased from 81 to 153. Major changes in the PPS model

for 2008 include four different equations based on early episodes, later episodes, and the number of therapy visits. *Note:* The term *adjacent* refers to whether the patient received home care within the 60 previous days:

- early episodes (1st or 2nd adjacent episode) with fewer than 14 therapy visits
- early episodes (1st or 2nd adjacent episode) with 14 or more therapy visits
- later episode (3rd and later) with fewer than 14 therapy visits
- later episode (3rd and later) with 14 or more therapy visits

In essence, the scoring, and thus the amount of reimbursement, changes based on the episode timing and number of therapy visits.

Although the patient assessment questions that determine the episode payment do not vary, the episode payment is adjusted slightly depending on the geographic region, secondary to labor and wage index adjustments. Rural agencies have also been given consideration, and some slight increases have been made to their episode payments. Other than these two adjustments, the Medicare payment formula for home health services does not vary. Although episodic payment does not dictate service levels, it does limit the amount that Medicare will pay for home health services. At first glance, an episodic payment system may seem entirely appropriate and easy to manage; however, consider what happens if the patient

- is discharged before the end of the 60-day period
- is discharged and readmitted to the agency in the same 60-day period
- is hospitalized or dies before the end of the 60-day period
- gets unexpectedly worse or better during a 60-day episode.

The answers to these seemingly simple scenarios increase the complexity of the PPS.

In theory, a Medicare beneficiary is admitted to the agency, and based on the patient assessment, receives *five or more* clinically appropriate number of visits (as defined by the agency and certified by the physician). The patient is then discharged by the agency in an improved state of physical health and functional ability. The agency is in turn reimbursed a lump sum for the care that was provided.

The case of Mr. Dean discussed earlier illustrates what some might call an "ideal" home health care patient. He was admitted to the agency and required a minimal amount of visits to achieve his goals. He was discharged independent in medication and compliant with his dietary restrictions. He was able to state the emergency procedures to be implemented in case he needed them, and his surgical wound healed without incident. Therefore, the agency received a complete episode payment for the service it provided. In fact, an agency receives a complete episode payment whenever a patient has received at least five visits prior to being discharged whether the reason for discharge is achievement of goals, death, hospitalization, or transfer to a hospice program.

The reality of providing home health care to Medicare beneficiaries is that, depending on where the patient lives and the availability of hospital services in that geographic location, between 25% and 30% of them experience a hospitalization while they are under the care of the home health agency. Some patients get worse and are placed in a nursing home or are referred to hospice care, whereas others require equipment only available at outpatient therapy departments or even change agencies in the middle of a 60-day episode. You might say, "So what? Agencies should be flexible and adaptable enough to meet the changing needs of their patients." Fortunately, agencies are; however, the complexities of the PPS regulations require agencies to experience payment adjustments and reductions with almost every change in a patient's status.

Principle Three: Low Utilization Payments

The Centers for Medicare & Medicaid Services anticipated scenarios where a patient may only receive a few home visits and determined that the agency should not receive a full episode payment for these patients. As part of the original PPS regulations, the concept of a low utilization payment adjustment (LUPA) was introduced and, with the 2008 revisions, the LUPA was retained.

A LUPA payment is made to the agency for all 60-day episodes that require fewer than five visits. Like all PPS rates, the standardized LUPA payment is slightly adjusted based on the geographic location of the agency. The standardized (unadjusted for geographic labor costs) LUPA payment is approximately $100 per visit. Once again, the LUPA payment depends on the agency's cost per visit and mix of visits provided during the LUPA episode. With the 2008 PPS revisions, an additional amount of approximately $88 is given to agencies for LUPA episodes that occur as the only episode for the patient or for the first episode in a sequence of adjacent episodes. The rationale for the additional payment is based on the extra time it takes to perform the initial assessment. For example, the first home health care visit can be up to 2 hours long. The nurse admitting the patient sometimes requires an additional 30 to 40 minutes to complete paperwork in the office, phone the physician to verify the plan of care, and make referrals to other disciplines. It is reasonable to assume that the cost of the first home health care visit is the most expensive of all visits provided to the patient.

A LUPA episode can be comprised of any mix of home health care services or disciplines. A LUPA episode may be four nursing visits; one nursing and three HCA visits; two PT, one medical social worker, and one HCA visit; or any combination of visits as long as it is fewer than five visits.

If a LUPA episode can have a negative financial impact on the agency, why would agencies have them? It is reasonable to ask why the agency does not "make sure" that no LUPA episodes occur. Why would a clinician provide three or four visits and then discharge a patient? The occurrence of LUPA episodes is not always in the agency's control or inappropriate. This scenario can happen for a few reasons. The first is the patient may have met their goals and no longer needs home health care services. Second, the patient may have returned to the hospital very early in the 60-day episode, and the agency did not get a subsequent referral to revisit the patient after the patient returned home. Third, the patient's plan of care may only require a monthly visit for an injection of vitamin B12 or a urinary catheter change every 6 to 8 weeks.

Although in some instances LUPA episodes are unavoidable, there are also instances where a LUPA episode was the result of inefficient management of the patient's plan of treatment. Take for example the case of Mrs. Spooner.

Mrs. Spooner

Mrs. Spooner is a 73-year-old patient who was admitted to My Town VNA after a right mastectomy. She was discharged home with two Jackson-Pratt (JP) drains in the lateral aspect of her incision. The home health care nurse taught Mrs. Spooner drain management and the signs and symptoms of infection that should be reported. Approximately 1 week after the surgery, the JP drains were removed and occupational therapy began to strengthen her affected arm. The therapist continued to see Mrs. Spooner twice weekly. During the fifth week, Mrs. Spooner reported a "lump" in her right axilla; dark-red, foul-smelling drainage from the incision; and a temperature of 100.8° F.

Mrs. Spooner returned to her surgeon, who opened the incision, evacuated a hematoma, placed her on an antibiotic, and ordered daily dressing changes for 2 weeks. At this point, the wound

measured 3 cm long, 1 cm wide, and approximately 2 cm deep. The physician-ordered plan of treatment required the nurse to pack the wound with gauze to prevent it from closing prematurely and to continue to assess for worsening of the infection. Mrs. Spooner's plan of treatment continued until she returned to the surgeon during week 7.

At week 7, the surgeon changed his orders and requested that the nurse reduce the visits to every other day. The wound care was changed to alginate packing and a dry sterile dressing to facilitate moist wound healing and closure of the wound.

Midway through week 8 (day 53), the home health care nurse discussed with Mr. and Mrs. Spooner the feasibility of teaching Mr. Spooner the wound care. Once he agreed, the nurse obtained a physician order to begin teaching Mr. Spooner to perform the wound care.

On day 55, the nurse began demonstrating and teaching the wound care to Mr. Spooner. When the nurse visited on day 57, Mr. Spooner attempted to provide a return demonstration of the wound care; however, he was not able to complete the dressing without verbal cueing and assistance from the nurse.

On the 59th day of the episode, Mr. Spooner was able to complete the dressing care independently. He required no verbal cueing or physical assistance from the nurse. He admitted to still being a little nervous about performing the dressing change and stated that after one more "perfect" change he felt he would be able to perform the dressing changes without the nurse. Since the nurse would be returning for one additional visit to validate Mr. Spooner's ability to change the dressing, the OASIS regulations required that the nurse complete a recertification OASIS to plan for the additional visit.

On day 61 (or day 1 of the second episode), the nurse returned to the patient's home to find out the patient had gone to the surgeon on the previous day, and the wound care was discontinued. Mr.

Spooner was instructed to cover the wound with a dressing only to protect it from being irritated by Mrs. Spooner's bra or other clothing. The wound had well-approximated edges and no drainage. Both he and Mrs. Spooner were able to list the signs and symptoms that should be reported to the physician and were discharged from agency services.

Since the dressing was being changed every other day and the teaching of Mr. Spooner began late in the first episode, one additional visit into the second episode became necessary. The nurse felt that although Mr. Spooner was able to demonstrate appropriate technique once, a second return demonstration was necessary to be sure. This "extra" visit resulted in an avoidable LUPA episode and payment for the agency.

Principle Four: Supplies and Outpatient Therapy

As part of the episodic payment, Medicare requires agencies to provide the beneficiaries with all of the disposable medical supplies that they require. The agency is required to provide items such as ostomy supplies, dressings, catheters, and other supplies – whether or not the agency is actually using the supplies as part of the physician-ordered plan of treatment. For example, a patient with a well-established colostomy is admitted to the agency for cardiac or respiratory care. During the assessment process, the nurse discusses the patient's ability to manage the colostomy. The patient has and will continue to manage the colostomy independently. The nurse established a plan of treatment that does not include any interventions related to colostomy, yet the agency is required to provide all of these supplies and pay for them from the episode payment. In the 2008 PPS changes, supplies are covered and case-mix adjusted separately based on 6 non-routine supply severity groups' payments that range from $14.12 to $551 per episode.

In an attempt to manage supply costs, some agencies have implemented strict supply management systems, protocols, and formularies that restrict the types of supplies available to staff. If careful attention is not paid, the cost of supplies can insidiously or, depending on the volume of supplies ordered, abruptly diminish the profitability of the agency.

The PPS regulations also bundled outpatient therapy services. The bundling of these services requires home health agencies to be financially responsible for all of the services a patient may receive in an outpatient rehabilitation facility. There are few limitations on the provision of physical, occupational, and speech therapy in a patient's home, and the majority of home health care patients are able to meet their rehabilitation goals without returning to an outpatient therapy department. However, in some instances, a patient may require a piece of equipment that cannot be brought into the home. For example, a patient may return to the outpatient therapy department for the development or adjustment of a prosthetic devise, debridement of a wound in a whirlpool tank, or a test to evaluate swallowing. Because the PPS makes the agency financially responsible for patient-related supplies and outpatient therapy services, many agencies have negotiated contracts with suppliers of these services. Not only is a contractual relationship required for most agencies, it also provides that agency with some control over these expenses.

As part of most agencies' admission process, Medicare beneficiaries are notified both verbally and in writing of an agency's responsibility to provide these bundled services at no cost. Patients are often asked to sign, acknowledging that they have received this information. As part of this notification process, patients are informed of their financial responsibility if they choose to use a vendor for services with whom the agency does not have a contract.

For patients who have relationships with vendors that are not contracted with the agency, the bundling of supplies may create a problem. For example, the patient who has a colostomy, feeding tube, or catheter may refuse to have the agency assume the management of his or her supplies if that means the disruption of a preexisting relationship. In this case, the patient may be asked to sign a form that outlines his or her refusal of this service, or the agency may decide to negotiate with the patient's supply vendor. In any event, the bundling of supplies has made it easier for the agency to obtain the supplies necessary to appropriately manage patient care. Agencies no longer face barriers because a patient cannot or will not pay for supplies. On the other hand, the bundling of supplies and outpatient therapy services has added to the complexity of the home health PPS.

Principle Five: Therapy Services

The provision of physical, occupational, and speech therapy is crucial to many home health patients. The architects of the Medicare PPS system recognized the importance of these services to home care patients. In addition, they recognized that the utilization of these services significantly adds cost to the management of the patient. In an attempt to fairly reimburse the agency for the provision of these services, a therapy add-on provision was built into the PPS.

Like all Medicare home health reimbursement, the determination for a therapy add-on payment adjustment is based on the OASIS assessment and the physician-ordered plan of treatment. OASIS M2200 specifically asks the clinician (nurse or therapist) to project the number of anticipated therapy visits for the episode.

(M2200) Therapy Need: In the home health plan of care for the Medicare payment episode for which this assessment will define a case mix group, what is the indicated need for therapy visits (total number of reasonable and necessary physical,

occupational, and speech-language pathology visits combined?)

Reimbursement for therapy is based on threshold numbers of 6, 14, and 20 visits, with a gradual increment in payment between the first and third therapy threshold. It is important to remember that episodes are discrete; they are only 60 days in length. Added reimbursement for patients requiring therapy can be seen in the service utilization of the CFS scoring. In essence, under the 2008 PPS, the S score comes from the answer to M2200.

Principle Six: Outlier Payments

The sixth and final principle of PPS is the outlier payment. Although the PPS payment structure provides adequate reimbursement for most Medicare beneficiaries, there is an entire contingent of patients who require such an intensive level of service that, even with the therapy add-on, the agency will lose a significant amount of money providing their care.

The outlier payment is an additional payment above the episode payment that is intended to reduce the losses the agency experiences, not eliminate them all together. In other words, catastrophic cases that are eligible for an outlier payment remain losing cases for the agency, but the additional payment makes the loss smaller.

As stated at the beginning of this chapter, the PPS is based on averages and the assumption that the agency will have more profitable episodes than losing episodes; therefore, the financial losses associated with a catastrophic case should be offset by other cases that are profitable.

FEE-FOR-SERVICE

Unlike the PPS system, the fee-for-service payment mechanism generally pays the home health agency for every **authorized** visit the agency makes to a beneficiary. In this system, the number of visits provided to the patient are usually controlled by an insurance company through a case management system.

Agencies are usually required to make one home visit to assess the patient's needs in the home environment and then establish a plan of treatment that includes the type and frequency of service necessary to return the patient to optimal level of functioning. This information is then communicated to a case reviewer, who then authorizes a finite number of visits that must occur within a specified amount of time (e.g., skilled nursing two times a week for 2 weeks). At the end of the 2-week period, the agency has to obtain additional authorization to continue services. To make a decision to authorize additional visits and ongoing services, the case reviewer is dependent on the clinical documentation.

In this system, the home care agency and its staff are contracted by an insurance company to provide skilled home visits and not necessarily provide case management services. The agency is expected to communicate to the case reviewer barriers limiting the patient from achieving goals and preventing the return to independence. For example, the home health care nurse might find that a congestive heart failure patient does not own a bathroom scale. Recognizing that identification of subtle changes in a patient's weight might prevent a very expensive hospitalization, the insurance company may provide the patient with a bathroom scale if the patient does not have one or cannot afford to purchase one.

In essence, the home health care nurse becomes the eyes and ears of the insurance company, and all patient-related decisions must include input from the case reviewer. The agency is paid for every authorized visit made to the patient. Any unauthorized visits may not be reimbursed; therefore, the home health agency must diligently track both visits and authorizations to ensure reimbursement for services rendered to the patient.

SUMMARY

As noted earlier, in most other settings, the organization's fiscal soundness is not directly related to every nursing assessment and plan of care. The price for the autonomous practice of nursing in home health is accountability. The nurse's decision to provide unnecessary visits to patients can quickly add up to real financial losses for the agency.

EXAM QUESTIONS

CHAPTER 8
Questions 86-98

Note: Choose the one option that BEST answers each question.

86. Optimal Medicare reimbursement to an agency is ensured by

    a. increasing the number of unauthorized nurse visits provided to all patients.

    b. focusing on what the patient wants, not just what the patient needs.

    c. accurate diagnosis and coding of the primary and five secondary diagnoses.

    d. choosing the least expensive medical supplies to meet patient care needs.

87. Case mix management requires that

    a. agencies avoid patients that will result in financial losses.

    b. agencies understand exactly what type of patients are referred and how much service they typically require.

    c. minimized services be provided to the patient regardless of the patient's needs.

    d. not-for-profit agencies do not have to pay close attention to their case mix.

88. Agencies can legitimately maximize their profits under the Medicare PPS by

    a. providing expert and efficient management of patients' plans of care.

    b. only accepting patients who are profitable.

    c. providing a minimum of services regardless of patients' documented needs.

    d. increasing the per-visit charge to Medicare.

89. Extra and unnecessary visits provided to a Medicare beneficiary will likely

    a. improve the patient's satisfaction with the agency's services.

    b. maintain referral source satisfaction.

    c. result in improved patient outcomes.

    d. negatively impact the agency's financial condition.

90. The individual patient's Medicare episodic payment is based on the

    a. patient's clinical and functional status.

    b. patient's clinical severity, functional status, and service utilization indicators.

    c. geographic location of the agency.

    d. number of visits the patient requires.

91. Which statement is correct regarding Medicare PPS reimbursement for home services?

    a. The amount of reimbursement is fixed and never varies.

    b. Medicare payment is based on the number of anticipated nursing visits.

    c. An episode payment may be adjusted slightly based on geographic region.

    d. Medicare payment is based on the number of anticipated HCA visits.

92. Regardless of the patient's discharge disposition, the agency will receive a full episode payment whenever the patient receives

    a. one visit.

    b. at least two visits.

    c. at least five visits.

    d. a phone call from the agency to arrange services.

93. A situation that can result in a LUPA is

    a. a patient who receives three nursing and one PT visit.

    b. a patient who receives one PT, two social work visits, one nursing visit for intravenous therapy, and one nursing visit for wound care.

    c. four HCA visits and one nursing visit, which occur before the patient is discharged.

    d. one medical social worker visit, one occupational therapy visit, and three nursing visits in the first 5 days of the episode, which result in the patient being transferred to a long-term care facility.

94. The Mrs. Spooner case presented in this chapter demonstrates which type of episode payment?

    a. Partial episode payment

    b. Full episode payment

    c. A significant change in condition adjustment

    d. Avoidable LUPA episode

95. The bundling provision of PPS reimbursement

    a. only requires the patient to be financially responsible for outpatient therapy services received.

    b. requires the agency to be financially responsible for services that the patient receives in an outpatient facility.

    c. requires the agency to only provide supplies that are directly related to the physician-certified plan of treatment.

    d. only requires the agency to provide catheter and ostomy supplies.

96. In an attempt to manage the cost of medical supplies, agencies

    a. should refuse to care for patients who are known to have high supply costs.

    b. should request that the patient sign a waiver of liability and take the responsibility for the cost of supplies.

    c. have implemented strict supply management systems.

    d. should bill patients for the noncovered portion of their supply expenses.

97. To maximize the reimbursement associated with the therapy add-on, agencies should

    a. closely monitor the provision of therapy services and strive to have therapy services begin as soon as the need is identified.

    b. require therapists to establish plans of care that result in 14 visits, regardless of the patient's documented need.

    c. teach therapists nursing skills and substitute nursing visits with therapy visits.

    d. have the patient receive a visit from each of the therapy disciplines to uncover any unidentified needs, thereby increasing the likelihood that at least 20 therapy visits will be made.

98. Outlier payments

  a. are lucrative enough to change a financially losing episode to one that is profitable.

  b. are only available to not-for-profit agencies.

  c. are intended to reduce the agency's financial losses but not eliminate them all together.

  d. require the completion of an additional OASIS document.

CHAPTER 9

THE MEDICARE HOME HEALTH NURSING BENEFIT

CHAPTER OBJECTIVE

At the completion of this chapter, the reader will be able to identify the rules that govern the provision of Medicare home health services.

LEARNING OBJECTIVE

After studying this chapter, the reader will be able to

1. recognize the characteristics of a homebound patient.

2. identify services that meet the skilled nursing standards.

INTRODUCTION

Medicare is a federally funded health insurance program that generally provides coverage to all Americans who are age 65 or older. The Medicare Trust Fund is administered by the Centers for Medicare & Medicaid Services (CMS). In addition to providing health coverage, the CMS also provides regulation and oversight to the majority of health providers in the United States.

Like all health insurance providers, Medicare has an explicit set of criteria that must be met before the patient can qualify for services. Once a beneficiary meets the qualifying criteria for services, the home health agency must ensure that all of the services billed to Medicare are actually covered by the Medicare home health benefit. Virtually every nurse who works in an agency that cares for Medicare beneficiaries must have a working knowledge of the guidelines that will be discussed in this chapter.

MEDICARE BENEFIT POLICY MANUAL

The *Medicare Benefit Policy Manual* requires an agency to ensure that the patient is entitled to receive Medicare benefits. It is incumbent on the agency to ensure that the patient is eligible for Medicare-covered home health services *before* services are provided. To ensure compliance with this condition, the nurse conducting the start of care/admission visit is usually responsible to verify, to the best of his or her ability, the patient's eligibility (CMS, 2005).

All agencies providing services to Medicare beneficiaries are required to be certified to participate in the Medicare program (CMS, 2005). This concept was discussed in-depth in Chapter 5 and will not be reiterated here, other than to say that an attempt to receive reimbursement from Medicare without being a certified provider is considered illegal and is likely to result in accusations of Medicare fraud, which could result in fines, other penalties, or incarceration.

An agency's intake process usually requires the referral source to provide information about who will be paying for the patient's services. If the patient is a Medicare beneficiary, the agency will document the patient's Medicare number and forward it to the nurse who will be making the home visit for verification. This is simply accomplished by matching the numbers provided by the Intake department to the numbers on the patient's Medicare card (see Figure 9-1). Discrepancies are usually reported back to the agency, and further investigations are conducted.

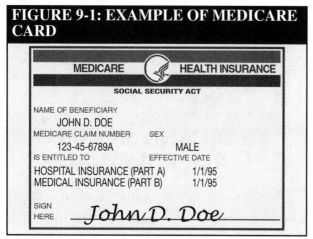

FIGURE 9-1: EXAMPLE OF MEDICARE CARD

During the admission process, the nurse must be sure that the services to be provided are covered under the Medicare benefit. Section 204 in the *Medicare Benefit Policy Manual* provides a detailed description of the conditions that the patient must meet to qualify for Medicare home health services (CMS, 2005). Qualifications include the expectation that the services are provided to a beneficiary who is confined to the home (homebound) and under the care of a physician. Medicare only covers services that are established under a physician-certified plan of care and are provided on an intermittent basis (CMS, 2005). The details of these conditions will be covered later in this chapter.

In addition to the conditions outlined above, the agency is responsible for ensuring that the care provided to the Medicare beneficiary is reasonable and necessary (CMS, 2005). Although physician certification of the plan of care provides support in determinations of reasonable and necessary care, not all care ordered by the physician is reasonable or necessary. Consider the case of Mrs. Obenchain.

Mrs. Obenchain

Mrs. Obenchain is an 82-year-old patient admitted to home health. Her physician-ordered plan requires the nurse to evaluate Mrs. Obenchain's diabetes status three times a week. During the admission process, the nurse has a physician order to check a fasting blood sugar; to evaluate Mrs. Obenchain's compliance with her diabetic diet; to teach Mrs. Obenchain the proper techniques to prepare and administer her insulin; and to teach Mrs. Obenchain the proper disposal of her used syringes.

Mrs. Obenchain tells the nurse that she has been a diabetic for over 20 years and is confident in her ability to manage her diabetes. When the nurse asks Mrs. Obenchain about why she thinks a home health referral was made, she tells the nurse, "I have been cheating quite a lot over the holidays, and my blood sugars have been running high."

Her fasting blood sugar level is 117 mg/dl. She demonstrates her ability to fill her syringe with the proper dose of mixed insulin. She easily and skillfully administers the insulin and then shows you that she disposes of all of her used syringes in a hard plastic bottle that she keeps under her sink. She states, "When it is half full, I close the cover and tape it real tight before I throw it away. I wouldn't want somebody to get stuck with my needle. That would be a terrible thing."

Mrs. Obenchain shows the nurse her glucose diary and is able to recall her diet for the last day and a half. All of her choices seem appropriate, yet the nurse reviews the agency's diet teaching instruction sheet. Mrs. Obenchain states, "I know all of this honey. I could be teaching you."

At the completion of this visit, should the nurse determine that Mrs. Obenchain needs home health services to teach her to manage her diabetes? Would the services be reasonable and necessary? As an experienced home health nurse, who has been "duped" by patients in the past, the nurse decides that a few visits should be provided to Mrs. Obenchain just to make sure she is as proficient as she seems. Would these services be reasonable and necessary?

When a Medicare reviewer evaluates the medical record to determine if the services provided were reasonable and necessary, he or she looks at the entire case, not just one or two visit notes. The *Medicare Benefit Policy Manual* requires the reviewer to make coverage determinations that take into account the individualized and unique needs of the patient (CMS, 2005). In addition to evaluating the nurse's notes, the reviewer assesses the supporting documentation found in the patient's medical record, such as the physician-certified plan of treatment/485 and the Outcome and Assessment Information Set.

Now, if you were a reviewer looking at the medical record of Mrs. Obenchain, would you think that continued home health services would be reasonable and necessary? What goals has the clinician documented that would support ongoing services? Are there new or different goals you would expect the nurse to establish? As a custodian of the Medicare trust fund, do you think that providing additional services to Mrs. Obenchain is money well spent?

PATIENT CONDITIONS

Four basic conditions must be met for a patient to qualify for the Medicare home health benefit. The patient must:

- be homebound;

- require skilled services;

- have his or her plan of care established and certified by a physician

- require care on an intermittent basis.

When establishing a home health plan of care, it is the agency's responsibility to ensure that the patient meets these qualifications. Failure to be in compliance with these conditions could be construed as fraud or abuse of the Medicare benefit.

Although it might seem that determining a patient's homebound status is an easy process, the language that guides the home health nurse to make this determination is vague at best. The issue of homebound status is an ongoing point of contention between the home health industry and Medicare. As a result, Medicare has attempted to clarify this language.

In July of 2002, Medicare released a "clarification" of the language related to the term *homebound.* It states that a patient can leave his or her home for the purposes of receiving health, treatment, or services without jeopardizing the homebound status. Regular absences from the home to attend outpatient rehabilitation, dialysis, or adult day care are considered therapeutic in nature and would not disqualify the patient from receiving Medicare home health services (CMS, 2005).

For many years, agencies considered a patient who was able to drive not homebound and would disqualify the patient from receiving Medicare benefits. However, the July 2002 clarification prohibits agencies from using the ability to drive as the only factor that determines the patient's homebound status. In fact, as long as the patient's absence from the home is infrequent or relatively short in duration or requires a taxing effort, the patient is to be considered homebound (CMS, 2005).

A patient does not jeopardize his or her homebound status if he or she attends a religious service or has an occasional absence for other nonmedical purposes, such as "an occasional trip to the barber, a walk around the block, a drive, attendance at a family reunion, funeral, graduation, or other infrequent or unique event" (CMS, 2005).

If the patient leaves the home, he or she is also still eligible for Medicare home health benefits as long as leaving requires a considerable and taxing effort, the assistance of a person or device, or supervision. The following examples demonstrate patients who meet these criteria and would not be disqualified from accessing Medicare home health services:

- a patient who is bedbound and requires the use of a Hoyer lift to transfer to a wheelchair

- a patient with severe dementia who cannot leave the home without close supervision and assistance for safety

- a patient with a hip replacement who has stairs leading outside of the home and requires a walker for safe ambulation

- a patient with chronic obstructive pulmonary disease who requires continuous oxygen therapy and exhibits dyspnea on exertion of less than 20 feet

- a patient with severe peripheral vascular disease and venous stasis ulcers on the lower extremities whose physician restricts activity by requiring the patient to minimize ambulation and keep the legs elevated.

On occasion, the patient's place of residence might create some confusion about whether the patient is entitled to receive Medicare home health services. The *Medicare Benefit Policy Manual* defines the patient's residence as anywhere the patient lives, including a private home, apartment, or rooming house (CMS, 2005). A patient is not entitled to receive Medicare home health services if the residence is part of an institution or facility. Certainly, a patient who lives in a nursing home would not be eligible to receive home health services; however, if the patient lives in an assisted living facility, he or she might be eligible (CMS, 2005).

The second condition the patient must meet is to be under the care of a physician who will take responsibility for the certification of the home health plan of care. The plan of care must include such information as the patient's medical diagnoses, medications, functional limitations, activities permitted, and safety measures. Appendix A provides an example of the home health plan of treatment/485 that is used to communicate this information to the physician.

Box 21 on the 485 found in Appendix A is the place where the nurse should document complete and specific treatment orders. For the purposes of home health, a complete physician order includes the discipline, frequency, duration, and service, as described in Table 9-1.

TABLE 9-1: MEDICARE DEFINITIONS

Discipline – includes but is not limited to nursing, home health aide care, and physical, speech, and occupation therapy.

Frequency – the number of times per day, week, or month the agency will be providing the service.

Duration – the period of time for which the service will be provided.

Service or Treatment – specifically which procedure will be performed (e.g., assessment, teaching, or intervention).

(CMS, 2005)

The following are examples of complete physician orders:

- skilled nursing bid x 5 days to administer Lovenox injections as ordered

- skilled nursing 2 x week x 1 week, then every other week x 8 to assess patient's cardiopulmonary status and evaluate medication compliance

- skilled nursing 1 x month to administer vitamin B_{12} subcutaneously or intramuscularly as ordered, home health aide 2 x week to assist patient with shower and personal care needs.

In addition to establishing a plan of treatment at the patient's start of care, the agency is required to recertify the plan of care every 60 days for as long as the patient continues to need home health services. Because the status of a home health patient can and often does change frequently, the nurse is required to prepare a comprehensive, up-to-date 485 that will be sent to the physician for signature.

Examples of changes in the patient's status include, but are not limited to, adjustments to the patient's medication plan, additional or discontinued services, or treatment changes based on an improvement or deterioration. The *Medicare Benefit Policy Manual* requires the nurse to obtain a physician-signed interim order whenever a patient's plan of care needs to be amended (CMS, 2005).

The recertification of a home health plan of care/485 requires the nurse to ensure that the medications, diagnosis, and orders are all up-to-date and reflect the patient's current status. Fortunately, most agencies have a computer system that makes amendments to the plan of care as they occur. When the nurse has to send the recertification plan of care to the physician, all the nurse has to do is verify that the computer-generated 485 is correct. Once the physician receives the 485, he or she is required to sign and date in Box 27 (see Appendix A). The physician's signature is intended to: "Certify/recertify that this patient is confined to his/her home and needs intermittent skilled nursing care, physical therapy and /or speech therapy or continues to need occupational therapy. The patient is under my care, and I have authorized the services on this plan of care and will periodically review the plan" (CMS, 1994, p. 1).

In addition to meeting the conditions and criteria discussed above, Section 205 requires the patient to demonstrate the need for skilled nursing and physical or speech therapy on an intermittent basis or a continuing need for occupational therapy (CMS, 2005). For the purposes of Medicare coverage, skilled nursing is classified as:

- observation and assessment of the patient's status when the skills of a professional nurse are required to identify a change in the patient's status

- management and evaluation of the patient's plan of care

- teaching and training activities

- administration of medications, medical gases, or tube feedings

- maintenance of the patient's airway or catheter

- wound or ostomy care

- rehabilitation nursing procedures and heat treatments.

Endless examples can be provided to illustrate the home health services covered by Medicare. In fact, just about every case discussed in this course exemplifies Medicare-covered services. At this point, it is more appropriate to illustrate the services that are not covered.

The first and most obvious is daily skilled services that do not have an end point in sight. Medicare only provides for **intermittent** skilled care. For example, if a patient has an extensive wound that, despite daily dressing changes, does not show any sign of improvement, Medicare will not pay for service to go on ad infinitum. If the nurse anticipates that the wound will show signs of healing in 2 or 3 months, daily visits will be covered.

Medicare will not pay for a skilled nurse to prefill a patient's medications. It will pay for the administration of oral, subcutaneous, intravenous, intramuscular, and other methods of medication administration. Medicare will pay for a nurse to administer a daily insulin injection to a patient, but it will not pay for the nurse to prefill the syringes and leave them for the patient to self-administer. The nurse can provide medication prefill services as long as that is not the sole reason that the nurse is visiting the patient. Once the patient no longer has a skilled need, the nurse cannot continue to visit the patient to prefill medications and charge Medicare for the visits.

For these reasons, many agencies prefer to identify a caregiver who can be taught to prefill the patient's medication. Because teaching is a Medicare-covered skill, teaching a patient or a caregiver to prefill a medication box or take all medications as part of a physician-certified plan of care are considered skilled and are covered by the patient's Medicare benefit.

For the most part, Medicare will not reimburse for the nurse to reinforce teaching that has already been accomplished. It will provide short-term benefits for the nurse to assess compliance with material that was taught or to evaluate the comprehension of the patient. For example, if a patient was discharged from the hospital independent in the administration of insulin and could verbalize an understanding of his or her dietary restrictions, Medicare will not pay for the home health nurse to reteach this information to the patient unless the nurse assesses that the patient does not demonstrate the same level of independence at home. Although these two examples might induce more questions than answers, it is unlikely that anyone can master the intricacies of the *Medicare Benefit Policy Manual* until he or she has the opportunity to apply them to real-life patient scenarios.

SUMMARY

Some agencies provide a copy of the HIM-II as part of an orientation program and require all staff to read it. Until a nurse has the opportunity to apply these regulations to the actual nuances of real-live patient care, he or she cannot begin to recognize the ambiguities and unanswered questions that remain. For some, the regulations might not make sense or seem contradictory when applied to patient situations. However, the *Medicare Benefit Policy Manual* is the proverbial "bible" of Medicare eligibility, and it is in the best interest of the patient that the nurse and the agency follow these regulations stringently.

EXAM QUESTIONS

CHAPTER 9
Questions 99-100

Note: Choose the option that BEST answers each question.

99. A patient who is able to drive a car

    a. is disqualified from receiving Medicare home health benefits.

    b. is qualified to receive Medicare home health benefits regardless of his or her home-bound status.

    c. may be eligible to receive a prorated portion of Medicare home health benefits.

    d. may be eligible to receive Medicare home health benefits if it requires a taxing effort to leave home and if the patient only does so for periods of infrequent and short duration.

100. Daily nursing visits for the administration of insulin injections to a patient who is blind, is diabetic, and has no caregiver; and nursing visits three times a week to teach another patient to take oral medications correctly are examples of

    a. services that exceed the reasonable and necessary standard.

    b. care that is too costly to be provided by Medicare-certified agencies.

    c. services that are considered nonskilled and disqualify the patient from receiving Medicare home health benefits.

    d. skilled services.

This concludes the final examination.

After reading the Summary on page 175, please answer the evaluation questions found on page v of this course book.

SUMMARY

The intent of this course was to provide the home health care nurse with an overview of the clinical practice realities. For some, home health care is considered the area where a nurse can go and "take a break" from the demands of practice. The home health care nurse is often thought of as one who visits with elderly patients and takes a blood pressure or changes a dressing. Certainly, both of those tasks are completed every day by thousands of home health care nurses across the country. However, practicing in home health care provides the nurse with challenges that cannot be conceived by nurses who have never ventured into community-based nursing.

The most successful home health care nurses are those who are comfortable functioning in an autonomous practice environment. Although there are surely other autonomous practice settings, for some patients, the skills and competencies of the home health care nurse can mean the difference between dependence and independence, life and death.

Unlike facility-based practice, home health care does not have a second or third shift that can act as a safety net for something missed. If the home health care nurse does not complete a comprehensive and thorough assessment of the patient on every visit, subtle symptoms or problems could be missed. When the patient complains of being tired or states, "I slept in the chair last night," the home health care nurse must investigate the implications of these comments. Every patient interaction provides clues to the patient's physical and emotional well-being. The presence of a monitor that will "beep" when the patient is becoming unstable is almost unheard of. Every patient's home represents a new set of issues, barriers, and hurdles to be overcome. Control is the patient's. Flexibility, creativity, empathy, and patience are mandatory nursing skills.

By in large, the majority of home health care is the delivery of nursing care. Agencies are structured by nurses to support the provision of nursing care. Nurses at all levels have an opportunity to not only connect with patients to assist them with achieving their desired outcomes but also to collaborate with other disciplines and participate in the development of new nursing knowledge.

In 2007, shrinking financial and human resources forced home health agencies to identify ways to continue to provide care to some of our most vulnerable friends and neighbors. Reductions in reimbursement have challenged nurses to identify creative teaching strategies to assist patients to become independent more quickly. The aging of the population has required home health agencies to employ multidisciplinary strategies to meet the needs of patients with severe chronic illnesses, comorbities, and disabilities. The implementation of new technologies, such as telemedicine, and best clinician practices assist clinicians to care for patients more efficiently, allowing agencies to extend their services to even more patients. Finally, the diversity of American culture and the melting pot of new and unfamiliar cultures will continue to provide the nurses who choose home health care with opportunities for ongoing growth and development of their professional skills. The question is, are you up to the challenge?

APPENDIX A

HOME HEALTH CERTIFICATION AND PLAN OF CARE

Department of Health and Human Services
Centers for Medicare & Medicaid Services

Form Approved
OMB No. 0938-0357

HOME HEALTH CERTIFICATION AND PLAN OF CARE

1. Patient's HI Claim No.	2. Start of Care Date	3. Certification Period From: To:	4. Medical Record No.	Provider No.

6. Patient's Name and Address	7. Provider's Name, Address and Telephone Number

8. Date of Birth	9. Sex M F	10. Medications: Dose/Frequency/Route (N) new (C) changed

11. ICD-9-CM	Principal Diagnosis	Date	
12. ICD-9-CM	Surgical Procedure	Date	
13. ICD-9-CM	Other Pertinent Diagnoses	Date	

14. DME and Supplies	15. Safety Measures
16. Nutrition Req.	17. Allergies

18.A. Functional Limitations			18.B. Activities Permitted		
1. Amputation	5. Paralysis	9. Legally Blind	1. Complete Bedrest	6. Partial Weight Bearing	A Wheelchair
2. Bowel/Bladder (incontinence)	6. Endurance	A Dyspnea With Minimal Exertion	2. Bedrest BRP	7. Independent at Home	B Walker
3. Contracture	7. Ambulation		3. Up As Tolerated	8. Crutches	C No Restrictions
4. Hearing	8. Speech	B Other (Specify)	5. Exercises Prescribed	9. Cane	D Other (Specify)

19. Mental Status:	1. Oriented 2. Comatose	3. Forgetful 4. Depressed	5. Disoriented 6. Lethargic	7. Agitated 8. Other	
20. Prognosis	1. Poor	2. Guarded	3. Fair	4. Good	5. Excellent

21. Orders for Discipline and Treatments (Specify Amount/Frequency/Duration)

22. Goals/Rehabilitation Potential/Discharge Plans

23. Nurse's Signature and Date of Verbal SOC Where Applicable	25. Date HHA Received Signed POT

24. Physician's Name and Address	26. I certify/recertify that this patient is confined to his/her home and needs intermittent skilled nursing care, physical therapy and/or speech therapy or continues to need occupational therapy. The patient is under my care, and I have authorized the services on this plan of care will periodically review the plan.
27. Attending Physician's Signature and Date Signed	required for payment of Federal funds may be subject to fine, imprisonment, or civil penalty under applicable Federal laws.

Form CMS-485 (C-3) (02-94) (Formerly HCFA-485) (Print Aligned)

177

APPENDIX B

OMB #0938-0760

Expiration date 7/31/2012

Outcome and Assessment Information Set

Items to be Used at Specific Time Points

Start of Care --- M0010-M0030, M0040-M0150, M1000-M1036, M1100-M1242, M1300-M1302, M1306, M1308-M1324, M1330-

    Start of care—further visits planned   M1350, M1400, M1410, M1600-M1730, M1740-M1910, M2000, M2002, M2010, M2020-M2250

Resumption of Care --- M0032, M0080-M0110, M1000-M1036, M1100-M1242, M1300-M1302, M1306, M1308-M1324, M1330-M1350,

    Resumption of care (after inpatient stay)   M1400, M1410, M1600-M1730, M1740-M1910, M2000, M2002, M2010, M2020-M2250

Follow-Up -- M0080-M0100, M0110, M1020-M1030, M1200, M1242, M1306, M1308, M1322-M1324, M1330-M1350, M1400,

    Recertification (follow-up) assessment   M1610, M1620, M1630, M1810-M1840, M1850, M1860,
    Other follow-up assessment   M2030, M2200

Transfer to an Inpatient Facility -------------------------------- M0080-M0100, M1040-M1055, M1500, M1510, M2004, M2015, M2300-M2410, M2430-M2440, M0903, M0906

    Transferred to an inpatient facility—patient not discharged from an agency
    Transferred to an inpatient facility—patient discharged from agency

Discharge from Agency — Not to an Inpatient Facility

    Death at home-- M0080-M0100, M0903, M0906
    Discharge from agency--- M0080-M0100, M1040-M1055, M1230, M1242, M1306-M1350, M1400-M1620, M1700-M1720, M1740, M1745, M1800-M1890, M2004, M2015-M2030, M2100-M2110, M2300-M2420, M0903, M0906

CLINICAL RECORD ITEMS

(M0080) Discipline of Person Completing Assessment:

    ☐ 1-RN   ☐ 2-PT   ☐ 3-SLP/ST   ☐ 4-OT

(M0090) Date Assessment Completed: _ _ / _ _ / _ _ _ _

                                   month / day / year

(M0100) This Assessment is Currently Being Completed for the Following Reason:

    Start/Resumption of Care
    ☐ 1 – Start of care—further visits planned
    ☐ 3 – Resumption of care (after inpatient stay)
    Follow-Up
    ☐ 4 – Recertification (follow-up) reassessment [*Go to M0110*]
    ☐ 5 – Other follow-up [*Go to M0110*]
    Transfer to an Inpatient Facility
    ☐ 6 – Transferred to an inpatient facility—patient not discharged from agency [*Go to M1040*]
    ☐ 7 – Transferred to an inpatient facility—patient discharged from agency [*Go to M1040*]
    Discharge from Agency — Not to an Inpatient Facility
    ☐ 8 – Death at home [*Go to M0903*]
    ☐ 9 – Discharge from agency [*Go to M1040*]

OMB #0938-0760

Expiration date 7/31/2012

(M0102) Date of Physician-ordered Start of Care (Resumption of Care): If the physician indicated a specific start of care (resumption of care) date when the patient was referred for home health services, record the date specified.

__ __ / __ __ / __ __ __ __   *(Go to M0110, if date entered)*
month / day / year

☐ NA –No specific SOC date ordered by physician

(M0104) Date of Referral: Indicate the date that the written or verbal referral for initiation or resumption of care was received by the HHA.

__ __ / __ __ / __ __ __ __
month / day / year

(M0110) Episode Timing: Is the Medicare home health payment episode for which this assessment will define a case mix group an "early" episode or a "later" episode in the patient's current sequence of adjacent Medicare home health payment episodes?

☐ 1 - Early

☐ 2 - Later

☐ UK - Unknown

☐ NA - Not Applicable: No Medicare case mix group to be defined by this assessment.

PATIENT HISTORY AND DIAGNOSES

(M1000) From which of the following **Inpatient Facilities** was the patient discharged <u>during the past 14 days</u>? **(Mark all that apply.)**

☐ 1 - Long-term nursing facility (NF)

☐ 2 - Skilled nursing facility (SNF / TCU)

☐ 3 - Short-stay acute hospital (IPP S)

☐ 4 - Long-term care hospital (LTCH)

☐ 5 - Inpatient rehabilitation hospital or unit (IRF)

☐ 6 - Psychiatric hospital or unit

☐ 7 - Other (specify) _____

☐ NA - Patient was not discharged from an inpatient facility [*Go to M1016*]

(M1005) Inpatient Discharge Date (most recent):

__ __ / __ __ / __ __ __ __
month / day / year

☐ UK - Unknown

(M1010) List each **Inpatient Diagnosis** and ICD-9-C M code at the level of highest specificity for only those conditions treated during an inpatient stay within the last 14 days (no E-codes, or V-codes):

Inpatient Facility Diagnosis	ICD-9-C M Code
a. _____	__ __ __ . __ __
b. _____	__ __ __ . __ __
c. _____	__ __ __ . __ __
d. _____	__ __ __ . __ __
e. _____	__ __ __ . __ __
f. _____	__ __ __ . __ __

OMB #0938-0760   Expiration date 7/31/2012

(M1012) List each **Inpatient Procedure** and the associated ICD-9-C M procedure code relevant to the plan of care.

<u>Inpatient Procedure</u>   <u>Procedure Code</u>

   a. _____   — — · — —
   b. _____   — — · — —
   c. _____   — — · — —
   d. _____   — — · — —

☐ NA - Not applicable
☐ UK - Unknown

(M1016) **Diagnoses Requiring Medical or Treatment Regimen Change Within Past 14 Days:** List the patient's Medical Diagnoses and ICD-9-C M codes at the level of highest specificity for those conditions requiring changed medical or treatment regimen within the past 14 days (no surgical, E-codes, or V-codes):

<u>Changed Medical Regimen Diagnosis</u>   <u>ICD-9-C M Code</u>

   a. _____   — — — · — —
   b. _____   — — — · — —
   c. _____   — — — · — —
   d. _____   — — — · — —
   e. _____   — — — · — —
   f. _____   — — — · — —

☐ NA - Not applicable (no medical or treatment regimen changes within the past 14 days)

(M1018) **Conditions Prior to Medical or Treatment Regimen Change or Inpatient Stay Within Past 14 Days**: If this patient experienced an inpatient facility discharge or change in medical or treatment regimen within the past 14 days, indicate any conditions which existed <u>prior to</u> the inpatient stay or change in medical or treatment regimen. **(Mark all that apply.)**

☐ 1 - Urinary incontinence
☐ 2 - Indwelling/suprapubic catheter
☐ 3 - Intractable pain
☐ 4 - Impaired decision-making
☐ 5 - Disruptive or socially inappropriate behavior
☐ 6 - Memory loss to the extent that supervision required
☐ 7 - None of the above
☐ NA - No inpatient facility discharge <u>and</u> no change in medical or treatment regimen in past 14 days
☐ UK - Unknown

OMB #0938-0760

Expiration date 7/31/2012

(M1020/1022/1024)   Diagnoses, Symptom Control, and Payment Diagnoses: List each diagnosis for which the patient is receiving home care (Column 1) and enter its ICD-9-C M code at the level of highest specificity (no surgical/procedure codes) (Column 2). Diagnoses are listed in the order that best reflect the seriousness of each condition and support the disciplines and services provided. Rate the degree of symptom control for each condition (Column 2). Choose one value that represents the degree of symptom control appropriate for each diagnosis: V-codes (for M1020 or M1022) or E-codes (for M1022 only) may be used. ICD-9-C M sequencing requirements must be followed if multiple coding is indicated for any diagnoses. If a V-code is reported in place of a case mix diagnosis, then optional item M1024 Payment Diagnoses (Columns 3 and 4) may be completed. A case mix diagnosis is a diagnosis that determines the Medicare P P S case mix group. Do not assign symptom control ratings for V- or E-codes.

Code each row according to the following directions for each column:

Column 1:   Enter the description of the diagnosis.

Column 2:   Enter the ICD-9-C M code for the diagnosis described in Column 1;

Rate the degree of symptom control for the condition listed in Column 1 using the following scale:

0 - Asymptomatic, no treatment needed at this time

1 - Symptoms well controlled with current therapy

2 - Symptoms controlled with difficulty, affecting daily functioning; patient needs ongoing monitoring

3 - Symptoms poorly controlled; patient needs frequent adjustment in treatment and dose monitoring

4 - Symptoms poorly controlled; history of re-hospitalizations

Note that in Column 2 the rating for symptom control of each diagnosis should not be used to determine the sequencing of the diagnoses listed in Column 1. These are separate items and sequencing may not coincide. Sequencing of diagnoses should reflect the seriousness of each condition and support the disciplines and services provided.

Column 3:   (OPTIONAL) If a V-code is assigned to any row in Column 2, in place of a case mix diagnosis, it may be necessary to complete optional item M1024 Payment Diagnoses (Columns 3 and 4). See OASIS-C Guidance Manual.

Column 4:   (OPTIONAL) If a V-code in Column 2 is reported in place of a case mix diagnosis that requires multiple diagnosis codes under ICD-9-C M coding guidelines, enter the diagnosis descriptions and the ICD-9-C M codes in the same row in Columns 3 and 4. For example, if the case mix diagnosis is a manifestation code, record the diagnosis description and ICD-9-C M code for the underlying condition in Column 3 of that row and the diagnosis description and ICD-9-C M code for the manifestation in Column 4 of that row. Otherwise, leave Column 4 blank in that row.

(Form on next page)

OMB #0938-0760   Expiration date 7/31/2012

(M1020) Primary Diagnosis & (M1022) Other Diagnoses		(M1024) Payment Diagnoses (OPTIONAL)	
Column 1	Column 2	Column 3	Column 4
Diagnoses (Sequencing of diagnoses should reflect the seriousness of each condition and support the disciplines and services provided.)	ICD-9-C M and symptom control rating for each condition. Note that the sequencing of these ratings may not match the sequencing of the diagnoses	Complete if a V-code is assigned under certain circumstances to Column 2 in place of a case mix diagnosis.	Complete **only if** the V-code in Column 2 is reported in place of a case mix diagnosis that is a multiple coding situation (e.g., a manifestation code).
Description	ICD-9-C M / Symptom Control Rating	Description/ ICD-9-C M	Description/ ICD-9-C M
(M1020) Primary Diagnosis a. _____	**(V-codes are allowed)** a. (__ __ __ . __ __) ☐0 ☐1 ☐2 ☐3 ☐4	**(V- or E-codes NOT allowed)** a._____ (__ __ __ . __ __)	**(V- or E-codes NOT allowed)** a._____ (__ __ __ . __ __)
(M1022) Other Diagnoses b. _____	**(V- or E-codes are allowed)** b. (__ __ __ . __ __) ☐0 ☐1 ☐2 ☐3 ☐4	**(V- or E-codes NOT allowed)** b._____ (__ __ __ . __ __)	**(V- or E-codes NOT allowed)** b._____ (__ __ __ . __ __)
c. _____	c. (__ __ __ . __ __) ☐0 ☐1 ☐2 ☐3 ☐4	c._____ (__ __ __ . __ __)	c._____ (__ __ __ . __ __)
d. _____	d. (__ __ __ . __ __) ☐0 ☐1 ☐2 ☐3 ☐4	d._____ (__ __ __ . __ __)	d._____ (__ __ __ . __ __)
e. _____	e. (__ __ __ . __ __) ☐0 ☐1 ☐2 ☐3 ☐4	e._____ (__ __ __ . __ __)	e._____ (__ __ __ . __ __)
f. _____	f. (__ __ __ . __ __) ☐0 ☐1 ☐2 ☐3 ☐4	f._____ (__ __ __ . __ __)	f._____ (__ __ __ . __ __)

(M1030) **Therapies** the patient receives <u>at home</u>: **(Mark all that apply.)**

    ☐ 1 - Intravenous or infusion therapy (excludes TPN)

    ☐ 2 - Parenteral nutrition (TPN or lipids)

    ☐ 3 - Enteral nutrition (nasogastric, gastrostomy, jejunostomy, or any other artificial entry into the alimentary canal)

    ☐ 4 - None of the above

(M1032) **Risk for Hospitalization:** Which of the following signs or symptoms characterize this patient as at risk for hospitalization? **(Mark all that apply.)**

    ☐ 1 - Recent decline in mental, emotional, or behavioral status

    ☐ 2 - Multiple hospitalizations (2 or more) in the past 12 months

    ☐ 3 - History of falls (2 or more falls - or any fall with an injury - in the past year)

    ☐ 4 - Taking five or more medications

    ☐ 5 - Frailty indicators, e.g., weight loss, self-reported exhaustion

    ☐ 6 - Other

    ☐ 7 - None of the above

OMB #0938-0760

Expiration date 7/31/2012

(M1034) Overall Status: Which description best fits the patient's overall status? **(Check one)**

☐ 0 - The patient is stable with no heightened risk(s) for serious complications and death (beyond those typical of the patient's age).

☐ 1 - The patient is temporarily facing high health risk(s) but is likely to return to being stable without heightened risk(s) for serious complications and death (beyond those typical of the patient's age).

☐ 2 - The patient is likely to remain in fragile health and have ongoing high risk(s) of serious complications and death.

☐ 3 - The patient has serious progressive conditions that could lead to death within a year.

☐ UK - The patient's situation is unknown or unclear.

(M1036) Risk Factors, either present or past, likely to affect current health status and/or outcome: **(Mark all that apply.)**

☐ 1 - Smoking

☐ 2 - Obesity

☐ 3 - Alcohol dependency

☐ 4 - Drug dependency

☐ 5 - None of the above

☐ UK - Unknown

LIVING ARRANGEMENTS

(M1100) Patient Living Situation: Which of the following best describes the patient's residential circumstance and availability of assistance? **(Check one box only.)**

Living Arrangement	Availability of Assistance				
	Around the clock	Regular daytime	Regular nighttime	Occasional / short-term assistance	No assistance available
a. Patient lives alone	☐ 01	☐ 02	☐ 03	☐ 04	☐ 05
b. Patient lives with other person(s) in the home	☐ 06	☐ 07	☐ 08	☐ 09	☐ 10
c. Patient lives in congregate situation (e.g., assisted living)	☐ 11	☐ 12	☐ 13	☐ 14	☐ 15

SENSORY STATUS

(M1200) Vision (with corrective lenses if the patient usually wears them):

☐ 0 - Normal vision: sees adequately in most situations; can see medication labels, newsprint.

☐ 1 - Partially impaired: cannot see medication labels or newsprint, but can see obstacles in path, and the surrounding layout; can count fingers at arm's length.

☐ 2 - Severely impaired: cannot locate objects without hearing or touching them or patient nonresponsive.

(M1210) Ability to hear (with hearing aid or hearing appliance if normally used):

☐ 0 - Adequate: hears normal conversation without difficulty.

☐ 1 - Mildly to Moderately Impaired: difficulty hearing in some environments or speaker may need to increase volume or speak distinctly.

☐ 2 - Severely Impaired: absence of useful hearing.

☐ UK - Unable to assess hearing.

OMB #0938-0760   Expiration date 7/31/2012

(M1220) Understanding of Verbal Content in patient's own language (with hearing aid or device if used):

- ☐ 0 - Understands: clear comprehension without cues or repetitions.
- ☐ 1 - Usually Understands: understands most conversations, but misses some part/intent of message. Requires cues at times to understand.
- ☐ 2 - Sometimes Understands: understands only basic conversations or simple, direct phrases. Frequently requires cues to understand.
- ☐ 3 - Rarely/Never Understands
- ☐ UK - Unable to assess understanding.

(M1230) Speech and Oral (Verbal) Expression of Language (in patient's own language):

- ☐ 0 - Expresses complex ideas, feelings, and needs clearly, completely, and easily in all situations with no observable impairment.
- ☐ 1 - Minimal difficulty in expressing ideas and needs (may take extra time; makes occasional errors in word choice, grammar or speech intelligibility; needs minimal prompting or assistance).
- ☐ 2 - Expresses simple ideas or needs with moderate difficulty (needs prompting or assistance, errors in word choice, organization or speech intelligibility). Speaks in phrases or short sentences.
- ☐ 3 - Has severe difficulty expressing basic ideas or needs and requires maximal assistance or guessing by listener. Speech limited to single words or short phrases.
- ☐ 4 - Unable to express basic needs even with maximal prompting or assistance but is not comatose or unresponsive (e.g., speech is nonsensical or unintelligible).
- ☐ 5 - Patient nonresponsive or unable to speak.

(M1240) Has this patient had a formal **Pain Assessment** using a standardized pain assessment tool (appropriate to the patient's ability to communicate the severity of pain)?

- ☐ 0 - No standardized assessment conducted
- ☐ 1 - Yes, and it does not indicate severe pain
- ☐ 2 - Yes, and it indicates severe pain

(M1242) Frequency of Pain Interfering with patient's activity or movement:

- ☐ 0 - Patient has no pain
- ☐ 1 - Patient has pain that does not interfere with activity or movement
- ☐ 2 - Less often than daily
- ☐ 3 - Daily, but not constantly
- ☐ 4 - All of the time

INTEGUMENTARY STATUS

(M1300) Pressure Ulcer Assessment: Was this patient assessed for **Risk of Developing Pressure Ulcers**?

- ☐ 0 - No assessment conducted [*Go to M1306*]
- ☐ 1 - Yes, based on an evaluation of clinical factors, e.g., mobility, incontinence, nutrition, etc., without use of standardized tool
- ☐ 2 - Yes, using a standardized tool, e.g., Braden, Norton, other

(M1302) Does this patient have a **Risk of Developing Pressure Ulcers**?

- ☐ 0 - No
- ☐ 1 - Yes

(M1306) Does this patient have at least one **Unhealed Pressure Ulcer at Stage II or Higher** or designated as "unstageable"?

- ☐ 0 - No [*Go to M1322*]
- ☐ 1 - Yes

OMB #0938-0760   Expiration date 7/31/2012

(M1308)   Current Number of Unhealed (non-epithelialized) Pressure Ulcers at Each Stage:
(Enter "0" if none; excludes Stage I pressure ulcers)

Stage description – unhealed pressure ulcers	Column 1 Complete at SOC/ROC/FU & D/C Number Currently Present	Column 2 Complete at FU & D/C Number of those listed in Column 1 that were present on admission (most recent SOC / ROC)
a. **Stage II:** Partial thickness loss of dermis presenting as a shallow open ulcer with red pink wound bed, without slough. May also present as an intact or open/ruptured serum-filled blister.	____	____
b. **Stage III:** Full thickness tissue loss. Subcutaneous fat may be visible but bone, tendon, or muscles are not exposed. Slough may be present but does not obscure the depth of tissue loss. May include undermining and tunneling.	____	____
c. **Stage IV:** Full thickness tissue loss with visible bone, tendon, or muscle. Slough or eschar may be present on some parts of the wound bed. Often includes undermining and tunneling.	____	____
d.1 Unstageable: Known or likely but unstageable due to non-removable dressing or device	____	____
d.2 Unstageable: Known or likely but unstageable due to coverage of wound bed by slough and/or eschar.	____	____
d.3 Unstageable: Suspected deep tissue injury in evolution.	____	____

Directions for M1310, M1312, and M1314: If the patient has one or more unhealed (non-epithelialized) Stage III or IV pressure ulcers, identify the **Stage III or IV pressure ulcer with the largest surface dimension (length x width)** and record in centimeters. If no Stage III or Stage IV pressure ulcers, go to M1320.

(M1310)   Pressure Ulcer Length: Longest length "head-to-toe" | ___ | ___ | . | ___ | (cm)

(M1312)   Pressure Ulcer Width: Width of the same pressure ulcer; greatest width perpendicular to the length

| ___ | ___ | . | ___ | (cm)

(M1314)   Pressure Ulcer Depth: Depth of the same pressure ulcer; from visible surface to the deepest area

| ___ | ___ | . | ___ | (cm)

(M1320)   Status of Most Problematic (Observable) Pressure Ulcer:

☐   0   -   Newly epithelialized
☐   1   -   Fully granulating
☐   2   -   Early/partial granulation
☐   3   -   Not healing
☐   NA -   No observable pressure ulcer

OMB #0938-0760   Expiration date 7/31/2012

(M1322) Current Number of Stage I Pressure Ulcers: Intact skin with non-blanchable redness of a localized area usually over a bony prominence. The area may be painful, firm, soft, warmer or cooler as compared to adjacent tissue.

☐ 0   ☐ 1   ☐ 2   ☐ 3   ☐ 4 or more

(M1324) Stage of Most Problematic Unhealed (Observable) Pressure Ulcer:

☐   1 -   Stage I
☐   2 -   Stage II
☐   3 -   Stage III
☐   4 -   Stage IV
☐   NA -   No observable pressure ulcer or unhealed pressure ulcer

(M1330) Does this patient have a **Stasis Ulcer?**

☐   0 -   No [*Go to M1340*]
☐   1 -   Yes, patient has BOTH observable and unobservable stasis ulcers
☐   2 -   Yes, patient has observable stasis ulcers ONLY
☐   3 -   Yes, patient has unobservable stasis ulcers ONLY (known but not observable due to non-removable dressing) [*Go to M1340*]

(M1332) Current Number of (Observable) Stasis Ulcer(s):

☐   1 -   One
☐   2 -   Two
☐   3 -   Three
☐   4 -   Four or more

(M1334) Status of Most Problematic (Observable) Stasis Ulcer:

☐   0 -   Newly epithelialized
☐   1 -   Fully granulating
☐   2 -   Early/partial granulation
☐   3 -   Not healing

(M1340) Does this patient have a **Surgical Wound?**

☐   0 -   No [*Go to M1350*]
☐   1 -   Yes, patient has at least one (observable) surgical wound
☐   2 -   Surgical wound known but not observable due to non-removable dressing [*Go to M1350*]

(M1342) Status of Most Problematic (Observable) Surgical Wound:

☐   0 -   Newly epithelialized
☐   1 -   Fully granulating
☐   2 -   Early/partial granulation
☐   3 -   Not healing

(M1350) Does this patient have a **Skin Lesion** or **Open Wound,** excluding bowel ostomy, other than those described above that is receiving intervention by the home health agency?

☐   0 -   No
☐   1 -   Yes

OMB #0938-0760

Expiration date 7/31/2012

RESPIRATORY STATUS

(M1400) When is the patient dyspneic or noticeably **Short of Breath**?

- ☐ 0 - Patient is not short of breath
- ☐ 1 - When walking more than 20 feet, climbing stairs
- ☐ 2 - With moderate exertion (e.g., while dressing, using commode or bedpan, walking distances less than 20 feet)
- ☐ 3 - With minimal exertion (e.g., while eating, talking, or performing other ADLs) or with agitation
- ☐ 4 - At rest (during day or night)

(M1410) **Respiratory Treatments** utilized at home: **(Mark all that apply.)**

- ☐ 1 - Oxygen (intermittent or continuous)
- ☐ 2 - Ventilator (continually or at night)
- ☐ 3 - Continuous / Bi-level positive airway pressure
- ☐ 4 - None of the above

ELIMINATION STATUS

(M1600) Has this patient been treated for a **Urinary Tract Infection** in the past 14 days?

- ☐ 0 - No
- ☐ 1 - Yes
- ☐ NA - Patient on prophylactic treatment
- ☐ UK - Unknown **[Omit "UK" option on DC]**

(M1610) **Urinary Incontinence or Urinary Catheter Presence:**

- ☐ 0 - No incontinence or catheter (includes anuria or ostomy for urinary drainage) [*Go to M1620*]
- ☐ 1 - Patient is incontinent
- ☐ 2 - Patient requires a urinary catheter (i.e., external, indwelling, intermittent, suprapubic) [*Go to M1620*]

(M1615) **When** does **Urinary Incontinence** occur?

- ☐ 0 - Timed-voiding defers incontinence
- ☐ 1 - Occasional stress incontinence
- ☐ 2 - During the night only
- ☐ 3 - During the day only
- ☐ 4 - During the day and night

(M1620) **Bowel Incontinence Frequency:**

- ☐ 0 - Very rarely or never has bowel incontinence
- ☐ 1 - Less than once weekly
- ☐ 2 - One to three times weekly
- ☐ 3 - Four to six times weekly
- ☐ 4 - On a daily basis
- ☐ 5 - More often than once daily
- ☐ NA - Patient has ostomy for bowel elimination
- ☐ UK - Unknown **[Omit "UK" option on FU, DC]**

OMB #0938-0760

Expiration date 7/31/2012

(M1630) Ostomy for Bowel Elimination: Does this patient have an ostomy for bowel elimination that (within the last 14 days): a) was related to an inpatient facility stay, or b) necessitated a change in medical or treatment regimen?

☐ 0 - Patient does <u>not</u> have an ostomy for bowel elimination.

☐ 1 - Patient's ostomy was <u>not</u> related to an inpatient stay and did <u>not</u> necessitate change in medical or treatment regimen.

☐ 2 - The ostomy <u>was</u> related to an inpatient stay or <u>did</u> necessitate change in medical or treatment regimen.

<u>NEURO/EMOTIONAL/BEHAVIORAL STATUS</u>

(M1700) Cognitive Functioning: Patient's current (day of assessment) level of alertness, orientation, comprehension, concentration, and immediate memory for simple commands.

☐ 0 - Alert/oriented, able to focus and shift attention, comprehends and recalls task directions independently.

☐ 1 - Requires prompting (cuing, repetition, reminders) only under stressful or unfamiliar conditions.

☐ 2 - Requires assistance and some direction in specific situations (e.g., on all tasks involving shifting of attention), or consistently requires low stimulus environment due to distractibility.

☐ 3 - Requires considerable assistance in routine situations. Is not alert and oriented or is unable to shift attention and recall directions more than half the time.

☐ 4 - Totally dependent due to disturbances such as constant disorientation, coma, persistent vegetative state, or delirium.

(M1710) When Confused (Reported or Observed Within the Last 14 Days):

☐ 0 - Never

☐ 1 - In new or complex situations only

☐ 2 - On awakening or at night only

☐ 3 - During the day and evening, but not constantly

☐ 4 - Constantly

☐ NA - Patient nonresponsive

(M1720) When Anxious (Reported or Observed Within the Last 14 Days):

☐ 0 - None of the time

☐ 1 - Less often than daily

☐ 2 - Daily, but not constantly

☐ 3 - All of the time

☐ NA - Patient nonresponsive

OMB #0938-0760

Expiration date 7/31/2012

(M1730) Depression Screening: Has the patient been screened for depression, using a standardized depression screening tool?

☐   0 -   No

☐   1 -   Yes, patient was screened using the PHQ-2©* scale. (Instructions for this two-question tool: Ask patient: "Over the last two weeks, how often have you been bothered by any of the following problems")

PHQ-2©*	Not at all 0 - 1 day	Several days 2 - 6 days	More than half of the days 7 – 11 days	Nearly every day 12 – 14 days	N/A Unable to respond
a) Little interest or pleasure in doing things	☐0	☐1	☐2	☐3	☐na
b) Feeling down, depressed, or hopeless?	☐0	☐1	☐2	☐3	☐na

☐   2 -   Yes, with a different standardized assessment-and the patient meets criteria for further evaluation for depression.

☐   3 -   Yes, patient was screened with a different standardized assessment-and the patient does not meet criteria for further evaluation for depression.

Copyright© Pfizer Inc. All rights reserved. Reproduced with permission.

(M1740) Cognitive, behavioral, and psychiatric symptoms that are demonstrated at least once a week (Reported or Observed): **(Mark all that apply.)**

☐   1 -   Memory deficit: failure to recognize familiar persons/places, inability to recall events of past 24 hours, significant memory loss so that supervision is required

☐   2 -   Impaired decision-making: failure to perform usual ADLs or IADLs, inability to appropriately stop activities, jeopardizes safety through actions

☐   3 -   Verbal disruption: yelling, threatening, excessive profanity, sexual references, etc.

☐   4 -   Physical aggression: aggressive or combative to self and others (e.g., hits self, throws objects, punches, dangerous maneuvers with wheelchair or other objects)

☐   5 -   Disruptive, infantile, or socially inappropriate behavior (**excludes** verbal actions)

☐   6 -   Delusional, hallucinatory, or paranoid behavior

☐   7 -   None of the above behaviors demonstrated

(M1745) Frequency of Disruptive Behavior Symptoms (Reported or Observed) Any physical, verbal, or other disruptive/dangerous symptoms that are injurious to self or others or jeopardize personal safety.

☐   0 -   Never

☐   1 -   Less than once a month

☐   2 -   Once a month

☐   3 -   Several times each month

☐   4 -   Several times a week

☐   5 -   At least daily

(M1750) Is this patient receiving **Psychiatric Nursing Services** at home provided by a qualified psychiatric nurse?

☐   0 -   No

☐   1 -   Yes

OMB #0938-0760   Expiration date 7/31/2012

ADL/IADLs

(M1800) Grooming: Current ability to tend safely to personal hygiene needs (i.e., washing face and hands, hair care, shaving or make up, teeth or denture care, fingernail care).

- ☐ 0 - Able to groom self unaided, with or without the use of assistive devices or adapted methods.
- ☐ 1 - Grooming utensils must be placed within reach before able to complete grooming activities.
- ☐ 2 - Someone must assist the patient to groom self.
- ☐ 3 - Patient depends entirely upon someone else for grooming needs.

(M1810) Current **Ability to Dress Upper Body** safely (with or without dressing aids) including undergarments, pullovers, front-opening shirts and blouses, managing zippers, buttons, and snaps:

- ☐ 0 - Able to get clothes out of closets and drawers, put them on and remove them from the upper body without assistance.
- ☐ 1 - Able to dress upper body without assistance if clothing is laid out or handed to the patient.
- ☐ 2 - Someone must help the patient put on upper body clothing.
- ☐ 3 - Patient depends entirely upon another person to dress the upper body.

(M1820) Current **Ability to Dress Lower Body** safely (with or without dressing aids) including undergarments, slacks, socks or nylons, shoes:

- ☐ 0 - Able to obtain, put on, and remove clothing and shoes without assistance.
- ☐ 1 - Able to dress lower body without assistance if clothing and shoes are laid out or handed to the patient.
- ☐ 2 - Someone must help the patient put on undergarments, slacks, socks or nylons, and shoes.
- ☐ 3 - Patient depends entirely upon another person to dress lower body.

(M1830) Bathing: Current ability to wash entire body safely. **Excludes grooming (washing face, washing hands, and shampooing hair).**

- ☐ 0 - Able to bathe self in shower or tub independently, including getting in and out of tub/shower.
- ☐ 1 - With the use of devices, is able to bathe self in shower or tub independently, including getting in and out of the tub/shower.
- ☐ 2 - Able to bathe in shower or tub with the intermittent assistance of another person:
     (a) for intermittent supervision or encouragement or reminders, OR
     (b) to get in and out of the shower or tub, OR
     (c) for washing difficult to reach areas.
- ☐ 3 - Able to participate in bathing self in shower or tub, but requires presence of another person throughout the bath for assistance or supervision.
- ☐ 4 - Unable to use the shower or tub, but able to bathe self independently with or without the use of devices at the sink, in chair, or on commode.
- ☐ 5 - Unable to use the shower or tub, but able to participate in bathing self in bed, at the sink, in bedside chair, or on commode, with the assistance or supervision of another person throughout the bath.
- ☐ 6 - Unable to participate effectively in bathing and is bathed totally by another person.

(M1840) Toilet Transferring: Current ability to get to and from the toilet or bedside commode safely and transfer on and off toilet/commode.

- ☐ 0 - Able to get to and from the toilet and transfer independently with or without a device.
- ☐ 1 - When reminded, assisted, or supervised by another person, able to get to and from the toilet and transfer.
- ☐ 2 - Unable to get to and from the toilet but is able to use a bedside commode (with or without assistance).
- ☐ 3 - Unable to get to and from the toilet or bedside commode but is able to use a bedpan/urinal independently.
- ☐ 4 - Is totally dependent in toileting.

OMB #0938-0760

Expiration date 7/31/2012

(M1845) Toileting Hygiene: Current ability to maintain perineal hygiene safely, adjust clothes and/or incontinence pads before and after using toilet, commode, bedpan, urinal. If managing ostomy, includes cleaning area around stoma, but not managing equipment.

☐ 0 - Able to manage toileting hygiene and clothing management without assistance.

☐ 1 - Able to manage toileting hygiene and clothing management without assistance if supplies/implements are laid out for the patient.

☐ 2 - Someone must help the patient to maintain toileting hygiene and/or adjust clothing.

☐ 3 - Patient depends entirely upon another person to maintain toileting hygiene.

(M1850) Transferring: Current ability to move safely from bed to chair, or ability to turn and position self in bed if patient is bedfast.

☐ 0 - Able to independently transfer.

☐ 1 - Able to transfer with minimal human assistance or with use of an assistive device.

☐ 2 - Able to bear weight and pivot during the transfer process but unable to transfer self.

☐ 3 - Unable to transfer self and is unable to bear weight or pivot when transferred by another person.

☐ 4 - Bedfast, unable to transfer but is able to turn and position self in bed.

☐ 5 - Bedfast, unable to transfer and is unable to turn and position self.

(M1860) Ambulation/Locomotion: Current ability to walk safely, once in a standing position, or use a wheelchair, once in a seated position, on a variety of surfaces.

☐ 0 - Able to independently walk on even and uneven surfaces and negotiate stairs with or without railings (i.e., needs no human assistance or assistive device).

☐ 1 - With the use of a one-handed device (e.g. cane, single crutch, hemi-walker), able to independently walk on even and uneven surfaces and negotiate stairs with or without railings.

☐ 2 - Requires use of a two-handed device (e.g., walker or crutches) to walk alone on a level surface and/or requires human supervision or assistance to negotiate stairs or steps or uneven surfaces.

☐ 3 - Able to walk only with the supervision or assistance of another person at all times.

☐ 4 - Chairfast, unable to ambulate but is able to wheel self independently.

☐ 5 - Chairfast, unable to ambulate and is unable to wheel self.

☐ 6 - Bedfast, unable to ambulate or be up in a chair.

(M1870) Feeding or Eating: Current ability to feed self meals and snacks safely. Note: This refers only to the process of eating, chewing, and swallowing, not preparing the food to be eaten.

☐ 0 - Able to independently feed self.

☐ 1 - Able to feed self independently but requires:

(a) meal set-up; OR
(b) intermittent assistance or supervision from another person; OR
(c) a liquid, pureed or ground meat diet.

☐ 2 - Unable to feed self and must be assisted or supervised throughout the meal/snack.

☐ 3 - Able to take in nutrients orally and receives supplemental nutrients through a nasogastric tube or gastrostomy.

☐ 4 - Unable to take in nutrients orally and is fed nutrients through a nasogastric tube or gastrostomy.

☐ 5 - Unable to take in nutrients orally or by tube feeding.

(M1880) Current **Ability to Plan and Prepare Light Meals** (e.g., cereal, sandwich) or reheat delivered meals safely:

☐ 0 - (a) Able to independently plan and prepare all light meals for self or reheat delivered meals; OR
(b) Is physically, cognitively, and mentally able to prepare light meals on a regular basis but has not routinely performed light meal preparation in the past (i.e., prior to this home care admission).

☐ 1 - Unable to prepare light meals on a regular basis due to physical, cognitive, or mental limitations.

☐ 2 - Unable to prepare any light meals or reheat any delivered meals.

OMB #0938-0760

Expiration date 7/31/2012

(M1890) **Ability to Use Telephone:** Current ability to answer the phone safely, including dialing numbers, and <u>effectively</u> using the telephone to communicate.

☐ 0 - Able to dial numbers and answer calls appropriately and as desired.

☐ 1 - Able to use a specially adapted telephone (i.e., large numbers on the dial, teletype phone for the deaf) and call essential numbers.

☐ 2 - Able to answer the telephone and carry on a normal conversation but has difficulty with placing calls.

☐ 3 - Able to answer the telephone only some of the time or is able to carry on only a limited conversation.

☐ 4 - <u>Unable</u> to answer the telephone at all but can listen if assisted with equipment.

☐ 5 - Totally unable to use the telephone.

☐ NA - Patient does not have a telephone.

(M1900) **Prior Functioning ADL/IADL:** Indicate the patient's usual ability with everyday activities prior to this current illness, exacerbation, or injury. Check only **one** box in each row.

Functional Area	Independent	Needed Some Help	Dependent
a. Self-Care (e.g., grooming, dressing, and bathing)	☐0	☐1	☐2
b. Ambulation	☐0	☐1	☐2
c. Transfer	☐0	☐1	☐2
d. Household tasks (e.g., light meal preparation, laundry, shopping)	☐0	☐1	☐2

(M1910) Has this patient had a multi-factor **Fall Risk Assessment** (such as falls history, use of multiple medications, mental impairment, toileting frequency, general mobility/transferring impairment, environmental hazards)?

☐ 0 - No multi-factor falls risk assessment conducted.

☐ 1 - Yes, and it does not indicate a risk for falls.

☐ 2 - Yes, and it indicates a risk for falls.

MEDICATIONS

(M2000) **Drug Regimen Review:** Does a complete drug regimen review indicate potential clinically significant medication issues, e.g., drug reactions, ineffective drug therapy, side effects, drug interactions, duplicate therapy, omissions, dosage errors, or noncompliance?

☐ 0 - Not assessed/reviewed [*Go to M2010*]

☐ 1 - No problems found during review [*Go to M2010*]

☐ 2 - Problems found during review

☐ NA - Patient is not taking any medications [*Go to M2040*]

(M2002) **Medication Follow-up:** Was a physician or the physician-designee contacted within one calendar day to resolve clinically significant medication issues, including reconciliation?

☐ 0 - No

☐ 1 - Yes

OMB #0938-0760

Expiration date 7/31/2012

(M2010) Patient/Caregiver High Risk Drug Education: Has the patient/caregiver received instruction on special precautions for all high-risk medications (such as hypoglycemics, anticoagulants, etc.) and how and when to report problems that may occur?

☐   0 -   No

☐   1 -   Yes

☐ NA -   Patient not taking any high risk drugs OR patient/caregiver fully knowledgeable about special precautions associated with all high-risk medications

(M2020) Management of Oral Medications: Patient's current ability to prepare and take all oral medications reliably and safely, including administration of the correct dosage at the appropriate times/intervals. **Excludes injectable and IV medications. (NOTE: This refers to ability, not compliance or willingness.)**

☐   0 -   Able to independently take the correct oral medication(s) and proper dosage(s) at the correct times.

☐   1 -   Able to take medication(s) at the correct times if:

(a) individual dosages are prepared in advance by another person; OR
(b) another person develops a drug diary or chart.

☐   2 -   Able to take medication(s) at the correct times if given reminders by another person at the appropriate times

☐   3 -   Unable to take medication unless administered by another person.

☐ NA -   No oral medications prescribed.

(M2030) Management of Injectable Medications: Patient's current ability to prepare and take all prescribed injectable medications reliably and safely, including administration of correct dosage at the appropriate times/intervals. **Excludes IV medications.**

☐   0 -   Able to independently take the correct medication(s) and proper dosage(s) at the correct times.

☐   1 -   Able to take injectable medication(s) at the correct times if:

(a) individual syringes are prepared in advance by another person; OR
(b) another person develops a drug diary or chart.

☐   2 -   Able to take medication(s) at the correct times if given reminders by another person based on the frequency of the injection

☐   3 -   Unable to take injectable medication unless administered by another person.

☐ NA -   No injectable medications prescribed.

(M2040) Prior Medication Management: Indicate the patient's usual ability with managing oral and injectable medications prior to this current illness, exacerbation, or injury. Check only **one** box in each row.

Functional Area	Independent	Needed Some Help	Dependent	Not Applicable
a. Oral medications	☐0	☐1	☐2	☐na
b. Injectable medications	☐0	☐1	☐2	☐na

OMB #0938-0760

Expiration date 7/31/2012

CARE MANAGEMENT

(M2100) **Types and Sources of Assistance:** Determine the level of caregiver ability and willingness to provide assistance for the following activities, if assistance is needed. (Check only **one** box in each row.)

Type of Assistance	No assistance needed in this area	Caregiver(s) currently provide assistance	Caregiver(s) need training/ supportive services to provide assistance	Caregiver(s) not likely to provide assistance	Unclear if Caregiver(s) will provide assistance	Assistance needed, but no Caregiver(s) available
a. **ADL assistance** (e.g., transfer/ ambulation, bathing, dressing, toileting, eating/feeding)	☐0	☐1	☐2	☐3	☐4	☐5
b. **IADL assistance** (e.g., meals, housekeeping, laundry, telephone, shopping, finances)	☐0	☐1	☐2	☐3	☐4	☐5
c. **Medication administration** (e.g., oral, inhaled or injectable)	☐0	☐1	☐2	☐3	☐4	☐5
d. **Medical procedures/ treatments** (e.g., changing wound dressing)	☐0	☐1	☐2	☐3	☐4	☐5
e. **Management of Equipment** (includes oxygen, IV/infusion equipment, enteral/ parenteral nutrition, ventilator therapy equipment or supplies)	☐0	☐1	☐2	☐3	☐4	☐5
f. **Supervision and safety** (e.g., due to cognitive impairment)	☐0	☐1	☐2	☐3	☐4	☐5
g. **Advocacy or facilitation** of patient's participation in appropriate medical care (includes transportation to or from appointments)	☐0	☐1	☐2	☐3	☐4	☐5

OMB #0938-0760

Expiration date 7/31/2012

(M2110) How Often does the patient receive **ADL or IADL assistance** from any caregiver(s) (other than home health agency staff)?

- ☐ 1 - At least daily
- ☐ 2 - Three or more times per week
- ☐ 3 - One to two times per week
- ☐ 4 - Received, but less often than weekly
- ☐ 5 - No assistance received
- ☐ UK - Unknown **[Omit "UK" option on DC]**

THERAPY NEED AND PLAN OF CARE

(M2200) **Therapy Need:** In the home health plan of care for the Medicare payment episode for which this assessment will define a case mix group, what is the indicated need for therapy visits (total of reasonable and necessary physical, occupational, and speech-language pathology visits combined)? **(Enter zero ["000"] if no therapy visits indicated.)**

(__ __ __) Number of therapy visits indicated (total of physical, occupational and speech-language pathology combined).

☐ NA - Not Applicable: No case mix group defined by this assessment.

(M2250) **Plan of Care Synopsis:** (Check only **one** box in each row.) Does the physician-ordered plan of care include the following:

Plan / Intervention	No	Yes	Not Applicable	
a. Patient-specific parameters for notifying physician of changes in vital signs or other clinical findings	☐0	☐1	☐na	Physician has chosen not to establish patient-specific parameters for this patient. Agency will use standardized clinical guidelines accessible for all care providers to reference
b. Diabetic foot care including monitoring for the presence of skin lesions on the lower extremities and patient/caregiver education on proper foot care	☐0	☐1	☐na	Patient is not diabetic or is bilateral amputee
c. Falls prevention interventions	☐0	☐1	☐na	Patient is not assessed to be at risk for falls
d. Depression intervention(s) such as medication, referral for other treatment, or a monitoring plan for current treatment	☐0	☐1	☐na	Patient has no diagnosis or symptoms of depression
e. Intervention(s) to monitor and mitigate pain	☐0	☐1	☐na	No pain identified
f. Intervention(s) to prevent pressure ulcers	☐0	☐1	☐na	Patient is not assessed to be at risk for pressure ulcers
g. Pressure ulcer treatment based on principles of moist wound healing OR order for treatment based on moist wound healing has been requested from physician	☐0	☐1	☐na	Patient has no pressure ulcers with need for moist wound healing

APPENDIX C

OMB #0938-0760

Expiration date 7/31/2012

Outcome and Assessment Information Set

Items to be Used at Specific Time Points

Start of Care --
   Start of care—further visits planned

M0010-M0030, M0040-M0150, M1000-M1036, M1100-M1242, M1300-M1302, M1306, M1308-M1324, M1330-M1350, M1400, M1410, M1600-M1730, M1740-M1910, M2000, M2002, M2010, M2020-M2250

Resumption of Care --
   Resumption of care (after inpatient stay)

M0032, M0080-M0110, M1000-M1036, M1100-M1242, M1300-M1302, M1306, M1308-M1324, M1330-M1350, M1400, M1410, M1600-M1730, M1740-M1910, M2000, M2002, M2010, M2020-M2250

Follow-Up ---
   Recertification (follow-up) assessment
   Other follow-up assessment

M0080-M0100, M0110, M1020-M1030, M1200, M1242, M1306, M1308, M1322-M1324, M1330-M1350, M1400, M1610, M1620, M1630, M1810-M1840, M1850, M1860, M2030, M2200

Transfer to an Inpatient Facility----------------------------------
   Transferred to an inpatient facility—patient not discharged from an agency
   Transferred to an inpatient facility—patient discharged from agency

M0080-M0100, M1040-M1055, M1500, M1510, M2004, M2015, M2300-M2410, M2430-M2440, M0903, M0906

Discharge from Agency — Not to an Inpatient Facility
   Death at home--
   Discharge from agency--

M0080-M0100, M0903, M0906
M0080-M0100, M1040-M1055, M1230, M1242, M1306-M1350, M1400-M1620, M1700-M1720, M1740, M1745, M1800-M1890, M2004, M2015-M2030, M2100-M2110, M2300-M2420, M0903, M0906

CLINICAL RECORD ITEMS

(M0080) **Discipline of Person Completing Assessment:**

   ☐ 1-RN   ☐ 2-PT   ☐ 3-SLP/ST   ☐ 4-OT

(M0090) **Date Assessment Completed:**   _ _ /_ _ /_ _ _ _
                                          month / day / year

(M0100) **This Assessment is Currently Being Completed for the Following Reason:**

   Start/Resumption of Care
   ☐   1 – Start of care—further visits planned
   ☐   3 – Resumption of care (after inpatient stay)

   Follow-Up
   ☐   4 – Recertification (follow-up) reassessment [*Go to M0110*]
   ☐   5 – Other follow-up [*Go to M0110*]

   Transfer to an Inpatient Facility
   ☐   6 – Transferred to an inpatient facility—patient not discharged from agency [*Go to M1040*]
   ☐   7 – Transferred to an inpatient facility—patient discharged from agency [*Go to M1040*]

   Discharge from Agency — Not to an Inpatient Facility
   ☐   8 – Death at home [*Go to M0903*]
   ☐   9 – Discharge from agency [*Go to M1040*]

OMB #0938-0760

Expiration date 7/31/2012

PATIENT HISTORY AND DIAGNOSES

(M1040) Influenza Vaccine: Did the patient receive the influenza vaccine from your agency for this year's influenza season (October 1 through March 31) during this episode of care?

☐ 0 - No

☐ 1 - Yes [*Go to M1050*]

☐ NA - Does not apply because entire episode of care (SOC/ROC to Transfer/Discharge) is outside this influenza season. [*Go to M1050*]

(M1045) Reason Influenza Vaccine not received: If the patient did not receive the influenza vaccine from your agency during this episode of care, state reason:

☐ 1 - Received from another health care provider (e.g., physician)

☐ 2 - Received from your agency previously during this year's flu season

☐ 3 - Offered and declined

☐ 4 - Assessed and determined to have medical contraindication(s)

☐ 5 - Not indicated; patient does not meet age/condition guidelines for influenza vaccine

☐ 6 - Inability to obtain vaccine due to declared shortage

☐ 7 - None of the above

(M1050) Pneumococcal Vaccine: Did the patient receive pneumococcal polysaccharide vaccine (PPV) from your agency during this episode of care (SOC/ROC to Transfer/Discharge)?

☐ 0 - No

☐ 1 - Yes [*Go to M1500 at TRN; Go to M1230 at DC*]

(M1055) Reason PPV not received: If patient did not receive the pneumococcal polysaccharide vaccine (PPV) from your agency during this episode of care (SOC/ROC to Transfer/Discharge), state reason:

☐ 1 - Patient has received PPV in the past

☐ 2 - Offered and declined

☐ 3 - Assessed and determined to have medical contraindication(s)

☐ 4 - Not indicated; patient does not meet age/condition guidelines for PPV

☐ 5 - None of the above

CARDIAC STATUS

(M1500) Symptoms in Heart Failure Patients: If patient has been diagnosed with heart failure, did the patient exhibit symptoms indicated by clinical heart failure guidelines (including dyspnea, orthopnea, edema, or weight gain) at any point since the previous OASIS assessment?

☐ 0 - No [*Go to M2004 at TRN; Go to M1600 at DC*]

☐ 1 - Yes

☐ 2 - Not assessed [*Go to M2004 at TRN; Go to M1600 at DC*]

☐ NA - Patient does not have diagnosis of heart failure [*Go to M2004 at TRN; Go to M1600 at DC*]

OMB #0938-0760   Expiration date 7/31/2012

(M1510) Heart Failure Follow-up: If patient has been diagnosed with heart failure and has exhibited symptoms indicative of heart failure since the previous OASIS assessment, what action(s) has (have) been taken to respond? **(Mark all that apply.)**

- ☐ 0 - No action taken
- ☐ 1 - Patient's physician (or other primary care practitioner) contacted the same day
- ☐ 2 - Patient advised to get emergency treatment (e.g., call 911 or go to emergency room)
- ☐ 3 - Implemented physician-ordered patient-specific established parameters for treatment
- ☐ 4 - Patient education or other clinical interventions
- ☐ 5 - Obtained change in care plan orders (e.g., increased monitoring by agency, change in visit frequency, telehealth, etc.)

MEDICATIONS

(M2004) Medication Intervention: If there were any clinically significant medication issues since the previous OASIS assessment, was a physician or the physician-designee contacted within one calendar day of the assessment to resolve clinically significant medication issues, including reconciliation?

- ☐ 0 - No
- ☐ 1 - Yes
- ☐ NA - No clinically significant medication issues identified since the previous OASIS assessment

(M2015) Patient/Caregiver Drug Education Intervention: Since the previous OASIS assessment, was the patient/caregiver instructed by agency staff or other health care provider to monitor the effectiveness of drug therapy, drug reactions, and side effects, and how and when to report problems that may occur?

- ☐ 0 - No
- ☐ 1 - Yes
- ☐ NA - Patient not taking any drugs

EMERGENT CARE

(M2300) Emergent Care: Since the last time OASIS data were collected, has the patient utilized a hospital emergency department (includes holding/observation)?

- ☐ 0 - No [*Go to M2400*]
- ☐ 1 - Yes, used hospital emergency department WITHOUT hospital admission
- ☐ 2 - Yes, used hospital emergency department WITH hospital admission
- ☐ UK - Unknown [*Go to M2400*]

OMB #0938-0760

Expiration date 7/31/2012

(M2310) **Reason for Emergent Care**: For what reason(s) did the patient receive emergent care (with or without hospitalization)? **(Mark all that apply.)**

- ☐ 1 - Improper medication administration, medication side effects, toxicity, anaphylaxis
- ☐ 2 - Injury caused by fall
- ☐ 3 - Respiratory infection (e.g., pneumonia, bronchitis)
- ☐ 4 - Other respiratory problem
- ☐ 5 - Heart failure (e.g., fluid overload)
- ☐ 6 - Cardiac dysrhythmia (irregular heartbeat)
- ☐ 7 - Myocardial infarction or chest pain
- ☐ 8 - Other heart disease
- ☐ 9 - Stroke (CVA) or TIA
- ☐ 10 - Hypo/Hyperglycemia, diabetes out of control
- ☐ 11 - GI bleeding, obstruction, constipation, impaction
- ☐ 12 - Dehydration, malnutrition
- ☐ 13 - Urinary tract infection
- ☐ 14 - IV catheter-related infection or complication
- ☐ 15 - Wound infection or deterioration
- ☐ 16 - Uncontrolled pain
- ☐ 17 - Acute mental/behavioral health problem
- ☐ 18 - Deep vein thrombosis, pulmonary embolus
- ☐ 19 - Other than above reasons
- ☐ UK - Reason unknown

OMB #0938-0760   Expiration date 7/31/2012

DATA ITEMS COLLECTED AT INPATIENT FACILITY ADMISSION OR AGENCY DISCHARGE ONLY

(M2400) **Intervention Synopsis:** (Check only **one** box in each row.) Since the previous OASIS assessment, were the following interventions BOTH included in the physician-ordered plan of care AND implemented?

Plan / Intervention	No	Yes	Not Applicable	
a. Diabetic foot care including monitoring for the presence of skin lesions on the lower extremities and patient/caregiver education on proper foot care	☐0	☐1	☐na	Patient is not diabetic or is bilateral amputee
b. Falls prevention interventions	☐0	☐1	☐na	Formal multi-factor Fall Risk Assessment indicates the patient was not at risk for falls since the last OASIS assessment
c. Depression intervention(s) such as medication, referral for other treatment, or a monitoring plan for current treatment	☐0	☐1	☐na	Formal assessment indicates patient did not meet criteria for depression AND patient did not have diagnosis of depression since the last OASIS assessment
d. Intervention(s) to monitor and mitigate pain	☐0	☐1	☐na	Formal assessment did not indicate pain since the last OASIS assessment
e. Intervention(s) to prevent pressure ulcers	☐0	☐1	☐na	Formal assessment indicates the patient was not at risk of pressure ulcers since the last OASIS assessment
f. Pressure ulcer treatment based on principles of moist wound healing	☐0	☐1	☐na	Dressings that support the principles of moist wound healing not indicated for this patient's pressure ulcers OR patient has no pressure ulcers with need for moist wound healing

(M2410) To which **Inpatient Facility** has the patient been admitted?

☐ 1 - Hospital [*Go to M2430*]

☐ 2 - Rehabilitation facility [*Go to M0903*]

☐ 3 - Nursing home [*Go to M2440*]

☐ 4 - Hospice [*Go to M0903*]

☐ NA - No inpatient facility admission **[Omit "NA" option on TRN]**

OMB #0938-0760

Expiration date 7/31/2012

(M2430) **Reason for Hospitalization**: For what reason(s) did the patient require hospitalization? **(Mark all that apply.)**

- ☐   1 -   Improper medication administration, medication side effects, toxicity, anaphylaxis
- ☐   2 -   Injury caused by fall
- ☐   3 -   Respiratory infection (e.g., pneumonia, bronchitis)
- ☐   4 -   Other respiratory problem
- ☐   5 -   Heart failure (e.g., fluid overload)
- ☐   6 -   Cardiac dysrhythmia (irregular heartbeat)
- ☐   7 -   Myocardial infarction or chest pain
- ☐   8 -   Other heart disease
- ☐   9 -   Stroke (CVA) or TIA
- ☐   10 -   Hypo/Hyperglycemia, diabetes out of control
- ☐   11 -   GI bleeding, obstruction, constipation, impaction
- ☐   12 -   Dehydration, malnutrition
- ☐   13 -   Urinary tract infection
- ☐   14 -   IV catheter-related infection or complication
- ☐   15 -   Wound infection or deterioration
- ☐   16 -   Uncontrolled pain
- ☐   17 -   Acute mental/behavioral health problem
- ☐   18 -   Deep vein thrombosis, pulmonary embolus
- ☐   19 -   Scheduled treatment or procedure
- ☐   20 -   Other than above reasons
- ☐ UK -   Reason unknown

[*Go to M0903*]

(M2440) For what **Reason(s)** was the patient **Admitted** to a **Nursing Home**? **(Mark all that apply.)**

- ☐   1 -   Therapy services
- ☐   2 -   Respite care
- ☐   3 -   Hospice care
- ☐   4 -   Permanent placement
- ☐   5 -   Unsafe for care at home
- ☐   6 -   Other
- ☐ UK -   Unknown

[*Go to M0903*]

(M0903) **Date of Last (Most Recent) Home Visit:**

__ __ / __ __ / __ __ __ __
month / day /   year

(M0906) **Discharge/Transfer/Death Date:** Enter the date of the discharge, transfer, or death (at home) of the patient.

__ __ / __ __ / __ __ __ __
month / day /   year

APPENDIX D

OMB #0938-0760

Expiration date 7/31/2012

Outcome and Assessment Information Set

Items to be Used at Specific Time Points

Start of Care	M0010-M0030, M0040-M0150, M1000-M1036, M1100-M1242, M1300-M1302, M1306, M1308-M1324, M1330-M1350, M1400, M1410, M1600-M1730, M1740-M1910, M2000, M2002, M2010, M2020-M2250
Start of care—further visits planned	
Resumption of Care	M0032, M0080-M0110, M1000-M1036, M1100-M1242, M1300-M1302, M1306, M1308-M1324, M1330-M1350, M1400, M1410, M1600-M1730, M1740-M1910, M2000, M2002, M2010, M2020-M2250
Resumption of care (after inpatient stay)	
Follow-Up	M0080-M0100, M0110, M1020-M1030, M1200, M1242, M1306, M1308, M1322-M1324, M1330-M1350, M1400, M1610, M1620, M1630, M1810-M1840, M1850, M1860, M2030, M2200
Recertification (follow-up) assessment Other follow-up assessment	
Transfer to an Inpatient Facility	M0080-M0100, M1040-M1055, M1500, M1510, M2004, M2015, M2300-M2410, M2430-M2440, M0903, M0906
Transferred to an inpatient facility—patient not discharged from an agency Transferred to an inpatient facility—patient discharged from agency	
Discharge from Agency — Not to an Inpatient Facility	
Death at home	M0080-M0100, M0903, M0906
Discharge from agency	M0080-M0100, M1040-M1055, M1230, M1242, M1306-M1350, M1400-M1620, M1700-M1720, M1740, M1745, M1800-M1890, M2004, M2015-M2030, M2100-M2110, M2300-M2420, M0903, M0906

CLINICAL RECORD ITEMS

(M0080) Discipline of Person Completing Assessment:

☐ 1-RN   ☐ 2-PT   ☐ 3-SLP/ST   ☐ 4-OT

(M0090) Date Assessment Completed: __ __ / __ __ / __ __ __ __
  month / day / year

(M0100) This Assessment is Currently Being Completed for the Following Reason:

Start/Resumption of Care
☐   1 – Start of care—further visits planned
☐   3 – Resumption of care (after inpatient stay)

Follow-Up
☐   4 – Recertification (follow-up) reassessment [*Go to M0110*]
☐   5 – Other follow-up [*Go to M0110*]

Transfer to an Inpatient Facility
☐   6 – Transferred to an inpatient facility—patient not discharged from agency [*Go to M1040*]
☐   7 – Transferred to an inpatient facility—patient discharged from agency [*Go to M1040*]

Discharge from Agency — Not to an Inpatient Facility
☐   8 – Death at home [*Go to M0903*]
☐   9 – Discharge from agency [*Go to M1040*]

OMB #0938-0760

Expiration date 7/31/2012

(M0110) **Episode Timing:** Is the Medicare home health payment episode for which this assessment will define a case mix group an "early" episode or a "later" episode in the patient's current sequence of adjacent Medicare home health payment episodes?

☐ 1 - Early

☐ 2 - Later

☐ UK - Unknown

☐ NA - Not Applicable: No Medicare case mix group to be defined by this assessment.

PATIENT HISTORY AND DIAGNOSES

(M1020/1022/1024) **Diagnoses, Symptom Control, and Payment Diagnoses:** List each diagnosis for which the patient is receiving home care (Column 1) and enter its ICD-9-C M code at the level of highest specificity (no surgical/procedure codes) (Column 2). Diagnoses are listed in the order that best reflect the seriousness of each condition and support the disciplines and services provided. Rate the degree of symptom control for each condition (Column 2). Choose one value that represents the degree of symptom control appropriate for each diagnosis: V-codes (for M1020 or M1022) or E-codes (for M1022 only) may be used. ICD-9-C M sequencing requirements must be followed if multiple coding is indicated for any diagnoses. If a V-code is reported in place of a case mix diagnosis, then optional item M1024 Payment Diagnoses (Columns 3 and 4) may be completed. A case mix diagnosis is a diagnosis that determines the Medicare P P S case mix group. Do not assign symptom control ratings for V- or E-codes.

Code each row according to the following directions for each column:

Column 1:   Enter the description of the diagnosis.

Column 2:   Enter the ICD-9-C M code for the diagnosis described in Column 1;

Rate the degree of symptom control for the condition listed in Column 1 using the following scale:

0 - Asymptomatic, no treatment needed at this time

1 - Symptoms well controlled with current therapy

2 - Symptoms controlled with difficulty, affecting daily functioning; patient needs ongoing monitoring

3 - Symptoms poorly controlled; patient needs frequent adjustment in treatment and dose monitoring

4 - Symptoms poorly controlled; history of re-hospitalizations

Note that in Column 2 the rating for symptom control of each diagnosis should not be used to determine the sequencing of the diagnoses listed in Column 1. These are separate items and sequencing may not coincide. Sequencing of diagnoses should reflect the seriousness of each condition and support the disciplines and services provided.

Column 3:   (OPTIONAL) If a V-code is assigned to any row in Column 2, in place of a case mix diagnosis, it may be necessary to complete optional item M1024 Payment Diagnoses (Columns 3 and 4). See OASIS-C Guidance Manual.

Column 4:   (OPTIONAL) If a V-code in Column 2 is reported in place of a case mix diagnosis that requires multiple diagnosis codes under ICD-9-C M coding guidelines, enter the diagnosis descriptions and the ICD-9-C M codes in the same row in Columns 3 and 4. For example, if the case mix diagnosis is a manifestation code, record the diagnosis description and ICD-9-C M code for the underlying condition in Column 3 of that row and the diagnosis description and ICD-9-C M code for the manifestation in Column 4 of that row. Otherwise, leave Column 4 blank in that row.

(Form on next page)

OMB #0938-0760   Expiration date 7/31/2012

(M1020) Primary Diagnosis & (M1022) Other Diagnoses		(M1024) Payment Diagnoses (OPTIONAL)	
Column 1	Column 2	Column 3	Column 4
Diagnoses (Sequencing of diagnoses should reflect the seriousness of each condition and support the disciplines and services provided.)	ICD-9-C M and symptom control rating for each condition. Note that the sequencing of these ratings may not match the sequencing of the diagnoses	Complete if a V-code is assigned under certain circumstances to Column 2 in place of a case mix diagnosis.	Complete **only if** the V-code in Column 2 is reported in place of a case mix diagnosis that is a multiple coding situation (e.g., a manifestation code).
Description	ICD-9-C M / Symptom Control Rating	Description/ ICD-9-C M	Description/ ICD-9-C M
(M1020) Primary Diagnosis	**(V-codes are allowed)**	**(V- or E-codes NOT allowed)**	**(V- or E-codes NOT allowed)**
a. _____	a. (__ __ __ . __ __) ☐0 ☐1 ☐2 ☐3 ☐4	a._____ (__ __ __ . __ __)	a._____ (__ __ __ . __ __)
(M1022) Other Diagnoses	**(V- or E-codes are allowed)**	**(V- or E-codes NOT allowed)**	**(V- or E-codes NOT allowed)**
b. _____	b. (__ __ __ . __ __) ☐0 ☐1 ☐2 ☐3 ☐4	b._____ (__ __ __ . __ __)	b._____ (__ __ __ . __ __)
c. _____	c. (__ __ __ . __ __) ☐0 ☐1 ☐2 ☐3 ☐4	c._____ (__ __ __ . __ __)	c._____ (__ __ __ . __ __)
d. _____	d. (__ __ __ . __ __) ☐0 ☐1 ☐2 ☐3 ☐4	d._____ (__ __ __ . __ __)	d._____ (__ __ __ . __ __)
e. _____	e. (__ __ __ . __ __) ☐0 ☐1 ☐2 ☐3 ☐4	e._____ (__ __ __ . __ __)	e._____ (__ __ __ . __ __)
f. _____	f. (__ __ __ . __ __) ☐0 ☐1 ☐2 ☐3 ☐4	f._____ (__ __ __ . __ __)	f._____ (__ __ __ . __ __)

(M1030) **Therapies** the patient receives <u>at home</u>: **(Mark all that apply.)**

- ☐ 1 - Intravenous or infusion therapy (excludes TPN)
- ☐ 2 - Parenteral nutrition (TPN or lipids)
- ☐ 3 - Enteral nutrition (nasogastric, gastrostomy, jejunostomy, or any other artificial entry into the alimentary canal)
- ☐ 4 - None of the above

SENSORY STATUS

(M1200) **Vision** (with corrective lenses if the patient usually wears them):

- ☐ 0 - Normal vision: sees adequately in most situations; can see medication labels, newsprint.
- ☐ 1 - Partially impaired: cannot see medication labels or newsprint, but <u>can</u> see obstacles in path, and the surrounding layout; can count fingers at arm's length.
- ☐ 2 - Severely impaired: cannot locate objects without hearing or touching them or patient nonresponsive.

OMB #0938-0760

Expiration date 7/31/2012

(M1242) **Frequency of Pain Interfering** with patient's activity or movement:

- ☐ 0 - Patient has no pain
- ☐ 1 - Patient has pain that does not interfere with activity or movement
- ☐ 2 - Less often than daily
- ☐ 3 - Daily, but not constantly
- ☐ 4 - All of the time

INTEGUMENTARY STATUS

(M1306) Does this patient have at least one **Unhealed Pressure Ulcer at Stage II or Higher** or designated as "unstageable"?

- ☐ 0 - No [*Go to M1322*]
- ☐ 1 - Yes

(M1308) **Current Number of Unhealed (non-epithelialized) Pressure Ulcers at Each Stage:**
(Enter "0" if none; excludes Stage I pressure ulcers)

Stage description – unhealed pressure ulcers	Column 1 Complete at SOC/ROC/FU & D/C Number Currently Present	Column 2 Complete at FU & D/C Number of those listed in Column 1 that were present on admission (most recent SOC / ROC)
a. **Stage II:** Partial thickness loss of dermis presenting as a shallow open ulcer with red pink wound bed, without slough. May also present as an intact or open/ruptured serum-filled blister.	⎯⎯	⎯⎯
b. **Stage III:** Full thickness tissue loss. Subcutaneous fat may be visible but bone, tendon, or muscles are not exposed. Slough may be present but does not obscure the depth of tissue loss. May include undermining and tunneling.	⎯⎯	⎯⎯
c. **Stage IV:** Full thickness tissue loss with visible bone, tendon, or muscle. Slough or eschar may be present on some parts of the wound bed. Often includes undermining and tunneling.	⎯⎯	⎯⎯
d.1 Unstageable: Known or likely but unstageable due to non-removable dressing or device	⎯⎯	⎯⎯
d.2 Unstageable: Known or likely but unstageable due to coverage of wound bed by slough and/or eschar.	⎯⎯	⎯⎯
d.3 Unstageable: Suspected deep tissue injury in evolution.	⎯⎯	⎯⎯

(M1322) **Current Number of Stage I Pressure Ulcers:** Intact skin with non-blanchable redness of a localized area usually over a bony prominence. The area may be painful, firm, soft, warmer or cooler as compared to adjacent tissue.

☐ 0   ☐ 1   ☐ 2   ☐ 3   ☐ 4 or more

OMB #0938-0760

Expiration date 7/31/2012

(M1324) Stage of Most Problematic Unhealed (Observable) Pressure Ulcer:

- ☐ 1 - Stage I
- ☐ 2 - Stage II
- ☐ 3 - Stage III
- ☐ 4 - Stage IV
- ☐ NA - No observable pressure ulcer or unhealed pressure ulcer

(M1330) Does this patient have a **Stasis Ulcer?**

- ☐ 0 - No [*Go to M1340*]
- ☐ 1 - Yes, patient has BOTH observable and unobservable stasis ulcers
- ☐ 2 - Yes, patient has observable stasis ulcers ONLY
- ☐ 3 - Yes, patient has unobservable stasis ulcers ONLY (known but not observable due to non-removable dressing) [*Go to M1340*]

(M1332) Current Number of (Observable) Stasis Ulcer(s):

- ☐ 1 - One
- ☐ 2 - Two
- ☐ 3 - Three
- ☐ 4 - Four or more

(M1334) Status of Most Problematic (Observable) Stasis Ulcer:

- ☐ 0 - Newly epithelialized
- ☐ 1 - Fully granulating
- ☐ 2 - Early/partial granulation
- ☐ 3 - Not healing

(M1340) Does this patient have a **Surgical Wound?**

- ☐ 0 - No [*Go to M1350*]
- ☐ 1 - Yes, patient has at least one (observable) surgical wound
- ☐ 2 - Surgical wound known but not observable due to non-removable dressing [*Go to M1350*]

(M1342) Status of Most Problematic (Observable) Surgical Wound:

- ☐ 0 - Newly epithelialized
- ☐ 1 - Fully granulating
- ☐ 2 - Early/partial granulation
- ☐ 3 - Not healing

(M1350) Does this patient have a **Skin Lesion** or **Open Wound,** excluding bowel ostomy, other than those described above that is receiving intervention by the home health agency?

- ☐ 0 - No
- ☐ 1 - Yes

RESPIRATORY STATUS

(M1400) When is the patient dyspneic or noticeably **Short of Breath?**

- ☐ 0 - Patient is not short of breath
- ☐ 1 - When walking more than 20 feet, climbing stairs
- ☐ 2 - With moderate exertion (e.g., while dressing, using commode or bedpan, walking distances less than 20 feet)
- ☐ 3 - With minimal exertion (e.g., while eating, talking, or performing other ADLs) or with agitation
- ☐ 4 - At rest (during day or night)

OMB #0938-0760

Expiration date 7/31/2012

ELIMINATION STATUS

(M1600) Has this patient been treated for a **Urinary Tract Infection** in the past 14 days?

- ☐ 0 - No
- ☐ 1 - Yes
- ☐ NA - Patient on prophylactic treatment
- ☐ UK - Unknown **[Omit "UK" option on DC]**

(M1610) Urinary Incontinence or Urinary Catheter Presence:

- ☐ 0 - No incontinence or catheter (includes anuria or ostomy for urinary drainage) [*Go to M1620*]
- ☐ 1 - Patient is incontinent
- ☐ 2 - Patient requires a urinary catheter (i.e., external, indwelling, intermittent, suprapubic)
      [*Go to M1620*]

(M1615) When does **Urinary Incontinence** occur?

- ☐ 0 - Timed-voiding defers incontinence
- ☐ 1 - Occasional stress incontinence
- ☐ 2 - During the night only
- ☐ 3 - During the day only
- ☐ 4 - During the day and night

(M1620) Bowel Incontinence Frequency:

- ☐ 0 - Very rarely or never has bowel incontinence
- ☐ 1 - Less than once weekly
- ☐ 2 - One to three times weekly
- ☐ 3 - Four to six times weekly
- ☐ 4 - On a daily basis
- ☐ 5 - More often than once daily
- ☐ NA - Patient has ostomy for bowel elimination
- ☐ UK - Unknown [Omit "UK" option on FU, DC]

NEURO/EMOTIONAL/BEHAVIORAL STATUS

(M1700) Cognitive Functioning: Patient's current (day of assessment) level of alertness, orientation, comprehension, concentration, and immediate memory for simple commands.

- ☐ 0 - Alert/oriented, able to focus and shift attention, comprehends and recalls task directions independently.
- ☐ 1 - Requires prompting (cuing, repetition, reminders) only under stressful or unfamiliar conditions.
- ☐ 2 - Requires assistance and some direction in specific situations (e.g., on all tasks involving shifting of attention), or consistently requires low stimulus environment due to distractibility.
- ☐ 3 - Requires considerable assistance in routine situations. Is not alert and oriented or is unable to shift attention and recall directions more than half the time.
- ☐ 4 - Totally dependent due to disturbances such as constant disorientation, coma, persistent vegetative state, or delirium.

OMB #0938-0760   Expiration date 7/31/2012

(M1830) **Bathing:** Current ability to wash entire body safely. **Excludes grooming (washing face, washing hands, and shampooing hair).**

- ☐ 0 - Able to bathe self in <u>shower or tub</u> independently, including getting in and out of tub/shower.
- ☐ 1 - With the use of devices, is able to bathe self in shower or tub independently, including getting in and out of the tub/shower.
- ☐ 2 - Able to bathe in shower or tub with the intermittent assistance of another person:
    - (a) for intermittent supervision or encouragement or reminders, <u>OR</u>
    - (b) to get in and out of the shower or tub, <u>OR</u>
    - (c) for washing difficult to reach areas.
- ☐ 3 - Able to participate in bathing self in shower or tub, <u>but</u> requires presence of another person throughout the bath for assistance or supervision.
- ☐ 4 - Unable to use the shower or tub, but able to bathe self independently with or without the use of devices at the sink, in chair, or on commode.
- ☐ 5 - Unable to use the shower or tub, but able to participate in bathing self in bed, at the sink, in bedside chair, or on commode, with the assistance or supervision of another person throughout the bath.
- ☐ 6 - Unable to participate effectively in bathing and is bathed totally by another person.

(M1840) **Toilet Transferring:** Current ability to get to and from the toilet or bedside commode safely <u>and</u> transfer on and off toilet/commode.

- ☐ 0 - Able to get to and from the toilet and transfer independently with or without a device.
- ☐ 1 - When reminded, assisted, or supervised by another person, able to get to and from the toilet and transfer.
- ☐ 2 - <u>Unable</u> to get to and from the toilet but is able to use a bedside commode (with or without assistance).
- ☐ 3 - <u>Unable</u> to get to and from the toilet or bedside commode but is able to use a bedpan/urinal independently.
- ☐ 4 - Is totally dependent in toileting.

(M1850) **Transferring:** Current ability to move safely from bed to chair, or ability to turn and position self in bed if patient is bedfast.

- ☐ 0 - Able to independently transfer.
- ☐ 1 - Able to transfer with minimal human assistance or with use of an assistive device.
- ☐ 2 - Able to bear weight and pivot during the transfer process but unable to transfer self.
- ☐ 3 - Unable to transfer self and is unable to bear weight or pivot when transferred by another person.
- ☐ 4 - Bedfast, unable to transfer but is able to turn and position self in bed.
- ☐ 5 - Bedfast, unable to transfer and is unable to turn and position self.

(M1860) **Ambulation/Locomotion:** Current ability to walk safely, once in a standing position, or use a wheelchair, once in a seated position, on a variety of surfaces.

- ☐ 0 - Able to independently walk on even and uneven surfaces and negotiate stairs with or without railings (i.e., needs no human assistance or assistive device).
- ☐ 1 - With the use of a one-handed device (e.g. cane, single crutch, hemi-walker), able to independently walk on even and uneven surfaces and negotiate stairs with or without railings.
- ☐ 2 - Requires use of a two-handed device (e.g., walker or crutches) to walk alone on a level surface and/or requires human supervision or assistance to negotiate stairs or steps or uneven surfaces.
- ☐ 3 - Able to walk only with the supervision or assistance of another person at all times.
- ☐ 4 - Chairfast, <u>unable</u> to ambulate but is able to wheel self independently.
- ☐ 5 - Chairfast, unable to ambulate and is <u>unable</u> to wheel self.
- ☐ 6 - Bedfast, unable to ambulate or be up in a chair.

OMB #0938-0760

Expiration date 7/31/2012

MEDICATIONS

(M2030) **Management of Injectable Medications:** <u>Patient's current ability</u> to prepare and take <u>all</u> prescribed injectable medications reliably and safely, including administration of correct dosage at the appropriate times/intervals. <u>**Excludes**</u> **IV medications.**

☐   0 -   Able to independently take the correct medication(s) and proper dosage(s) at the correct times.

☐   1 -   Able to take injectable medication(s) at the correct times if:

     (a) individual syringes are prepared in advance by another person; <u>OR</u>
     (b) another person develops a drug diary or chart.

☐   2 -   Able to take medication(s) at the correct times if given reminders by another person based on the frequency of the injection

☐   3 -   <u>Unable</u> to take injectable medication unless administered by another person.

☐ NA -   No injectable medications prescribed.

THERAPY NEED AND PLAN OF CARE

(M2200) **Therapy Need:** In the home health plan of care for the Medicare payment episode for which this assessment will define a case mix group, what is the indicated need for therapy visits (total of reasonable and necessary physical, occupational, and speech-language pathology visits combined)? **(Enter zero ["000"] if no therapy visits indicated.)**

(__ __ __)   Number of therapy visits indicated (total of physical, occupational and speech-language pathology combined).

☐ NA -   Not Applicable: No case mix group defined by this assessment.

APPENDIX E

OMB #0938-0760

Expiration date 7/31/2012

Outcome and Assessment Information Set

Items to be Used at Specific Time Points

Start of Care --
    Start of care—further visits planned

M0010-M0030, M0040-M0150, M1000-M1036, M1100-M1242, M1300-M1302, M1306, M1308-M1324, M1330-M1350, M1400, M1410, M1600-M1730, M1740-M1910, M2000, M2002, M2010, M2020-M2250

Resumption of Care ---
    Resumption of care (after inpatient stay)

M0032, M0080-M0110, M1000-M1036, M1100-M1242, M1300-M1302, M1306, M1308-M1324, M1330-M1350, M1400, M1410, M1600-M1730, M1740-M1910, M2000, M2002, M2010, M2020-M2250

Follow-Up --
    Recertification (follow-up) assessment
    Other follow-up assessment

M0080-M0100, M0110, M1020-M1030, M1200, M1242, M1306, M1308, M1322-M1324, M1330-M1350, M1400, M1610, M1620, M1630, M1810-M1840, M1850, M1860, M2030, M2200

Transfer to an Inpatient Facility -------------------------------
    Transferred to an inpatient facility—patient not discharged from an agency
    Transferred to an inpatient facility—patient discharged from agency

M0080-M0100, M1040-M1055, M1500, M1510, M2004, M2015, M2300-M2410, M2430-M2440, M0903, M0906

Discharge from Agency — Not to an Inpatient Facility

    Death at home-- M0080-M0100, M0903, M0906

    Discharge from agency--------------------------------------- M0080-M0100, M1040-M1055, M1230, M1242, M1306-M1350, M1400-M1620, M1700-M1720, M1740, M1745, M1800-M1890, M2004, M2015-M2030, M2100-M2110, M2300-M2420, M0903, M0906

CLINICAL RECORD ITEMS

(M0080) Discipline of Person Completing Assessment:
    ☐ 1-RN   ☐ 2-PT   ☐ 3-SLP/ST   ☐ 4-OT

(M0090) Date Assessment Completed: __ __ / __ __ / __ __ __ __
                             month / day / year

(M0100) This Assessment is Currently Being Completed for the Following Reason:

    Start/Resumption of Care
    ☐ 1 – Start of care—further visits planned
    ☐ 3 – Resumption of care (after inpatient stay)

    Follow-Up
    ☐ 4 – Recertification (follow-up) reassessment [*Go to M0110*]
    ☐ 5 – Other follow-up [*Go to M0110*]

    Transfer to an Inpatient Facility
    ☐ 6 – Transferred to an inpatient facility—patient not discharged from agency [*Go to M1040*]
    ☐ 7 – Transferred to an inpatient facility—patient discharged from agency [*Go to M1040*]

    Discharge from Agency — Not to an Inpatient Facility
    ☐ 8 – Death at home [*Go to M0903*]
    ☐ 9 – Discharge from agency [*Go to M1040*]

OMB #0938-0760

Expiration date 7/31/2012

(M1040) Influenza Vaccine: Did the patient receive the influenza vaccine from your agency for this year's influenza season (October 1 through March 31) during this episode of care?

☐   0 -   No

☐   1 -   Yes [*Go to M1050*]

☐   NA -   Does not apply because entire episode of care (SOC/ROC to Transfer/Discharge) is outside this influenza season. [*Go to M1050*]

(M1045) Reason Influenza Vaccine not received: If the patient did not receive the influenza vaccine from your agency during this episode of care, state reason:

☐   1 -   Received from another health care provider (e.g., physician)

☐   2 -   Received from your agency previously during this year's flu season

☐   3 -   Offered and declined

☐   4 -   Assessed and determined to have medical contraindication(s)

☐   5 -   Not indicated; patient does not meet age/condition guidelines for influenza vaccine

☐   6 -   Inability to obtain vaccine due to declared shortage

☐   7 -   None of the above

(M1050) Pneumococcal Vaccine: Did the patient receive pneumococcal polysaccharide vaccine (PPV) from your agency during this episode of care (SOC/ROC to Transfer/Discharge)?

☐   0 -   No

☐   1 -   Yes [*Go to M1500 at TRN; Go to M1230 at DC*]

(M1055) Reason PPV not received: If patient did not receive the pneumococcal polysaccharide vaccine (PPV) from your agency during this episode of care (SOC/ROC to Transfer/Discharge), state reason:

☐   1 -   Patient has received PPV in the past

☐   2 -   Offered and declined

☐   3 -   Assessed and determined to have medical contraindication(s)

☐   4 -   Not indicated; patient does not meet age/condition guidelines for PPV

☐   5 -   None of the above

SENSORY STATUS

(M1230) Speech and Oral (Verbal) Expression of Language (in patient's own language):

☐   0 -   Expresses complex ideas, feelings, and needs clearly, completely, and easily in all situations with no observable impairment.

☐   1 -   Minimal difficulty in expressing ideas and needs (may take extra time; makes occasional errors in word choice, grammar or speech intelligibility; needs minimal prompting or assistance).

☐   2 -   Expresses simple ideas or needs with moderate difficulty (needs prompting or assistance, errors in word choice, organization or speech intelligibility). Speaks in phrases or short sentences.

☐   3 -   Has severe difficulty expressing basic ideas or needs and requires maximal assistance or guessing by listener. Speech limited to single words or short phrases.

☐   4 -   <u>Unable</u> to express basic needs even with maximal prompting or assistance but is not comatose or unresponsive (e.g., speech is nonsensical or unintelligible).

☐   5 -   Patient nonresponsive or unable to speak.

(M1242) Frequency of Pain Interfering with patient's activity or movement:

☐   0 -   Patient has no pain

☐   1 -   Patient has pain that does not interfere with activity or movement

☐   2 -   Less often than daily

☐   3 -   Daily, but not constantly

☐   4 -   All of the time

OMB #0938-0760

Expiration date 7/31/2012

INTEGUMENTARY STATUS

(M1306) Does this patient have at least one **Unhealed Pressure Ulcer at Stage II or Higher** or designated as "unstageable"?

☐   0 - No [*Go to M1322*]

☐   1 - Yes

(M1307) The **Oldest Non-epithelialized Stage II Pressure Ulcer** that is present at discharge

☐   1 - Was present at the most recent SOC/ROC assessment

☐   2 - Developed since the most recent SOC/ROC assessment: record date pressure ulcer first identified:

__ __ / __ __ / ____ __ __
month / day / year

☐   NA - No non-epithelialized Stage II pressure ulcers are present at discharge

(M1308)   **Current Number of Unhealed (non-epithelialized) Pressure Ulcers at Each Stage:**
(Enter "0" if none; excludes Stage I pressure ulcers)

	Column 1 Complete at SOC/ROC/FU & D/C	Column 2 Complete at FU & D/C
Stage description – unhealed pressure ulcers	<u>Number Currently Present</u>	<u>Number of those listed in Column 1 that were present on admission (most recent SOC / ROC)</u>
a. **Stage II:** Partial thickness loss of dermis presenting as a shallow open ulcer with red pink wound bed, without slough. May also present as an intact or open/ruptured serum-filled blister.	____	____
b. **Stage III:** Full thickness tissue loss. Subcutaneous fat may be visible but bone, tendon, or muscles are not exposed. Slough may be present but does not obscure the depth of tissue loss. May include undermining and tunneling.	____	____
c. **Stage IV:** Full thickness tissue loss with visible bone, tendon, or muscle. Slough or eschar may be present on some parts of the wound bed. Often includes undermining and tunneling.	____	____
d.1 Unstageable: Known or likely but unstageable due to non-removable dressing or device	____	____
d.2 Unstageable: Known or likely but unstageable due to coverage of wound bed by slough and/or eschar.	____	____
d.3 Unstageable: Suspected deep tissue injury in evolution.	____	____

OMB #0938-0760

Expiration date 7/31/2012

Directions for M1310, M1312, and M1314: If the patient has one or more unhealed (non-epithelialized) Stage III or IV pressure ulcers, identify the **Stage III or IV pressure ulcer with the largest surface dimension (length x width)** and record in centimeters. If no Stage III or Stage IV pressure ulcers, go to M1320.

(M1310) **Pressure Ulcer Length:** Longest length "head-to-toe" | ___ | ___ | . | ___ | (cm)

(M1312) **Pressure Ulcer Width:** Width of the same pressure ulcer; greatest width perpendicular to the length

| ___ | ___ | . | ___ | (cm)

(M1314) **Pressure Ulcer Depth:** Depth of the same pressure ulcer; from visible surface to the deepest area

| ___ | ___ | . | ___ | (cm)

(M1320) **Status of Most Problematic (Observable) Pressure Ulcer:**

☐ 0 - Newly epithelialized
☐ 1 - Fully granulating
☐ 2 - Early/partial granulation
☐ 3 - Not healing
☐ NA - No observable pressure ulcer

(M1322) **Current Number of Stage I Pressure Ulcers:** Intact skin with non-blanchable redness of a localized area usually over a bony prominence. The area may be painful, firm, soft, warmer or cooler as compared to adjacent tissue.

☐ 0 ☐ 1 ☐ 2 ☐ 3 ☐ 4 or more

(M1324) **Stage of Most Problematic Unhealed (Observable) Pressure Ulcer:**

☐ 1 - Stage I
☐ 2 - Stage II
☐ 3 - Stage III
☐ 4 - Stage IV
☐ NA - No observable pressure ulcer or unhealed pressure ulcer

(M1330) Does this patient have a **Stasis Ulcer**?

☐ 0 - No [*Go to M1340*]
☐ 1 - Yes, patient has BOTH observable and unobservable stasis ulcers
☐ 2 - Yes, patient has observable stasis ulcers ONLY
☐ 3 - Yes, patient has unobservable stasis ulcers ONLY (known but not observable due to non-removable dressing) [*Go to M1340*]

(M1332) **Current Number of (Observable) Stasis Ulcer(s):**

☐ 1 - One
☐ 2 - Two
☐ 3 - Three
☐ 4 - Four or more

(M1334) **Status of Most Problematic (Observable) Stasis Ulcer:**

☐ 0 - Newly epithelialized
☐ 1 - Fully granulating
☐ 2 - Early/partial granulation
☐ 3 - Not healing

(M1340) Does this patient have a **Surgical Wound?**

☐ 0 - No [*Go to M1350*]
☐ 1 - Yes, patient has at least one (observable) surgical wound
☐ 2 - Surgical wound known but not observable due to non-removable dressing [*Go to M1350*]

OMB #0938-0760   Expiration date 7/31/2012

(M1342) Status of Most Problematic (Observable) Surgical Wound:

- ☐ 0 - Newly epithelialized
- ☐ 1 - Fully granulating
- ☐ 2 - Early/partial granulation
- ☐ 3 - Not healing

(M1350) Does this patient have a **Skin Lesion** or **Open Wound,** excluding bowel ostomy, other than those described above that is receiving intervention by the home health agency?

- ☐ 0 - No
- ☐ 1 - Yes

RESPIRATORY STATUS

(M1400) When is the patient dyspneic or noticeably **Short of Breath**?

- ☐ 0 - Patient is not short of breath
- ☐ 1 - When walking more than 20 feet, climbing stairs
- ☐ 2 - With moderate exertion (e.g., while dressing, using commode or bedpan, walking distances less than 20 feet)
- ☐ 3 - With minimal exertion (e.g., while eating, talking, or performing other ADLs) or with agitation
- ☐ 4 - At rest (during day or night)

(M1410) Respiratory Treatments utilized at home: **(Mark all that apply.)**

- ☐ 1 - Oxygen (intermittent or continuous)
- ☐ 2 - Ventilator (continually or at night)
- ☐ 3 - Continuous / Bi-level positive airway pressure
- ☐ 4 - None of the above

CARDIAC STATUS

(M1500) Symptoms in Heart Failure Patients: If patient has been diagnosed with heart failure, did the patient exhibit symptoms indicated by clinical heart failure guidelines (including dyspnea, orthopnea, edema, or weight gain) at any point since the previous OASIS assessment?

- ☐ 0 - No [*Go to M2004 at TRN; Go to M1600 at DC*]
- ☐ 1 - Yes
- ☐ 2 - Not assessed [*Go to M2004 at TRN; Go to M1600 at DC*]
- ☐ NA - Patient does not have diagnosis of heart failure [*Go to M2004 at TRN; Go to M1600 at DC*]

(M1510) Heart Failure Follow-up: If patient has been diagnosed with heart failure and has exhibited symptoms indicative of heart failure since the previous OASIS assessment, what action(s) has (have) been taken to respond? **(Mark all that apply.)**

- ☐ 0 - No action taken
- ☐ 1 - Patient's physician (or other primary care practitioner) contacted the same day
- ☐ 2 - Patient advised to get emergency treatment (e.g., call 911 or go to emergency room)
- ☐ 3 - Implemented physician-ordered patient-specific established parameters for treatment
- ☐ 4 - Patient education or other clinical interventions
- ☐ 5 - Obtained change in care plan orders (e.g., increased monitoring by agency, change in visit frequency, telehealth, etc.)

OMB #0938-0760

Expiration date 7/31/2012

ELIMINATION STATUS

(M1600) Has this patient been treated for a **Urinary Tract Infection** in the past 14 days?

☐   0 -   No

☐   1 -   Yes

☐   NA -   Patient on prophylactic treatment

☐   UK -   Unknown **[Omit "UK" option on DC]**

(M1610)   **Urinary Incontinence or Urinary Catheter Presence:**

☐   0 -   No incontinence or catheter (includes anuria or ostomy for urinary drainage) [*Go to M1620*]

☐   1 -   Patient is incontinent

☐   2 -   Patient requires a urinary catheter (i.e., external, indwelling, intermittent, suprapubic)
     [*Go to M1620*]

(M1615)   **When** does **Urinary Incontinence** occur?

☐   0 -   Timed-voiding defers incontinence

☐   1 -   Occasional stress incontinence

☐   2 -   During the night only

☐   3 -   During the day only

☐   4 -   During the day and night

(M1620) Bowel Incontinence Frequency:

☐   0 -   Very rarely or never has bowel incontinence

☐   1 -   Less than once weekly

☐   2 -   One to three times weekly

☐   3 -   Four to six times weekly

☐   4 -   On a daily basis

☐   5 -   More often than once daily

☐   NA -   Patient has ostomy for bowel elimination

☐   UK -   Unknown [Omit "UK" option on FU, DC]

NEURO/EMOTIONAL/BEHAVIORAL STATUS

(M1700)   **Cognitive Functioning:** Patient's current (day of assessment) level of alertness, orientation, comprehension, concentration, and immediate memory for simple commands.

☐   0 -   Alert/oriented, able to focus and shift attention, comprehends and recalls task directions independently.

☐   1 -   Requires prompting (cuing, repetition, reminders) only under stressful or unfamiliar conditions.

☐   2 -   Requires assistance and some direction in specific situations (e.g., on all tasks involving shifting of attention), or consistently requires low stimulus environment due to distractibility.

☐   3 -   Requires considerable assistance in routine situations. Is not alert and oriented or is unable to shift attention and recall directions more than half the time.

☐   4 -   Totally dependent due to disturbances such as constant disorientation, coma, persistent vegetative state, or delirium.

OMB #0938-0760

Expiration date 7/31/2012

(M1710) When Confused (Reported or Observed Within the Last 14 Days):

☐ 0 - Never

☐ 1 - In new or complex situations only

☐ 2 - On awakening or at night only

☐ 3 - During the day and evening, but not constantly

☐ 4 - Constantly

☐ NA - Patient nonresponsive

(M1720) When Anxious (Reported or Observed Within the Last 14 Days):

☐ 0 - None of the time

☐ 1 - Less often than daily

☐ 2 - Daily, but not constantly

☐ 3 - All of the time

☐ NA - Patient nonresponsive

(M1740) Cognitive, behavioral, and psychiatric symptoms that are demonstrated <u>at least once a week</u> (Reported or Observed): **(Mark all that apply.)**

☐ 1 - Memory deficit: failure to recognize familiar persons/places, inability to recall events of past 24 hours, significant memory loss so that supervision is required

☐ 2 - Impaired decision-making: failure to perform usual ADLs or IADLs, inability to appropriately stop activities, jeopardizes safety through actions

☐ 3 - Verbal disruption: yelling, threatening, excessive profanity, sexual references, etc.

☐ 4 - Physical aggression: aggressive or combative to self and others (e.g., hits self, throws objects, punches, dangerous maneuvers with wheelchair or other objects)

☐ 5 - Disruptive, infantile, or socially inappropriate behavior (**excludes** verbal actions)

☐ 6 - Delusional, hallucinatory, or paranoid behavior

☐ 7 - None of the above behaviors demonstrated

(M1745) Frequency of Disruptive Behavior Symptoms (Reported or Observed) Any physical, verbal, or other disruptive/dangerous symptoms that are injurious to self or others or jeopardize personal safety.

☐ 0 - Never

☐ 1 - Less than once a month

☐ 2 - Once a month

☐ 3 - Several times each month

☐ 4 - Several times a week

☐ 5 - At least daily

ADL/IADLs

(M1800) Grooming: Current ability to tend safely to personal hygiene needs (i.e., washing face and hands, hair care, shaving or make up, teeth or denture care, fingernail care).

☐ 0 - Able to groom self unaided, with or without the use of assistive devices or adapted methods.

☐ 1 - Grooming utensils must be placed within reach before able to complete grooming activities.

☐ 2 - Someone must assist the patient to groom self.

☐ 3 - Patient depends entirely upon someone else for grooming needs.

OMB #0938-0760

Expiration date 7/31/2012

(M1810) Current Ability to Dress Upper Body safely (with or without dressing aids) including undergarments, pullovers, front-opening shirts and blouses, managing zippers, buttons, and snaps:

☐ 0 - Able to get clothes out of closets and drawers, put them on and remove them from the upper body without assistance.

☐ 1 - Able to dress upper body without assistance if clothing is laid out or handed to the patient.

☐ 2 - Someone must help the patient put on upper body clothing.

☐ 3 - Patient depends entirely upon another person to dress the upper body.

(M1820) Current Ability to Dress Lower Body safely (with or without dressing aids) including undergarments, slacks, socks or nylons, shoes:

☐ 0 - Able to obtain, put on, and remove clothing and shoes without assistance.

☐ 1 - Able to dress lower body without assistance if clothing and shoes are laid out or handed to the patient.

☐ 2 - Someone must help the patient put on undergarments, slacks, socks or nylons, and shoes.

☐ 3 - Patient depends entirely upon another person to dress lower body.

(M1830) Bathing: Current ability to wash entire body safely. **Excludes grooming (washing face, washing hands, and shampooing hair).**

☐ 0 - Able to bathe self in shower or tub independently, including getting in and out of tub/shower.

☐ 1 - With the use of devices, is able to bathe self in shower or tub independently, including getting in and out of the tub/shower.

☐ 2 - Able to bathe in shower or tub with the intermittent assistance of another person:

    (a) for intermittent supervision or encouragement or reminders, OR
    (b) to get in and out of the shower or tub, OR
    (c) for washing difficult to reach areas.

☐ 3 - Able to participate in bathing self in shower or tub, but requires presence of another person throughout the bath for assistance or supervision.

☐ 4 - Unable to use the shower or tub, but able to bathe self independently with or without the use of devices at the sink, in chair, or on commode.

☐ 5 - Unable to use the shower or tub, but able to participate in bathing self in bed, at the sink, in bedside chair, or on commode, with the assistance or supervision of another person throughout the bath.

☐ 6 - Unable to participate effectively in bathing and is bathed totally by another person.

(M1840) Toilet Transferring: Current ability to get to and from the toilet or bedside commode safely and transfer on and off toilet/commode.

☐ 0 - Able to get to and from the toilet and transfer independently with or without a device.

☐ 1 - When reminded, assisted, or supervised by another person, able to get to and from the toilet and transfer.

☐ 2 - Unable to get to and from the toilet but is able to use a bedside commode (with or without assistance).

☐ 3 - Unable to get to and from the toilet or bedside commode but is able to use a bedpan/urinal independently.

☐ 4 - Is totally dependent in toileting.

(M1845) Toileting Hygiene: Current ability to maintain perineal hygiene safely, adjust clothes and/or incontinence pads before and after using toilet, commode, bedpan, urinal. If managing ostomy, includes cleaning area around stoma, but not managing equipment.

☐ 0 - Able to manage toileting hygiene and clothing management without assistance.

☐ 1 - Able to manage toileting hygiene and clothing management without assistance if supplies/implements are laid out for the patient.

☐ 2 - Someone must help the patient to maintain toileting hygiene and/or adjust clothing.

☐ 3 - Patient depends entirely upon another person to maintain toileting hygiene.

OMB #0938-0760   Expiration date 7/31/2012

(M1850) **Transferring:** Current ability to move safely from bed to chair, or ability to turn and position self in bed if patient is bedfast.

- ☐ 0 - Able to independently transfer.
- ☐ 1 - Able to transfer with minimal human assistance or with use of an assistive device.
- ☐ 2 - Able to bear weight and pivot during the transfer process but unable to transfer self.
- ☐ 3 - Unable to transfer self and is unable to bear weight or pivot when transferred by another person.
- ☐ 4 - Bedfast, unable to transfer but is able to turn and position self in bed.
- ☐ 5 - Bedfast, unable to transfer and is unable to turn and position self.

(M1860) **Ambulation/Locomotion:** Current ability to walk safely, once in a standing position, or use a wheelchair, once in a seated position, on a variety of surfaces.

- ☐ 0 - Able to independently walk on even and uneven surfaces and negotiate stairs with or without railings (i.e., needs no human assistance or assistive device).
- ☐ 1 - With the use of a one-handed device (e.g. cane, single crutch, hemi-walker), able to independently walk on even and uneven surfaces and negotiate stairs with or without railings.
- ☐ 2 - Requires use of a two-handed device (e.g., walker or crutches) to walk alone on a level surface and/or requires human supervision or assistance to negotiate stairs or steps or uneven surfaces.
- ☐ 3 - Able to walk only with the supervision or assistance of another person at all times.
- ☐ 4 - Chairfast, <u>unable</u> to ambulate but is able to wheel self independently.
- ☐ 5 - Chairfast, unable to ambulate and is <u>unable</u> to wheel self.
- ☐ 6 - Bedfast, unable to ambulate or be up in a chair.

(M1870) **Feeding or Eating:** Current ability to feed self meals and snacks safely. Note: This refers only to the process of <u>eating</u>, <u>chewing</u>, and <u>swallowing</u>, <u>not preparing</u> the food to be eaten.

- ☐ 0 - Able to independently feed self.
- ☐ 1 - Able to feed self independently but requires:
  (a) meal set-up; <u>OR</u>
  (b) intermittent assistance or supervision from another person; <u>OR</u>
  (c) a liquid, pureed or ground meat diet.
- ☐ 2 - <u>Unable</u> to feed self and must be assisted or supervised throughout the meal/snack.
- ☐ 3 - Able to take in nutrients orally <u>and</u> receives supplemental nutrients through a nasogastric tube or gastrostomy.
- ☐ 4 - <u>Unable</u> to take in nutrients orally and is fed nutrients through a nasogastric tube or gastrostomy.
- ☐ 5 - Unable to take in nutrients orally or by tube feeding.

(M1880) Current **Ability to Plan and Prepare Light Meals** (e.g., cereal, sandwich) or reheat delivered meals safely:

- ☐ 0 - (a) Able to independently plan and prepare all light meals for self or reheat delivered meals; <u>OR</u>
  (b) Is physically, cognitively, and mentally able to prepare light meals on a regular basis but has not routinely performed light meal preparation in the past (i.e., prior to this home care admission).
- ☐ 1 - <u>Unable</u> to prepare light meals on a regular basis due to physical, cognitive, or mental limitations.
- ☐ 2 - Unable to prepare any light meals or reheat any delivered meals.

(M1890) **Ability to Use Telephone:** Current ability to answer the phone safely, including dialing numbers, and <u>effectively</u> using the telephone to communicate.

- ☐ 0 - Able to dial numbers and answer calls appropriately and as desired.
- ☐ 1 - Able to use a specially adapted telephone (i.e., large numbers on the dial, teletype phone for the deaf) and call essential numbers.
- ☐ 2 - Able to answer the telephone and carry on a normal conversation but has difficulty with placing calls.
- ☐ 3 - Able to answer the telephone only some of the time or is able to carry on only a limited conversation.
- ☐ 4 - <u>Unable</u> to answer the telephone at all but can listen if assisted with equipment.
- ☐ 5 - Totally unable to use the telephone.
- ☐ NA - Patient does not have a telephone.

OMB #0938-0760

Expiration date 7/31/2012

MEDICATIONS

(M2004) **Medication Intervention:** If there were any clinically significant medication issues since the previous OASIS assessment, was a physician or the physician-designee contacted within one calendar day of the assessment to resolve clinically significant medication issues, including reconciliation?

☐   0   -   No
☐   1   -   Yes
☐   NA   -   No clinically significant medication issues identified since the previous OASIS assessment

(M2015) **Patient/Caregiver Drug Education Intervention**: Since the previous OASIS assessment, was the patient/caregiver instructed by agency staff or other health care provider to monitor the effectiveness of drug therapy, drug reactions, and side effects, and how and when to report problems that may occur?

☐   0   -   No
☐   1   -   Yes
☐   NA   -   Patient not taking any drugs

(M2020) **Management of Oral Medications:** <u>Patient's current ability</u> to prepare and take <u>all</u> oral medications reliably and safely, including administration of the correct dosage at the appropriate times/intervals. **Excludes injectable and IV medications. (NOTE: This refers to ability, not compliance or willingness.)**

☐   0   -   Able to independently take the correct oral medication(s) and proper dosage(s) at the correct times.
☐   1   -   Able to take medication(s) at the correct times if:
         (a) individual dosages are prepared in advance by another person; <u>OR</u>
         (b) another person develops a drug diary or chart.
☐   2   -   Able to take medication(s) at the correct times if given reminders by another person at the appropriate times
☐   3   -   <u>Unable</u> to take medication unless administered by another person.
☐   NA   -   No oral medications prescribed.

(M2030) **Management of Injectable Medications:** <u>Patient's current ability</u> to prepare and take <u>all</u> prescribed injectable medications reliably and safely, including administration of correct dosage at the appropriate times/intervals. **Excludes IV medications.**

☐   0   -   Able to independently take the correct medication(s) and proper dosage(s) at the correct times.
☐   1   -   Able to take injectable medication(s) at the correct times if:
         (a) individual syringes are prepared in advance by another person; <u>OR</u>
         (b) another person develops a drug diary or chart.
☐   2   -   Able to take medication(s) at the correct times if given reminders by another person based on the frequency of the injection
☐   3   -   <u>Unable</u> to take injectable medication unless administered by another person.
☐   NA   -   No injectable medications prescribed.

OMB #0938-0760   Expiration date 7/31/2012

CARE MANAGEMENT

(M2100)   Types and Sources of Assistance: Determine the level of caregiver ability and willingness to provide assistance for the following activities, if assistance is needed. (Check only **one** box in each row.)

Type of Assistance	No assistance needed in this area	Caregiver(s) currently provide assistance	Caregiver(s) need training/ supportive services to provide assistance	Caregiver(s) not likely to provide assistance	Unclear if Caregiver(s) will provide assistance	Assistance needed, but no Caregiver(s) available
a. **ADL assistance** (e.g., transfer/ ambulation, bathing, dressing, toileting, eating/feeding)	☐0	☐1	☐2	☐3	☐4	☐5
b. **IADL assistance** (e.g., meals, housekeeping, laundry, telephone, shopping, finances)	☐0	☐1	☐2	☐3	☐4	☐5
c. **Medication administration** (e.g., oral, inhaled or injectable)	☐0	☐1	☐2	☐3	☐4	☐5
d. **Medical procedures/ treatments** (e.g., changing wound dressing)	☐0	☐1	☐2	☐3	☐4	☐5
e. **Management of Equipment** (includes oxygen, IV/infusion equipment, enteral/ parenteral nutrition, ventilator therapy equipment or supplies)	☐0	☐1	☐2	☐3	☐4	☐5
f. **Supervision and safety** (e.g., due to cognitive impairment)	☐0	☐1	☐2	☐3	☐4	☐5
g. **Advocacy or facilitation** of patient's participation in appropriate medical care (includes transporta-tion to or from appointments)	☐0	☐1	☐2	☐3	☐4	☐5

OMB #0938-0760

Expiration date 7/31/2012

(M2110) **How Often** does the patient receive **ADL or IADL assistance** from any caregiver(s) (other than home health agency staff)?

☐ 1 - At least daily
☐ 2 - Three or more times per week
☐ 3 - One to two times per week
☐ 4 - Received, but less often than weekly
☐ 5 - No assistance received
☐ UK - Unknown **[Omit "UK" option on DC]**

EMERGENT CARE

(M2300) **Emergent Care:** Since the last time OASIS data were collected, has the patient utilized a hospital emergency department (includes holding/observation)?

☐ 0 - No [*Go to M2400*]
☐ 1 - Yes, used hospital emergency department WITHOUT hospital admission
☐ 2 - Yes, used hospital emergency department WITH hospital admission
☐ UK - Unknown [*Go to M2400*]

(M2310) **Reason for Emergent Care:** For what reason(s) did the patient receive emergent care (with or without hospitalization)? **(Mark all that apply.)**

☐ 1 - Improper medication administration, medication side effects, toxicity, anaphylaxis
☐ 2 - Injury caused by fall
☐ 3 - Respiratory infection (e.g., pneumonia, bronchitis)
☐ 4 - Other respiratory problem
☐ 5 - Heart failure (e.g., fluid overload)
☐ 6 - Cardiac dysrhythmia (irregular heartbeat)
☐ 7 - Myocardial infarction or chest pain
☐ 8 - Other heart disease
☐ 9 - Stroke (CVA) or TIA
☐ 10 - Hypo/Hyperglycemia, diabetes out of control
☐ 11 - GI bleeding, obstruction, constipation, impaction
☐ 12 - Dehydration, malnutrition
☐ 13 - Urinary tract infection
☐ 14 - IV catheter-related infection or complication
☐ 15 - Wound infection or deterioration
☐ 16 - Uncontrolled pain
☐ 17 - Acute mental/behavioral health problem
☐ 18 - Deep vein thrombosis, pulmonary embolus
☐ 19 - Other than above reasons
☐ UK - Reason unknown

OMB #0938-0760

Expiration date 7/31/2012

DATA ITEMS COLLECTED AT INPATIENT FACILITY ADMISSION OR AGENCY DISCHARGE ONLY

(M2400) **Intervention Synopsis:** (Check only **one** box in each row.) Since the previous OASIS assessment, were the following interventions BOTH included in the physician-ordered plan of care AND implemented?

Plan / Intervention	No	Yes	Not Applicable	
a. Diabetic foot care including monitoring for the presence of skin lesions on the lower extremities and patient/caregiver education on proper foot care	☐0	☐1	☐na	Patient is not diabetic or is bilateral amputee
b. Falls prevention interventions	☐0	☐1	☐na	Formal multi-factor Fall Risk Assessment indicates the patient was not at risk for falls since the last OASIS assessment
c. Depression intervention(s) such as medication, referral for other treatment, or a monitoring plan for current treatment	☐0	☐1	☐na	Formal assessment indicates patient did not meet criteria for depression AND patient did not have diagnosis of depression since the last OASIS assessment
d. Intervention(s) to monitor and mitigate pain	☐0	☐1	☐na	Formal assessment did not indicate pain since the last OASIS assessment
e. Intervention(s) to prevent pressure ulcers	☐0	☐1	☐na	Formal assessment indicates the patient was not at risk of pressure ulcers since the last OASIS assessment
f. Pressure ulcer treatment based on principles of moist wound healing	☐0	☐1	☐na	Dressings that support the principles of moist wound healing not indicated for this patient's pressure ulcers OR patient has no pressure ulcers with need for moist wound healing

(M2410) To which **Inpatient Facility** has the patient been admitted?

☐   1 - Hospital [*Go to M2430*]

☐   2 - Rehabilitation facility [*Go to M0903*]

☐   3 - Nursing home [*Go to M2440*]

☐   4 - Hospice [*Go to M0903*]

☐ NA - No inpatient facility admission **[Omit "NA" option on TRN]**

(M2420) **Discharge Disposition:** Where is the patient after discharge from your agency? **(Choose only one answer.)**

☐   1 - Patient remained in the community (without formal assistive services)

☐   2 - Patient remained in the community (with formal assistive services)

☐   3 - Patient transferred to a non-institutional hospice

☐   4 - Unknown because patient moved to a geographic location not served by this agency

☐ UK - Other unknown

[*Go to M0903*]

(M0903) **Date of Last (Most Recent) Home Visit:**

__ __ / __ __ / __ __ __ __
month / day /   year

(M0906) **Discharge/Transfer/Death Date:** Enter the date of the discharge, transfer, or death (at home) of the patient.

__ __ / __ __ / __ __ __ __
month / day /   year

APPENDIX F

WOUND OSTOMY CONTINENCE NURSES SOCIETY GUIDANCE ON OASIS-C INTEGUMENTARY ITEMS

OVERVIEW AND BACKGROUND

OASIS-C is a modification to the Outcome and Assessment Information Set (OASIS) that Home Health Agencies must collect in order to participate in the Medicare program. This is the first major update of the OASIS since it was implemented in 2000.

It includes removing items not used for payment or quality, adding items to address clinical domains not covered, modified wording for selected items and adding process items that support measurement of evidence based practices. The system for wound classification uses terms that lack universal definition and clinicians have verbalized concerns that they may be interpreting these terms incorrectly. The WOCN Society has therefore developed the following guidelines for the classification of wounds. These items were developed by consensus among the WOCN Society panel of content experts.

(M1300) Pressure Ulcer Assessment: Was this patient assessed for risk of developing pressure ulcers?

(M1302) Does this patient have a Risk of Developing Pressure Ulcers?

(M1306) Does this patient have at least one Unhealed Pressure Ulcer at Stage II or Higher or designated as "unstageable"?

Definitions:

○ **Unhealed:** The absence of the skin's original integrity.

○ **Non-epithelialized:** The absence of regenerated epidermis across a wound surface.

○ **Pressure Ulcer:** A *pressure ulcer* is localized injury to the skin and/or underlying tissue, usually over a bony prominence, as a result of pressure or pressure in combination with shear and/or friction. *A number of contributing or confounding factors are also associated with pressure ulcers; the significance of these factors is yet to be elucidated.*

○ **Pressure Ulcer Stages (NPUAP 2007):**

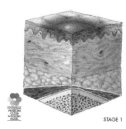

Stage I. A Stage I pressure ulcer presents as intact skin with non-blanchable redness of a localized area, usually over a bony prominence. Darkly pigmented skin may not have visible blanching; its color may differ from the surrounding area.

Further description. The area may be painful, firm, soft, and warmer or cooler as compared to adjacent tissue. Stage I ulcers may be difficult to detect in individuals with dark skin tones and may indicate "at risk" persons (a heralding sign of risk).

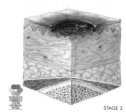

Stage II. A Stage II pressure ulcer is characterized by partial-thickness loss of dermis presenting as a shallow open ulcer with a red-pink wound bed without slough. It also may present as an intact or open/ruptured serum-filled blister.

Further description. A Stage II ulcer also may present as a shiny or dry shallow ulcer without slough or bruising.* This stage

OASIS-C Guidance Document – Content Validated - December, 2009   Page 2 of 8
Wound, Ostomy and Continence Nurses Society • 15000 Commerce Parkway, Suite C, Mount Laurel, NJ 08054

225

WOUND OSTOMY CONTINENCE NURSES SOCIETY
GUIDANCE ON OASIS-C INTEGUMENTARY ITEMS

*should not be used to describe skin tears, tape burns, perineal dermatitis, maceration, or excoriation. * Bruising indicates suspected deep tissue injury.*

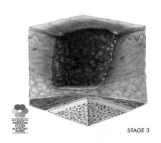

Stage III. A Stage III pressure ulcer is characterized by full-thickness tissue loss. Subcutaneous fat may be visible but bone, tendon, or muscle is not exposed. Slough may be present but does not obscure the depth of tissue loss. Stage III ulcers may include undermining and tunneling.

Further description. The depth of a Stage III pressure ulcer varies by anatomical location. The bridge of the nose, ear, occiput, and malleolus do not have subcutaneous tissue; Stage III ulcers in these locations can be shallow. In contrast, areas of significant adiposity can develop extremely deep Stage III pressure ulcers. Bone/tendon is not visible or directly palpable.

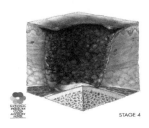

Stage IV. A Stage IV pressure ulcer presents with full-thickness tissue loss with exposed bone, tendon, or muscle. Slough or eschar may be present on some parts of the wound bed. These ulcers often include undermining and tunneling.

Further description. The depth of a Stage IV pressure ulcer varies by anatomical location. The bridge of the nose, ear, occiput, and malleolus do not have subcutaneous tissue; Stage IV ulcers in these locations can be shallow. Stage IV ulcers can extend into muscle and/or supporting structures (eg, fascia, tendon, or joint capsule); osteomyelitis is possible. Exposed bone/tendon is visible or directly palpable.

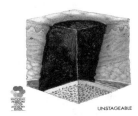

Unstageable. Full-thickness tissue loss in which the base of the ulcer is covered by slough (yellow, tan, gray, green or brown) and/or eschar (tan, brown or black) in the wound bed may render a wound unstageable.

Further description. Until enough slough and/or eschar is removed to expose the base of the wound, the true depth (and therefore, the stage) cannot be determined. Stable (dry, adherent, intact without erythema or fluctuance) eschar on the heels serves as "the body's natural (biological) cover" and should not be removed.

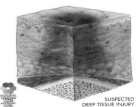

Suspected Deep Tissue Injury. Deep tissue injury may be characterized by a purple or maroon localized area of discolored intact skin or a blood-filled blister due to damage of underlying soft tissue from pressure and/or shear. Presentation may be preceded by tissue that is painful, firm, mushy, boggy, and warmer or cooler as compared to adjacent tissue.

Further description. Deep tissue injury may be difficult to detect in individuals with dark skin tones. Evolution may include a thin blister over a dark wound

WOUND OSTOMY CONTINENCE NURSES SOCIETY
GUIDANCE ON OASIS-C INTEGUMENTARY ITEMS

bed. The wound may further evolve and become covered by thin eschar. Evolution may be rapid, exposing additional layers of tissue even with optimal treatment.

(M1307) The Oldest Non-epithelialized Stage II Pressure Ulcer that is present at discharge

(M1308) Current Number of Unhealed (non-epithelialized) Pressure Ulcers at Each Stage

(M1310) Pressure Ulcer Length: Longest length "head-to-toe"

(M1312) Pressure Ulcer Width: Width of the same pressure ulcer; greatest width perpendicular to the length

(M1314) Pressure Ulcer Depth: Depth of the same pressure ulcer; from visible surface to the deepest area

(M1320) Status of Most Problematic (Observable) Pressure Ulcer
- 0 - Newly epithelialized
- 1 - Fully granulating
- 2 - Early/partial granulation
- 3 - Not healing
- NA - No observable pressure ulcer

Definitions:

- **Newly epithelialized**
  - wound bed completely covered with new epithelium
  - no exudate
  - no avascular tissue (eschar and/or slough)
  - no signs or symptoms of infection

- **Fully granulating**
  - wound bed filled with granulation tissue to the level of the surrounding skin
  - no dead space
  - no avascular tissue (eschar and/or slough)
  - no signs or symptoms of infection
  - wound edges are open

- **Early/partial granulation**
  - ≥25% of the wound bed is covered with granulation tissue
  - < 25% of the wound bed is covered with avascular tissue (eschar and/or slough)
  - no signs or symptoms of infection
  - wound edges open

- **3 - Not healing**
  - wound with ≥25% avascular tissue (eschar and/or slough) OR
  - signs/symptoms of infection OR
  - clean but non-granulating wound bed OR
  - closed/hyperkeratotic wound edges OR
  - persistent failure to improve despite appropriate comprehensive wound management

WOUND OSTOMY CONTINENCE NURSES SOCIETY
GUIDANCE ON OASIS-C INTEGUMENTARY ITEMS

(M1322) Current Number of Stage I Pressure Ulcers

(M1324) Stage of Most Problematic Unhealed (Observable) Pressure Ulcer

(M1330) Does this patient have a Stasis Ulcer?

(M1332) Current Number of (Observable) Stasis Ulcer(s)

(M1334) Status of Most Problematic (Observable) Stasis Ulcer
- 0 - Newly epithelialized
- 1 - Fully granulating
- 2 - Early/partial granulation
- 3 - Not healing
- NA - No observable stasis ulcer

Definitions:

o **Newly epithelialized**
  - o wound bed completely covered with new epithelium
  - o no exudate
  - o no avascular tissue (eschar and/or slough)
  - o no signs or symptoms of infection

o **Fully granulating**
  - o wound bed filled with granulation tissue to the level of the surrounding skin
  - o no dead space
  - o no avascular tissue (eschar and/or slough)
  - o no signs or symptoms of infection
  - o wound edges are open

o **Early/partial granulation**
  - o ≥25% of the wound bed is covered with granulation tissue
  - o < 25% of the wound bed is covered with avascular tissue (eschar and/or slough)
  - o no signs or symptoms of infection
  - o wound edges open

o **3 - Not healing**
  - o wound with ≥25% avascular tissue (eschar and/or slough) OR
  - o signs/symptoms of infection OR
  - o clean but non-granulating wound bed OR
  - o closed/hyperkeratotic wound edges OR
  - o persistent failure to improve despite appropriate comprehensive wound management

(M1340) Does this patient have a Surgical Wound?

WOUND OSTOMY CONTINENCE NURSES SOCIETY GUIDANCE ON OASIS-C INTEGUMENTARY ITEMS

(M1342) Status of Most Problematic (Observable) Surgical Wound:
>   0 -   Newly epithelialized
>   1 -   Fully granulating
>   2 -   Early/partial granulation
>   3 -   Not healing
>   NA - No observable surgical wound

Definitions:
- **Newly epithelialized**
  - wound bed completely covered with new epithelium
  - no exudate
  - no avascular tissue (eschar and/or slough)
  - no signs or symptoms of infection

- **Fully granulating**
  - wound bed filled with granulation tissue to the level of the surrounding skin
  - no dead space
  - no avascular tissue (eschar and/or slough)
  - no signs or symptoms of infection
  - wound edges are open

- **Early/partial granulation**
  - ≥25% of the wound bed is covered with granulation tissue
  - < 25% of the wound bed is covered with avascular tissue (eschar and/or slough)
  - no signs or symptoms of infection
  - wound edges open

- **3 - Not healing**
  - wound with ≥25% avascular tissue (eschar and/or slough) OR
  - signs/symptoms of infection OR
  - clean but non-granulating wound bed OR
  - closed/hyperkeratotic wound edges OR
  - persistent failure to improve despite appropriate comprehensive wound management

This guidance applies to surgical wounds closed by either primary intention (i.e. approximated incisions) or secondary intention (i.e. open surgical wounds).

(M1350) Does this patient have a Skin Lesion or Open Wound, excluding bowel ostomy, other than those described above that is receiving intervention by the home health agency?

WOUND OSTOMY CONTINENCE NURSES SOCIETY
GUIDANCE ON OASIS-C INTEGUMENTARY ITEMS

GLOSSARY

Avascular	Lacking in blood supply; synonyms are dead, devitalized, necrotic, and nonviable. Specific types include slough and eschar.
Clean Wound	Wound free of devitalized tissue, purulent drainage, foreign material or debris
Closed Wound Edges	Edges of top layers of epidermis have rolled down to cover lower edge of epidermis, including basement membrane, so that epithelial cells cannot migrate from wound edges; Also described as epibole or hyperkeratotic. Presents clinically as sealed edge of mature epithelium; and wound edge may present clinically as hard/thickened; and/or discolored (e.g., yellowish, gray, or white).
Dead Space	A defect or cavity
Dehisced / Dehiscence	Separation of surgical incision; loss of approximation of wound edges
Epidermis	Outermost layer of skin. New epidermis appears pink and dry and may look shiny. (Reference: Acute and Chronic Wounds, Nursing Management, Bryant Ruth, 2000, pg 21)
Epithelialization	Regeneration of epidermis across a wound surface
Eschar	Black or brown necrotic, devitalized tissue; tissue can be loose or firmly adherent, hard, soft, dry or wet.
Full Thickness	Tissue damage involving total loss of epidermis and dermis and extending into the subcutaneous tissue and possibly into the muscle or bone.
Granulation Tissue	The pink/red, moist tissue comprised of new blood vessels, connective tissue, fibroblasts, and inflammatory cells, which fills an open wound when it starts to heal; typically appears deep pink or red with an irregular, "berry-like" surface
Healing	A dynamic process involving synthesis of new tissue for repair of skin and soft tissue defects.
Hyperkeratosis	Hard, white/gray tissue surrounding a wound
Infection	The presence of bacteria or other microorganisms in sufficient quantity to damage tissue or impair healing. Wounds can be classified as infected when the wound tissue contains 100,000 or greater microorganisms per gram of tissue. Typical signs and symptoms of infection include purulent exudate, odor, erythema, induration, warmth, tenderness, edema, pain, fever, and elevated white cell count. However, clinical signs of infection may not be present, especially in the immuno-compromised patient or the patient with poor perfusion.
Necrotic Tissue	See avascular.
Newly epithelialized	The process of regeneration of the epidermis across a wound surface or regeneration of the epidermis across a wound surface
Non-epithelialized	The absence of regenerated epidermis across a wound surface.

WOUND OSTOMY CONTINENCE NURSES SOCIETY
GUIDANCE ON OASIS-C INTEGUMENTARY ITEMS

Non-granulating   Absence of granulation tissue; wound surface appears smooth as opposed to granular. For example, in a wound that is clean but non-granulating, the wound surface appears smooth and red as opposed to berry-like.

Partial Thickness   Confined to the skin layers; skin damage that does not penetrate below the dermis and may be limited to the epidermal layers only.

Scab   A crust of dried blood and serum.

Sinus Tract   Course or path of tissue destruction occurring in any direction from the surface or edge of the wound; results in dead space with potential for abscess formation. Also sometimes called "tunneling". (Can be distinguished from undermining by fact that sinus tract involves a small portion of the wound edge whereas undermining involves a significant portion of the wound edge.)

Slough   Soft moist avascular (devitalized) tissue; may be white, yellow, tan, grey or green; may be loose or firmly adherent.

Tunneling   See sinus tract

Undermining   Area of tissue destruction extending under intact skin along the periphery of a wound; commonly seen in shear injuries. Can be distinguished from sinus tract by fact that undermining involves a significant portion of the wound edge, whereas sinus tract involves only a small portion of the wound edge.

Unhealed   The absence of the skin's original integrity.

Note. Used with permission from WOCN.

APPENDIX G

Clinical Fact Sheet — Quick Assessment of Leg Ulcers

	Venous Insufficiency (STASIS)	Arterial Insufficiency	Peripheral Neuropathy
History	• Advanced Age • CHF • Lymphedema • Obesity • Orthopedic Procedures • Pain reduced by elevation • Pregnancy • Previous DVT with Phlebitis • Pulmonary Embolus • Reduced mobility • Sedentary Lifestyle • Traumatic Injury • Vascular Ulcers • Work History	• Arterial Disease • Cardiovascular Disease • Diabetes • Dyslipidemia • Hypertension • Increased pain with activity and/or elevation • Intermittent Claudication • Obesity • Painful Ulcer • Sickle Cell Anemia • Smoking • Vascular procedures/surgeries	• Advanced age • Alcoholism • Chemotherapy • Diabetes • Hansen's Disease • Heredity • HIV, AIDS and related drug therapies • Hypertension • Impaired glucose tolerance • Obesity • Raynaud's Disease, Scleroderma • Smoking • Spinal Cord Injury and neuromuscular diseases
Location	• Malleolus • Medial aspect of leg superior to medial malleolus	• Areas exposed to pressure or repetitive trauma, or rubbing of footwear • Lateral malleolus • Mid tibial • Phalangeal heads • Toe tips or web spaces	• Altered pressure points/sites of painless trauma/repetitive stress • Dorsal and distal toes • Heels • Inter-digital • Metatarsal heads • Mid-foot (dorsal and plantar) • Toe interphalangeal joints
Assessment	**WOUND** • Base: ruddy red; yellow adherent or loose slough; granulation tissue present; undermining or tunneling are uncommon • Depth: usually shallow • Margins: irregular • Exudate: moderate to heavy • Infection: less common **SURROUNDING SKIN** • Venous dermatitis (erythematic, weeping, scaling, crusting) • Hemosiderosis (brown staining) • Lipodermatosclerosis; Atrophy Blanche • Temperature: normal; warm to touch • Edema: pitting or non-pitting; possible induration and cellulitis • Scarring from previous ulcers, ankle flare, tinea pedis • Infection: Induration, cellulitis, inflamed, tender bulla	**WOUND** • Base: Pale; granulation rarely present; necrosis, eschar, gangrene (wet or dry) may be present • Depth: may be deep • Margins: edges rolled; punched out, smooth and undermining • Exudate: minimal • Infection: frequent (signs may be subtle) **SURROUNDING SKIN** • Pallor on elevation • Dependant rubor • Shiny, taut, thin, dry, • Hair loss over lower extremities • Atrophy of subcutaneous tissue • Edema: variable; atypical • Temperature: decreased/cold • Infection: Cellulitis • Necrosis, eschar, gangrene may be present **NAILS** • Dystrophic	**WOUND** • Base: pink/pale; necrotic tissue variable; • Depth: variable • Edges well defined • Exudate: usually small to moderate • Wound shape: usually rounded or oblong and found over bony prominence **SURROUNDING SKIN** • Normal skin tones • Trophic changes • Fissuring or callus formation • Edema: with erythema may indicate high pressure • Temperature: warm **NAILS** • Onychomycosis; dystrophic nails; paronychia, hypertrophy

WOCN ◆ 15000 Commerce Parkway, Suite C ◆ Mount Laurel, NJ 08054 ◆ (888) 224-WOCN ◆ Web site: www.wocn.org

Clinical Fact Sheet — Quick Assessment of Leg Ulcers

	Venous Insufficiency (STASIS)	Arterial Insufficiency	Peripheral Neuropathy
Perfusion	**PAIN** ◆ Minimal unless infected or dessicated ◆ Described as throbbing, sharp, itchy, sore, tender, heaviness ◆ Worsens with prolonged dependency **PERIPHERAL PULSES** ◆ Present/palpable **NON-INVASIVE VASCULAR TESTING** ◆ Capillary Refill: normal (less than 3 seconds) ◆ ABI to rule out arterial component **MEASURES TO IMPROVE VENOUS RETURN** ◆ (Provided vascular studies have ruled out significant arterial disease) ◆ Surgical obliteration of damaged veins ◆ Elevation of legs ◆ Medications ◆ Exercise ◆ Education ◆ Compression therapy to provide at least **30mm Hg compression at ankle'** ◆ **See WOCN Clinical Practice Guideline for Compression Therapy	**PAIN** ◆ Intermittent claudication ◆ Resting; positional; nocturnal ◆ Painful Ulcer ◆ Paresthesias **PERIPHERAL PULSES** ◆ Absent or diminished **NON-INVASIVE VASCULAR TESTING** ◆ Capillary refill: Delayed (more than 3 seconds) ◆ ABI <0.9 ◆ TcPO2 <40mmHG ◆ TP >30mm HG **MEASURES TO IMPROVE TISSUE PERFUSION** ◆ Revascularization if possible ◆ Medications to improve RBC transit through narrowed vessels ◆ Lifestyle changes (avoid tobacco, caffeine, restrictive garments, cold temperatures) ◆ Hydration ◆ Measures to prevent trauma to tissues (appropriate foot wear) ◆ Maintain legs in neutral or dependent position ◆ Pressure reduction for heels and toes	**PAIN** ◆ Decreased sensitivity to touch; if present, pain may be superficial, deep, aching, stabbing, dull, sharp, burning or cool; altered sensation not described as "pain" (numbness, warmth, prickling, tingling) **PERIPHERAL PULSES** ◆ Palpable/present **NON-INVASIVE VASCULAR TESTING** ◆ Capillary refill: Normal *NOTE: LEAD may co-exist with neuropathic disease* **MEASURES TO ELIMINATE TRAUMA** ◆ Reduction of shear stress and offloading of neuropathic wounds (bedrest, contact casting, orthopedic shoes) ◆ Use of assistive devices to provide support, balance and additional offloading ◆ Appropriate footwear ◆ Tight glucose/glycemic control ◆ Aggressive prevention/treatment of infection (debridement of callus and necrotic tissue; pharmacologic treatment when appropriate) ◆ Revascularizaton if ischemic ◆ Complications: Cellulitis, osteomyelitis, gangrene, Charcot fracture
Topical Therapy	◆ Goals: absorb exudates, maintain moist wound surface	**DRY, NON-INFECTED, NECROTIC WOUND** ◆ Keep dry **INFECTED WOUND/DRY OR MOIST NECROSIS** ◆ Referral for potential surgical debridement/antibiotic therapy **OPEN WOUND/NON-NECROTIC** ◆ Moist wound healing; ◆ Non-occlusive dressings ◆ Aggressive treatment of any infection	◆ Use dressings that maintain a moist surface, absorb exudates and allow easy visualization ◆ Cautious use of occlusive dressings

Note. Used with permission from WOCN.

APPENDIX H

Home Health Agency
Outcome and Assessment Information Set(OASIS)
STATEMENT OF PATIENT PRIVACY RIGHTS

As a home health patient, you have the privacy rights listed below.

● **You have the right to know why we need to ask you questions.**

We are required by law to collect health information to make sure:
1) you get quality health care, and
2) payment for Medicare and Medicaid patients is correct.

● **You have the right to have your personal health care information kept confidential.**

You may be asked to tell us information about yourself so that
we will know which home health services will be best for you.
We keep anything we learn about you confidential.
This means, only those who are legally authorized to know, or who
have a medical need to know, will see your personal health information.

● **You have the right to refuse to answer questions.**

We may need your help in collecting your health information.
If you choose not to answer, we will fill in the information as best we can.
You do not have to answer every question to get services.

● **You have the right to look at your personal health information.**

  ▪ We know how important it is that the information we collect about you is correct. If you think we made a mistake, ask us to correct it.
  ▪ If you are not satisfied with our response, you can ask the Centers for Medicare & Medicaid Services, the federal Medicare and Medicaid agency, to correct your information.

You can ask the Centers for Medicare & Medicaid Services to see, review, copy, or correct your personal health information which that Federal agency maintains in its HHA OASIS System of Records. See the back of this Notice for CONTACT INFORMATION. If you want a more detailed description of your privacy rights, see the back of this Notice: PRIVACY ACT STATEMENT - HEALTH CARE RECORDS.

This is a Medicare & Medicaid Approved Notice.

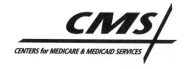

CENTERS for MEDICARE & MEDICAID SERVICES

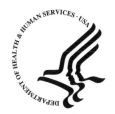

235

APPENDIX I

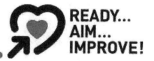

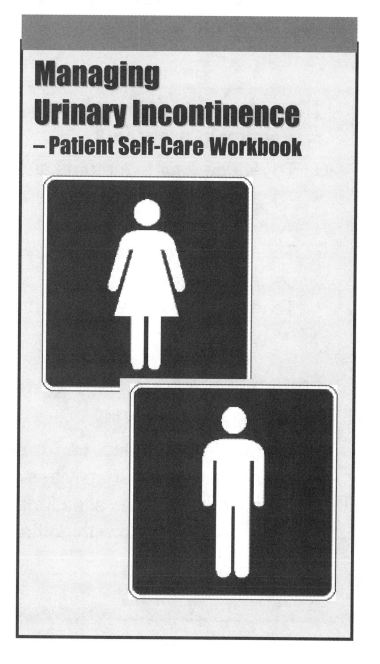

Page 2   **Incontinence Management :**

What is urinary incontinence ?

- Urinary incontinence is any unexpected loss or inability to control urine. Urinary incontinence often requires a person to change their habits and lifestyle to avoid an accident

What are the goals of an incontinence management program?

- To reduce your symptoms and accidents
- To provide exercises and tips to improve your bladder control
- To improve your ability to do physical and social activities
- To improve the quality of your life

When should I consider an incontinence management program?

- If your incontinence has caused you to change or limit your activities
- If you avoid social situations or limit the time you spend with others to avoid accidents

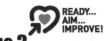

What is Urinary Incontinence?   Page 3

What causes urinary incontinence?

Temporary incontinence is caused by things like:

- Urinary tract infections
- Constipation
- Vaginal infections
- Mobility problems
- Medications for pain, high blood pressure or depression

Chronic incontinence is caused by things like:

- Weak pelvic floor muscles
- Overactive bladder
- Strokes, brain or spinal chord problems
- Prostate problems in men
- Gynecological or "female" problems

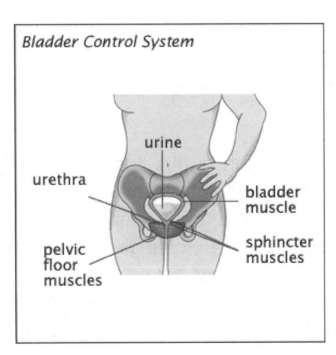

Bladder Control System

Page 4   **Am I Incontinent?**

I don't really have urinary incontinence... Do I?

Millions of Americans suffer with urinary incontinence years before they seek any help. If you answer yes to any of these questions your problem may be improved with an exercise program and changes in some of your habits.

- [ ] Do you leak urine on the way to the bathroom?
- [ ] Do you experience dribbling after you urinate?
- [ ] Do you leak urine when you cough, sneeze, laugh, bend or pick up heavy objects?
- [ ] Do you have pain or burning when you urinate?
- [ ] Do you have difficulty starting the flow of urine?

The information in this booklet will help you better understand urinary incontinence and get you started on a home program that includes exercises, changes in your diet and habits. Your home care nurse and therapist will teach you and answer questions you may have about urinary incontinence.

How is Incontinence Affecting You?:   Page 5

READY...
AIM...
IMPROVE!

How does your urinary incontinence affect you?			
Rate yourself using this table:			
Urinary Incontinence keeps me from: ↓	**At least Once a month**	**At least Once a week**	**Every day**
Attending social events			
Taking car or bus rides			
Having more company in my home			
Being able to Relax			
Doing housework			
Walking around inside my house			
Walking around outside my house			

Fact or Fiction ?

"Everybody experiences urinary incontinence, it is normal for somebody my age?"

Fiction: Urinary incontinence is not part of normal aging although as we get older there may be other factors that make it harder for us to control our urine.

Page 6   **Types of Incontinence:**

Types of incontinence

Before your nurse or therapist can make a plan to improve your incontinence, s/he must first try to understand what type of incontinence you have.

Stress Incontinence is leaking of urine that occurs when your normal activities put pressure on your bladder, squeezing it and causing it to leak.

Stress incontinence is usually improved by retraining your bladder and making the muscles that control urination stronger.

Urge incontinence happens because your bladder suddenly and unexpectedly contracts (squeezes) creating an immediate need to get to the bathroom or leaking occurs.

Urge incontinence is usually improved by retraining your bladder and teaching it to wait to be emptied.

Overflow Incontinence : Page 7

Overflow incontinence happens because your bladder does not get completely emptied when you go to the bathroom. The remaining urine causes the bladder to get filled up and overflow causing leaking.

Overflow incontinence is usually improved by retraining your bladder so that it gets completely emptied when you go to the bathroom and by increasing the amount of urine that it can hold.

Fact or Fiction ?

"There is nothing that can be done about urinary incontinence other than buy pads (or other products) at the grocery store?"

Fiction: There are some easy exercises, changes in diet, habits and medicines that can help you to improve your urinary incontinence. Once you begin an exercise program you should not expect to see an improvement for 6-8 weeks. Hang in there!

Page 8   **Your Bladder Diary:**

Date Time	Aware of urge to urinate?		Amount of leaking?			Activity when occured
	Yes	No	Sm	Med	Lg	
	Yes	No	Sm	Med	Lg	
	Yes	No	Sm	Med	Lg	
	Yes	No	Sm	Med	Lg	
	Yes	No	Sm	Med	Lg	
	Yes	No	Sm	Med	Lg	
	Yes	No	Sm	Med	Lg	
	Yes	No	Sm	Med	Lg	
	Yes	No	Sm	Med	Lg	
	Yes	No	Sm	Med	Lg	
	Yes	No	Sm	Med	Lg	
	Yes	No	Sm	Med	Lg	
	Yes	No	Sm	Med	Lg	
	Yes	No	Sm	Med	Lg	
	Yes	No	Sm	Med	Lg	

Where Are My Pelvic Muscles?   Page 9

Where are my pelvic muscles?

Sometimes people have difficulty finding exactly where their pelvic muscles are so before you exercise these muscles you have to learn to become aware of where they are.

- Both men and women can do this by sitting on the toilet.

- Once you begin to urinate squeeze the muscles that stop the flow of urine.

- You may have to do this a few times to see what it feels like to control those muscles.

- These are the muscles you will exercise to make stronger, but once you become familiar with where these pelvic muscles are, discontinue this activity of stopping your flow of urine, and progress with the following exercise plan:

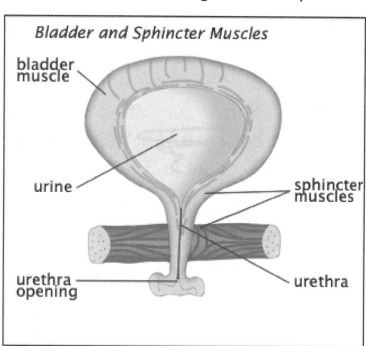

READY...
AIM...
IMPROVE!

Page 10   **Pelvic Muscle Exercises**

Pelvic Muscle Exercises:

Important!   Always empty your bladder before you begin your exercises.

- **Lay** on your back and **squeeze** your pelvic muscles while you slowly count to 3.

  1----- 2 ----- 3

- **Relax** your muscles while you slowly count to 3.   1----- 2 ----- 3

- **Sit** in a comfortable chair and **squeeze** your pelvic muscles while you slowly count to 3.   1----- 2 ----- 3

- **Relax** your muscles while you slowly count to 3.   1----- 2 ----- 3

- **Stand** with your arms and shoulders relaxed **squeeze** your pelvic muscles while you slowly count to 3.

  1----- 2 ----- 3

- **Relax** your muscles while you slowly count to 3.   1----- 2 ----- 3

Exercise Log: **Page 11**

READY...
AIM...
IMPROVE!

Exercise Log

To be most effective each exercise should be repeated 10 times, 3 times a day...

Day #1	Lying	Sitting	Standing
Morning	☐	☐	☐
Noon	☐	☐	☐
Night	☐	☐	☐

Day #2	Lying	Sitting	Standing
Morning	☐	☐	☐
Noon	☐	☐	☐
Night	☐	☐	☐

Day #3	Lying	Sitting	Standing
Morning	☐	☐	☐
Noon	☐	☐	☐
Night	☐	☐	☐

Day #4	Lying	Sitting	Standing
Morning	☐	☐	☐
Noon	☐	☐	☐
Night	☐	☐	☐

After two weeks - try increasing the hold/count to 5, and then to 10.

Page 12   **Controlling Urinary Urge:**

Controlling Urinary Urges

<u>Goal</u> is to try delay urination to no more frequently than every 3-4 hours

Try these techniques until the urge to urinate has passed:

Stop what you're doing and Sit or lie down

<u>Deep Breathing</u>
- Take slow deep breaths in through your nose out through your mouth

<u>Mental Distraction</u>
- Concentrate on mind games like singing a song or counting backward from 100

<u>Quick Flicks</u>
- Quickly and forcefully squeeze and relax your pelvic muscle

Remember: Do Not Urinate "Just in Case". This will eventually decrease the volume of urine your bladder can hold.
Try to wait until the next scheduled time.

Nutrition and Urinary Incontinence...   **Page 13**

Nutrition and Urinary Incontinence

It is important to eat a healthy diet and drink plenty of fluids when you have urinary incontinence. If you do not eat enough, you may experience constipation which could worsen your incontinence problem. Lack of fluids may cause your bladder to be irritated causing it to contract when you don't want it to and worsening your incontinence problem. If you are overweight, you may be putting extra pressure on your bladder. This squeezing of your bladder can make problems with bladder overflow worse.

☐ Eat a balanced diet with enough fiber to avoid constipation

☐ Drink enough fluids – 6-8 cups of caffeine-free fluids every day will help keep your bladder flushed

☐ Limit you intake of caffeine (be on alert for caffeine in soft drinks)

☐ Limit your intake of chocolate

☐ Limit your alcohol intake to not more than 1-2 drinks per day

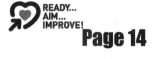

Page 14   **Scheduled Urination:**

Scheduled Urination

If the exercises and controlling urges hasn't helped improve your incontinence here are some tips that can help you to remain dry and avoid embarrassing accidents.

Create a reminder system to help you to remember to go to the bathroom on a schedule. Reminders might be based on:

- Time (8am, 11 am, 1pm ...)
- Activities (breakfast, snack, lunch...)
- Television programming
- Medication schedule

Write your schedule down and keep it handy.

Take your time getting to the bathroom
—Don't rush. If you need help getting to the bathroom don't wait until the last minute to ask for help.

Wear clothes that are easy for you get on and take off

For More Information: **Page 15**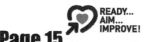

For More Information:

National Women's Health Information Center
(800) 994-9662
www.womenshealth.gov

National Kidney and Urologic Diseases
Information Clearinghouse
(800) 891-5390
 www.niddk.nih.gov/health/kidney/nkudic.htm

Tool Developed by:
Stephanie Mello Gaskell MSN, MBA RN COS-C &
Linda H. Krulish, PT MHS COS-C
OASIS Answers, Inc.

Content Sources:
Nursing Best Practice Guideline
Registered Nurses Association of Ontario Toronto, 2005.
http://www.rnao.org/bestpractices/PDF/BPG_Continence_rev05.pdf

Merck Institute of Aging and Health
http://www.miahonline.org/tools/UI/attachments/UI_06_diary.pdf

Talking together about bladder control: frequently asked questions
about urinary incontinence
The Canadian Continence Foundation (2001).
http://www.continence-fdn.ca/booklet/IncontBookletBlue.pdf
Illustrations www.4woman.gov

APPENDIX J

TABLE 1: SEVERITY SCORING TABLE

Episode Timing (M0110)	01 or UK ("Early")		02 ("Later")	
Therapy visits (M2200)	0-13	14+	0-13	14+
SCORING EQUATION:	1	2	3	4

TABLE 4: CLINICAL AND FUNCTIONAL SCORES (formerly Table 2a)
Updated by CMS for OASIS C effective January 1, 2010

CLINICAL DIMENSION

ROW	Episode Number from M0110 E=Early (Episodes 1 or 2) L=Later (Episodes ≥3)	E	E	L	L
	Number Therapy visits from M2200	0-13	14+	0-13	14+
	VARIABLE DESCRIPTION	POINTS by SCORING EQUATION:			
	(All diagnoses points come from those diagnoses being placed in M1020/1022/1024)	1	2	3	4
1	Primary or Other Diagnosis = **Blindness/Low Vision**	3	3	3	3
2	Primary or Other Diagnosis = **Blood disorders**	2	5	0	0
3	Primary or Other Diagnosis = **Cancer, selected benign neoplasms**	4	7	3	10
4	Primary Diagnosis = **Diabetes**	5	12	1	8
5	Other Diagnosis = **Diabetes**	2	4	1	4
6	Primary or Other Diagnosis = **Dysphagia** AND Primary or Other Diagnosis = Neuro 3 – Stroke	2	6	0	6
7	Primary or Other Diagnosis = **Dysphagia** AND M1030 (Therapy at home) = 3 (Enteral)	0	6	0	0
8	Primary or Other Diagnosis = **Gastrointestinal disorders**	2	6	1	4
9	Primary or Other Diagnosis = **Gastrointestinal disorders** AND M1630 (ostomy)= 1 or 2	3	0	0	0
10	Primary or Other Diagnosis = **Gastrointestinal disorders** AND Primary or Other Diagnosis = Neuro 1 – Brain disorders and paralysis, OR Neuro 2 – Peripheral neurological disorders, OR Neuro 3 – Stroke, OR Neuro 4 – Multiple Sclerosis	0	0	2	0
11	Primary or Other Diagnosis = **Heart Disease OR Hypertension**	3	7	1	8
12	Primary Diagnosis = **Neuro 1 – Brain disorders and paralysis**	3	8	5	8
13	Primary or Other Diagnosis = **Neuro 1 – Brain disorders and paralysis** AND M1840 (Toileting) = 2 or more	3	10	3	10
14	Primary or Other Diagnosis = **Neuro 1 – Brain disorders and paralysis** OR **Neuro 2 – Peripheral neurological disorders** AND M1810 or M1820 (Dressing upper or lower body)= 1, 2, or 3	2	4	2	2
15	Primary or Other Diagnosis = **Neuro 3 – Stroke**	0	1	0	0
16	Primary or Other Diagnosis = **Neuro 3 – Stroke** AND M1810 or M1820 (Dressing upper or lower body)= 1, 2, or 3	1	3	2	8
17	Primary or Other Diagnosis = **Neuro 3 – Stroke** AND M1860 (Ambulation) = **4** or more	1	5	0	0
18	Primary or Other Diagnosis = **Neuro 4 – Multiple Sclerosis** AND AT LEAST ONE OF THE FOLLOWING: M1830 (bathing) = 2 or more OR M1840 (Toileting) = 2 or more OR M1850 (Transferring) = 2 or more OR M1860 (Ambulation) = **4** or more	3	3	12	18
19	Primary or Other Diagnosis = **Ortho 1 – Leg Disorders** or **Gait Disorders** AND M1324 (most problematic pressure ulcer stage)= 1, 2, 3 or 4	2	0	0	0
20	Primary or Other Diagnosis = **Ortho 1 – Leg** OR **Ortho 2 – Other orthopedic disorders** AND M1030 (Therapy at home) = 1 (IV/Infusion) or 2 (Parenteral)	5	5	0	0
21	Primary or Other Diagnosis = **Psych 1 – Affective and other psychoses, depression**	3	5	2	5

continued on next page

22	Primary or Other Diagnosis = **Psych 2 – Degenerative and other organic psychiatric disorders**	1	2	0	2
23	Primary or Other Diagnosis = **Pulmonary disorders**	1	5	1	5
24	Primary or Other Diagnosis = **Pulmonary disorders** AND M1860 (Ambulation) = 1 or more	1	0	0	0
25	Primary Diagnosis = **Skin 1 –Traumatic wounds, burns, and post-operative complications**	10	20	8	20
26	Other Diagnosis = **Skin 1 – Traumatic wounds, burns, post-operative complications**	6	6	4	4
27	Primary or Other Diagnosis = **Skin 1 –Traumatic wounds, burns, and post-operative complications** OR **Skin 2 – Ulcers and other skin conditions** AND M1030 (Therapy at home) = 1 (IV/Infusion) or 2 (Parenteral)	2	0	2	0
28	Primary or Other Diagnosis = **Skin 2 – Ulcers and other skin conditions**	6	12	5	12
29	Primary or Other Diagnosis = **Tracheostomy**	4	4	4	0
30	Primary or Other Diagnosis = **Urostomy/Cystostomy**	6	23	4	23
31	M1030 (**Therapy at home**) = 1 (IV/Infusion) or 2 (Parenteral)	8	15	5	12
32	M1030 (**Therapy at home**) = 3 (Enteral)	4	12	0	12
33	M1200 (**Vision**) = 1 or more	1	0	0	1
34	M1242 (**Pain**) = 3 or 4	1	0	0	0
35	M1308 (**Number Pressure Ulcers**) = Two or more pressure ulcers at stage 3 or 4	3	3	5	5
36	M1324 (**Most problematic pressure ulcer stage**) = 1 or 2	5	11	5	11
37	M1324 (**Most problematic pressure ulcer stage**) = 3 or 4	16	26	12	23
38	M1334 (**Stasis ulcer status**) = 2	8	8	8	8
39	M1334 (**Stasis ulcer status**) = 3	11	11	11	11
40	M1342 (**Surgical wound status**) = 2	0	2	3	0
41	M1342 (**Surgical wound status**) = 3	4	4	4	4
42	M1400 (**Dyspnea**) = 2, 3, or 4	2	2	0	0
43	M1620 (**Bowel Incontinence**) = 2 to 5	1	2	1	0
44	M1630 (**Ostomy**) = 1 or 2	5	9	3	9
45	M2030 (**Injectable Drug Use**) = 0, 1, 2 **or 3**	1	1	2	4

FUNCTIONAL DIMENSION

46	M1810 or M1820 (**Dressing upper or lower body**) = 1, 2, or 3	2	4	2	2
47	M1830 (**Bathing**) = 2 or more	3	3	6	6
48	M1840 (**Toileting**) = 2 or more	2	3	2	0
49	M1850 (**Transferring**) = 2 or more	0	2	0	0
50	M1860 (**Ambulation**) = 1,2 **or 3**	1	0	1	0
51	M1860 (**Ambulation**) = **4** or more	3	4	4	5

CLINICAL SEVERITY LEVEL (By points)

Grouping Step:	1	2	3	4	5	HIPPS Value
C1 (Low)	0 to 4	0 to 6	0 to 2	0 to 8	0 to 7	A
C2 (Moderate)	5 to 8	7 to 14	3 to 5	9 to 16	8 to 14	B
C3 (High)	9+	15+	6+	17+	15+	C

FUNCTIONAL SEVERITY LEVEL (By points)

Grouping Step:	1	2	3	4	5	HIPPS Value
F1 (Low)	0 to 5	0 to 6	0 to 8	0 to 7	0 to 6	F
F2 (Moderate)	6	7	9	8	7	G
F3 (High)	7+	8+	10+	9+	8+	H

SERVICES UTILIZATION LEVEL (Therapy Visits)

Grouping Step:	1	2	3	4	5	HIPPS Value
S1	0 to 5	14 to 15	0 to 5	14 to 15	20	K
S2	6	16 to 17	6	16 to 17	N/A	L
S3	7 to 9	18 to 19	7 to 9	18 to 19	N/A	M
S4	10	N/A	10	N/A	N/A	N
S5	11 to 13	N/A	11 to 13	N/A	N/A	P

Note: Used with permission from Selman-Holman & Associates, LLC.
Source: CMS HHRG Overview January 2010.

RESOURCES

ASSOCIATIONS/ ORGANIZATIONS

American Nurses Association

8515 Georgia Ave.

Suite 400

Silver Spring, MD 20910

Tel: 301-628-5000

  800-274-4ANA (4262)

Fax: 301-628-5001

www.nursingworld.org

National Association for Home Care and Hospice

228 Seventh St., SE

Washington, DC 20003

Tel: 202-547-7424

Fax: 202-547-3540

www.nahc.com

Quality Insights of Pennsylvania

2601 Market Place St., Suite 320

Harrisburg, PA 17110

Tel: 717-671-5425

  877-346-6180

www.qipa.org/pa/

Visiting Nurse Associations of America

900 19th St., Suite 200

Washington, DC 20006

Tel: 202-384-1420

Fax: 202-384-1444

www.vnaa.org

Wound, Ostomy and Continence Nurses Society

1550 S. Coast Hwy.,

Suite 201

Laguna Beach, CA 92651

www.wocn.org

PUBLICATIONS

Home Healthcare Nurse

The Journal for the Home Care and Hospice Professional

16522 Hunters Green Parkway

Hagerstown, MD 21740-2116

Tel: 1-800-638-3030

Fax: 301-223-2400

Lippincott Williams & Wilkins

ISSN 0884-741X

www.lww.com

Instant OASIS Answers 2010: A CMS-Based Ready Reference for Data Collectors

PO Box 2768

Redmond, WA 98073

Tel: 425-868-2304

Fax: 425-868-5484

Email: info@oasisanswers.com

www.oasisanswers.com/products.htm

GLOSSARY

Adverse Event Outcome Report: A computer-generated report derived from the analysis of an agency's OASIS data. The report provides the agency with its incidence for each of the 13 adverse event outcomes. This report also provides a comparison of the agency's incidence rate to the incidence rate of the reference group.

benchmarking: The process by which the performance of one agency is compared to all others that have contributed data during the same time period. Agencies use the process of benchmarking to establish realistic goals for performance improvement activities.

best clinical practices: Standardized clinical strategies and interventions that, when applied consistently, result in desired, predictable patient outcomes.

care processes: The use of assessment tools or the planning and delivery of specific clinical interventions.

Case Mix Report: A report that provides an agency with a summary of OASIS data for all patients who appear on the agency's End Result Outcome Report.

Center for Medicare & Medicaid Services (CMS): Formerly known as the Health Care Financing Administration; part of the U.S. Department of Health and Human Services that is responsible for regulating and administering the Medicare benefit.

Conditions of Participation: The federal guidelines that provide health care providers with a detailed and extensive explanation of the minimum requirements to obtain and maintain Medicare certification.

End Result Outcome Report: Report that provides an agency with an aggregate level summary that details the agency's performance on each of the 41 patient outcomes measured. This report is the result of analysis of the agency's OASIS data by the Centers for Medicare & Medicaid Services.

end result outcomes: Measure the change in a patient's clinical and functional status between two points in time. The change in the patient's status can be positive (improved), negative (declined), or null (unchanged).

episode of care: Under Medicare, a 60-day period; all episodes are discrete and cannot overlap in any way.

level of significance: A statistical value that identifies the probability that the difference between an agency's performance and the national reference is due to chance.

low utilization payment adjustment (LUPA): An adjustment to the Medicare prospective payment system episode payment that is applied when a home health beneficiary receives less than five home visits.

negative outcome: The result achieved when a patient declines from a more functional status to a less functional status.

null outcome: The result when a patient's status neither improves nor declines but rather remains stable when compared at two points in time.

partial episode payment (PEP): A proportional adjustment to the Medicare prospective payment system episode payment that is applied when the patient does not complete an episode of care as a result of a transfer to another agency.

positive outcome: The result achieved when the patient improves from a less functional status to a more functional status.

Prospective Payment System (PPS): The Medicare home health care reimbursement system whereby the Centers for Medicare & Medicaid Services provides an agency with an episodic payment based on a patient's OASIS assessment.

risk adjustment: A statistical application that minimizes the influence of patient-related factors, such as age and functional ability, that might adversely impact an agency's outcomes.

REFERENCES

American Experience. (1997-2002). *Influenza 1918.* Accessed June 23, 2010, from http://www.pbs.org/wgbh/americanexperience/features/introduction/influenza-introduction/

American Heritage Dictionary of the English Language (4th ed.). (2000). Boston: Houghton Mifflin Company.

American Nurses Association. (1986). *Standards of home health nursing practice.* Kansas City, MO: Author.

American Nurses' Association. (1999). *Scope and standards of home health nursing practice.* Washington, DC: Author.

American Nurses Association. (2001). *Code of ethics for nurses with interpretive statements.* Washington, DC: Author.

American Nurses Association. (2008). *Home health nursing: Scope and standards of practice.* Silver Spring, MD: Author.

American Occupational Therapy Association. (n.d.). *Consumers.* Accessed June 23, 2010, from http://www.aota.org/Consumers.aspx

American Red Cross Nursing. (n.d.). Accessed June 23, 2010, from http://www.redcross.org/museum/history/brief.asp

American Red Cross (n.d.-a). *Early relief efforts respond to the bloodshed on the battlefield and the devastation of natural disasters.* Accessed June 23, 2010, from http://www.redcross.org/museum/history/pre1900_b.asp

American Red Cross (n.d.-b). *The Influenza Pandemic of 1918 and the Red Cross response.* Accessed June 23, 2010, from http://www.redcross.org/museum/history/influenza.asp

American Speech-Language-Hearing Association. (n.d.). *Swallowing disorders in adults.* Accessed June 23, 2010, from http://www.asha.org/public/speech/swallowing/SwallowingAdults.htm

Association for Computing Machinery. (1997). *ACM code of ethics and professional conduct.* Accessed June 23, 2010, from http://www.acm.org/constitution/code.html

Austin, T. (n.d.). *Dementia Tutorial: Diagnosis and Management in Primary Care.* A Primary Care Based, Education/Research Project. Retrieved June 23, 2010, from http://www.ehr.chime.ucl.ac.uk/display/demcare/Abbreviated+Mental+Test+Score

Benchmark of the week #38. (2002, March 29). *Home health line*, Vol. XXVIII, Number 13.

Bureau of Labor Statistics, U.S. Department of Labor. (2009a). *Occupational outlook handbook, 2010–11 edition.* Physical therapists. Accessed June 24, 2010, from http://www.bls.gov/oco/ocos080.htm

Bureau of Labor Statistics, U.S. Department of Labor. (2009b). *Occupational outlook handbook, 2010–11 edition.* Respiratory therapists. Accessed June 24, 2010, from http://www.bls.gov/oco/ocos084.htm

Bureau of Labor Statistics, U.S. Department of Labor. (2009c). *Occupational outlook handbook, 2010–11 edition.* Social workers. Accessed June 24, 2010, from http://www.bls.gov/oco/ocos060.htm

Bureau of Labor Statistics, U.S. Department of Labor. (2010). *Occupational outlook handbook, 2010–11 edition.* Dietitians and nutritionists. Accessed June 24, 2010, from http://www.bls.gov/oco/ocos077.htm

Centers for Medicare & Medicaid Services. (1994). *CMS form 485.* Available from www.medquest.us/PDFs/Appendix05/E1E2485HomeHealth CertiandPlanofCarev.4.pdf

Centers for Medicare and Medicaid Services. (2001). *Guidelines for Reviewing Case Mix and Adverse Event Outcome Reports.* Available from http://www.cms.gov/HomeHealth QualityInits/downloads/HHQIOASISOBQM Appendix.pdf

Centers for Medicare & Medicaid Services. (2002a). *Home health agency manual, chapter II coverage of services.* Accessed June 24, 2010, from http://www.mass.gov/?pageID=eohhs2terminal &L=6&L0=Home&L1=Government&L2= Laws%2C+Regulations+and+Policies&L3= MassHealth+Regulations+and+Other+ Publications&L4=Provider+Library&L5=Mass Health+Provider+Manuals&sid=Eeohhs2&b= terminalcontent&f=masshealth_provider_ manuals_pvman_homehealthagency&csid= Eeohhs2

Centers for Medicare and Medicaid Services. (2002b). Medicare program: update to the prospective payment system for home health agencies for Fiscal Year 2003. *Federal Register. June 28, 2002;67(125):43616-43629*

Centers for Medicare and Medicaid Services. (2005). Home Health Services, Chapter 7 in *Medicare Benefit Policy Manual.* Retrieved June 24, 2010 from http://www.cms.gov/ manuals/Downloads/bp102c07.pdf

Centers for Medicare & Medicaid Resources. (2007). *Medicare program: Home health prospective payment system refinement and rate update for calendar year 2008* (42 CFR Part 484). Federal Register, Part II, Vol. 72, No. 167, 8-29-07, Rules and Regulations. Accessed on June 30, 2010, from http://edocket.access .gpo.gov/2007/pdf/07-4184.pdf

Centers for Medicare & Medicaid Services. (2009). *OASIS-C Guidance Manual.* Accessed on March 20, 2010, from http://www.cms.hhs.gov/ homehealthqualityinits/14_hhqioasisuser manual.asp

Centers for Medicare and Medicaid Services. (2010). *Electronic Code of Federal Regulations.* Title 42: Public Health. Part 484: Home Health Services. Retrieved June 24, 2010, from http://ecfr.gpoaccess.gov/cgi/t/text/text-idx?c=ecfr&tpl=/ecfrbrowse/Title42/42cfr484_ main_02.tpl

Doty, P. (1919). A retrospect of the influenza epidemic. *The Public Health Nurse, 11*(12), 949-957. Available from http://ublib.buffalo.edu/ hsl/resources/guides/flu.html

Dowling-Castronovo, A. & Bradway, C. (2008). Urinary incontinence. In E. Capezuti, D. Zwicker, M. Mezey, & T. Fulmer, *Evidence-based geriatric nursing: Protocols for best practice* (pp. 309-336). New York, NY: Springer.

Dunn, D. (2005). *Substance abuse among nurses – defining the issue.* Retrieved June 24, 2010, from http://findarticles.com/p/articles/mi_ m0FSL /is_4_82/ai_n15754444

Fazzi Associates. (2000). The National PPS Expert Design Project. *Caring, 19*(10), 36-50,

Florence Nightingale Museum Trust. (n.d.). *Florence Nightingale.* Accessed June 24, 2010, from http://www.florence-nightingale.co.uk/ cms/index.php/florence-introduction

Greenleaf, R.W. (1898). *An historical report of the Boston Dispensary for one hundred and one years: 1796–1897.* Accessed June 24, 2010, from http://books.google.com/books?id= h9QhEwKSy_QC&dq=boston+dispensary& printsec=frontcover&source=web&ots=F9CeM z0a1e&sig=uhBNnka5bV-tkbq8gU6qkN60044

Home Health Resource Grouper. (2010). *Medicare Home Health Prospective Payment System Patient Classification Algorithm.* Retrieved June 24, 2010, from http://www.selmanholman .com/docs/HHRG_Overview_Jan2010.pdf

Joint Commission on Accreditation of Healthcare Organizations. (2006). *Comprehensive accreditation manual for home care, 2006-2007.* Oakbrook Terrace, IL: Author.

Lewis, J.J. (n.d.). *Florence Nightingale.* Accessed June 24, 2010, from http://womenshistory .about.com/od/nightingale/p/nightingale.htm

McDonald, C.J. (n.d.). *The "Nightingale Pledge."* Accessed June 24, 2010, from http://www. countryjoe.com/nightingale/pledge.htm

Medicare home health care: Payments to home health agencies are considerably higher than costs. (May, 2002). (Government Accounting Office, GAO-02-663). Washington, DC: U.S. Government Printing Office.

Medicare Payment Advisory Commission. (2009). *A data book: Healthcare spending and the Medicare program, June 2009.* Accessed June 24, 2010 from http://www.medpac.gov/ documents/Jun09DataBookEntireReport.pdf

MetLife. (n.d.). *Helping and healing people.* Accessed June 24, 2010, from http://www.metlife.com/ about/corporate-profile/metlife-history/helping- healing-people/index.html?SCOPE= Metlife&MSHiC=65001&L=10&W=and%20 healing%20helping%20people%20&Pre=%3CF ONT%20STYLE%3D%22background%3A%2 3ffff00%22%3E&Post=%3C/FONT%3E

Office of the Federal Register. (2007). *The Code of Federal Regulations, Title 42: Public Health, Part 484: Home Health Services.* Retrieved from http://www.access.gpo.gov/nara/cfr/ waisidx_05/42cfr484_05.html

Office of Inspector General. (2007). *List by exclusion type.* Accessed June 24, 2010, from http://oig.hhs.gov/fraud/exclusions.html

Pfizer, Inc. (2005). Patient Health Questionnaire. Accessed on June 24, 2010, from http://www.mapitrust.org/questionnaires/ download/66/PHQ9DepressionScreener.pdf

Profiles in caring: Lillian D. Wald. (n.d.). Accessed June 24, 2010, from http://www.nahc.org/ nahc/val/columns/sc10-4.html

Reichley, M. (1999). Advances in home care: Then, now and into the future. *Success in Home Care, 3*(6), 10, 12-18.

Schoen, C., Doty, M.M., Collins, S.R., & Holmgren, A.L. (2005). *Insured but not protected: How many adults are underinsured?* Retrieved June 24, 2010, from *Health Affairs* Web Exclusive, W5-289-W5-302: http://www.commonwealth fund.org/publications/publications_show.htm? doc_id=280812

Timeline of nursing history. (June 2010). Retrieved June 24, 2010, from Wikipedia: http://en .wikipedia.org/wiki/Timeline_of_nursing_ history#1870s

United States Department of Health & Human Services. Office of the Assistant Secretary for Planning and Evaluation. (2005). *Overview of the uninsured in the United States: An analysis of the 2005 current population survey.* Retrieved June 24, 2010, from http://aspe.hhs .gov/health/reports/05/uninsured-cps/index.htm

U.S. Department of Health & Human Services. (2008). *Home Health Compare.* Retrieved June 23, 2010, from http://www.medicare.gov/HH Compare/Home.asp?version=default&browser =IE%7C7%7CWinXP&language=English& defaultstatus=0&pagelist=Home&Cookies EnabledStatus=True

Vladeck, B. (March 5, 1997). *Testimony on Reforming the Medicare Home Health Benefit.* Accessed from http://www.hhs.gov/asl/testify/ t970305a.html

Wound Ostomy Continence Nurses Society. (2009). *Guidance on OASIS-C Integumentary Items.* Retrieved April 22, 2010 from http://www.wocn. org/pdfs/GuidanceOASIS-C.pdf

INDEX

Page references followed by *b* indicate a box; followed by *fig* indicate an illustrated figure; followed by *t* indicate a table.